W9-BIN-986

Nurse Practitioner's Business Practice and Legal Guide

SECOND EDITION

Carolyn Buppert, CRNP, JD

Attorney

Annapolis, Maryland

JONES AND BARTLETT PUBLISHERS

Sudbury, Massachusetts

BOSTON TORONTO LONDON SINGAPORE

World Headquarters
Jones and Bartlett Publishers
40 Tall Pine Drive
Sudbury, MA 01776
978-443-5000
info@jbpub.com
www.jbpub.com

Jones and Bartlett Publishers Canada
2406 Nikanna Road
Mississauga, ON L5C 2W6
CANADA

Jones and Bartlett Publishers International
Barb House, Barb Mews
London W6 7PA
UK

Library of Congress Cataloging-in-Publication Data

Buppert, Carolyn.
Nurse practitioner's business practice and legal guide / Carolyn Buppert.—2nd ed.
p. cm.
Includes index.
ISBN 0-7637-3341-5 (hardcover)
1. Nursing—Practice—United States. 2. Nurse practitioners—Legal status, laws, etc.—United States. I. Title.
RT86.73.B87 2004
610.73'06'92—dc22

2003019267

Production Credits
Acquisitions Editor: Penny Glynn
Production Manager: Amy Rose
Editorial Assistant: Amy Sibley
Production Assistant: Tracey Chapman
Marketing Manager: Joy Stark-Vancs
Marketing Associate: Elizabeth Waterfall
Manufacturing Buyer: Amy Bacus
Composition: Dartmouth Publishing, Inc.
Printing and Binding: Malloy, Inc.
Cover Printing: Malloy, Inc.

Printed in the United States of America
07 06 05 04 03 10 9 8 7 6 5 4 3 2 1

Table of Contents

Preface ... **ix**

Chapter 1 **What is a Nurse Practitioner?** ... **1**
- Definition of Nurse Practitioner ... 1
- A Nurse Practitioner, By Any Other Name ... 2
- Services Provided by NPs ... 3
- Preparation and License Requirements ... 5
- Initials ... 6
- Areas of Practice ... 6
- Legal History of NPs ... 6
- Demographics ... 7
- NPs in Primary Care ... 7
- NPs' Legal Authority to be Primary Care Providers ... 9
- NP Versus PA: What's the Difference? ... 10
- NP Versus Physician: What's the Difference? ... 12
- NP Versus RN: What's the Difference? ... 14
- NP Versus CNS: What's the Difference? ... 15
- Where Do Nurse Practitioners Practice? ... 17
- **Appendix 1-A:** State-by-State What is a Nurse Practitioner? 18
- **Appendix 1-B:** State-by-State Titles for Nurse Practitioners. 33

Chapter 2 **Legal Scope of Nurse Practitioner Practice** ... **37**
- Professional Association Definition of Scope of Practice ... 37
- Statutory Versus Regulatory Scope of NP Practice ... 38
- Physician Challenges to NPs' Scope of Practice ... 39
- Need for Clarity of Scope of Practice ... 39
- NP Scope of Practice Compared with RN Scope of Practice. 40
- NP and MD Scope of Practice Compared ... 43
- Mandated Physician Involvement with NP Practice ... 44
- **Appendix 2-A:** State-by-State Law Nurse Practitioner Scope of Practice ... 47
- **Appendix 2-B:** State-by-State Requirement, if any, of Physician Collaboration ... 75

Chapter 3 **State Regulation of Nurse Practitioner Practice** **111**
How Laws About NP Practice Evolve.................................... 111
What is Regulated?.................................... 112
Appendix 3-A: Agency That Regulates Nurse Practitioners, State-by-State.................................... 114
Appendix 3-B: State-by-State Nurse Practitioner Qualifications Required by Law 117

Chapter 4 **Federal Regulation of the Nurse Practitioner Profession....** **135**
Medicare.................................... 135
Medicaid.................................... 139
Nursing Homes.................................... 139
In-Office and Hospital Laboratories Under CLIA.................................... 140
Self-Referral by Health Care Providers, Under the Stark Acts.................................... 140
Prescription of Controlled Substances Under the DEA.......... 142
Reporting to the National Practitioner Data Bank 142
Patient Confidentiality.................................... 142
Discrimination in Hiring and Firing.................................... 145
People with Disabilities Under the ADA.................................... 145
Appendix 4-A: Documentation Guidelines for Evaluation and Management Services 146

Chapter 5 **Prescribing** **183**
Controlled Substances.................................... 183
Guidelines for Prescribing Legally.................................... 186
Appendix 5-A: State-by-State Law Prescriptive Authority... 188

Chapter 6 **Hospital Privileges** **227**
Are Hospital Privileges an Issue for NPs?.................................... 227
Do PCPs Need Hospital Privileges? 228
What if Health Plans Require PCPs to Have Admitting Privileges?.................................... 229
Do NPs Need Hospital Privileges for Advancement of the Profession?.................................... 229
Do Individual NPs Need Hospital Privileges? 229
Who has Hospital Privileges?.................................... 230
Does Federal Law Support Full Hospital Privileges for NPs?.................................... 232
What Does it Mean to Have Hospital Privileges?.................................... 232
Levels of Privilege 232
The Application Process 233
Expense.................................... 233
Denial of Privileges 233
Expect Change.................................... 234

Chapter 7 **Negligence and Malpractice** **235**
What Can Happen to an NP Who is Sued? 236
Life Cycle of a Lawsuit 236
What is Malpractice? 236
Elements of Malpractice 236
Examples of Lawsuits Against NPs 238
The National Practitioner Data Bank 242
Working with Practice Guidelines 243
How to Prevent Lawsuits 244
What to do if Sued 244
Communication 244
Liability of Collaborating Physicians 244
Malpractice Insurance 246

Chapter 8 **Risk Management** **249**
Risk of Making a Clinical Error 249
Risk of Being Sued for Malpractice When There Was No Clinical Error 252
Risk of Public Perception That the Individual NP Is a Poor-Quality Provider 253
Risk of Breaching Patient Confidentiality 253
Risk of Violating a Patient's Right to Informed Consent 255
Risk of Negligent Nondisclosure 260
Risk of Poor Quality Ratings 261
Risk of Disciplinary Action 261
Risk of Medicare Fraud 263
Business Risk Management 264
Dealing with High-Risk Patients 265

Chapter 9 **Reimbursement for Nurse Practitioner Services** **269**
Payers 269
Medicare 269
Medicaid 273
Indemnity Insurers 273
Managed-Care Organizations 274
Direct Contracts for Health Services 279
Billing Third-Party Payers 279
Billing Self-Paying Patients 284
Appendix 9-A: Credentialing Information 286

Chapter 10 **The Employed Nurse Practitioner** **289**
What Rights Does an Employed NP Have? 289
Does an NP Need a Contract? 290
Three Difficult Clauses 291
How to Negotiate a Reasonable Agreement 296

Interviewing 303
Responsibilities of an NP Employee 303
Employer's Evaluation of the NP's Performance 304
Malpractice Insurance 304
Collaborative Practice Agreements 304
Appendix 10-A: Sample Nurse Practitioner Collaborative Practice Agreement 306
Appendix 10-B: Sample Employment Agreement 310

Chapter 11 **Practice Ownership: Legal Business Considerations for the Nurse Practitioner Owner 321**
Advantages of Practice Ownership 321
Decisions Before Starting a Practice 322
Business Planning 338
Doing Business 343
Appendix 11-A: A Checklist for Setting Up a Practice 358
Appendix 11-B: Independent Contractor Agreement 372
Appendix 11-C: Sample Business Plan 377
Appendix 11-D: Professional Services Agreement 393

Chapter 12 **Lawmaking and Health Policy 399**
The Legal Process 399
The Judicial System 400
Health Policy 400
Laws and Rules That Affect NPs 401
Changing Laws 401
Understanding the Big Picture 402
The Process of Changing the Law 408
Conclusion 414

Chapter 13 **Promoting the Profession to the Public 417**
Public Relations Steps 418
Setting the Goal 418
Developing the Plan 418
Developing the Budget 419
Working the Plan 419
The Substance of the Message 420
Supporting Data 421
Collecting Impressive Facts 423
Present Barriers to Fact Collection 424
Not-So-Impressive Facts About NPs 424
Dealing with the Downside 425
Appendix 13-A: A Simple PR Plan for a State NP Organization 428

Appendix 13-B: Some Talking Points for NPs 430
Appendix 13-C: Sample Fact Sheets on NPs 433

Chapter 14 Standards of Care for Nurse Practitioner Practice 437
Definitions of Standard of Care 437
Who is Monitoring Standard of Care 437
How Should NPs Keep Current on Standard of Care? 446
Credentialing 446

Chapter 15 Measuring Nurse Practitioner Performance 449
Measuring Quality 449
Multiple Measures, Multiple Measurers 450
Productivity 450
Housekeeping Performance Measures 451
NCQA Measures of Clinical Performance 451
Other Measures 452
Formal Research 452
Patient Ratings 453
Peer Review 453
Utilization 453
How to Get an "A" on Performance Report Cards 454
Ensuring Compliance 454
Appendix 15-A: NPs' Self-Evaluation 456
Appendix 15-B: Health Maintenance Flowchart 457

Chapter 16 Resolving Ethical Dilemmas 459
Examples 459
Analyzing the Ethical Choices Inherent in These Situations. 460
Ethical Analyses 467

Chapter 17 Strategies for NPs 469
Opportunities in a Changing Field 469
Opponents of a See-A-Nurse-First System 470
What are the Challenges for NPs Attempting to Advance the Profession? 470
Strategies to Implement Collectively 471
Ten Organizational Strategies 471

Index 479

Preface

This book contains the answers to many questions asked of me in my 12 years of practice as an attorney. I specialize in legal issues affecting nurse practitioners. The questions came from nurse practitioners, employers of nurse practitioners, student nurse practitioners and their professors, other attorneys, bureaucrats, and legislators conducting hearings about bills that addressed nurse practitioners.

Nurse practitioners frequently ask questions such as:

- A physician (or hospital or group) wants to hire me to do [fill in a particular health care service]. Can I legally do that?
- An insurance company refuses to pay the bill for a patient's visit with me. What can I do?
- A big company bought my group's practice. The big company is not sure what to do with me. They know nothing about what nurse practitioners can do in our state. Can you tell them about nurse practitioners?
- What should be covered in my employment contract?
- Can I incorporate in a business with physicians?
- I have been working in a trauma center for 4 years. Now I hear that my notes need to be co-signed by a physician. Is that true?
- An internet-based pharmacist refuses to fill a prescription I wrote because I am not a physician. I have the legal authority to prescribe in my state. What can I do?
- I have been working without a contract. Now the company wants me to be on call three nights a week. Do I have to do it?
- I'm writing a paper for my "nurse practitioner role" class on legislative issues affecting nurse practitioners. What are these issues?
- How can I get on a managed care provider panel?
- A group wants to pay me a base salary plus a percentage of billings over $120,000. Is this reasonable?
- What does "incident to a physician's professional services" mean?
- How do I start my own practice?

- I know nothing about how billing is done. Can you tell me how to get reimbursed for my services?

Legislators and bureaucrats frequently ask such questions as:

- How is a nurse practitioner different from a registered nurse?
- Which states allow nurse practitioners to practice independently?
- How does a nurse practitioner know when to consult a physician?
- Doesn't a physician have to supervise everything a nurse practitioner does?
- In how many states can nurse practitioners write prescriptions?

Employers of nurse practitioners frequently ask such questions as:

- I want the nurse practitioner to see my hospitalized patients. Can we get reimbursed for that?
- How can we get paid by Medicare for patient visits to the nurse practitioner?
- We want to put nurse practitioners in nursing homes. Who has to sign and what has to be signed to get them started?
- Who is liable if the nurse practitioner makes a mistake? The nurse practitioner or the physician?

Other attorneys ask:

- A nursing home I represent has hired a nurse practitioner to do administrative work and to see patients. How can we bill for his or her services?
- My clients want to start a network of nurse practitioner practices. What can you tell me about that? Do you know anything about Florida law on nurse practitioners?

Some of the questioners have become clients, and I have done the necessary legal research to answer their questions and have completed the necessary legal documents to carry out their plans. Others will now benefit from those clients.

Nurse practitioners who read this book will have a solid knowledge base to use, whether it be in developing an employment relationship, undertaking a business venture, giving testimony before the state legislature, composing a letter to an insurance company about an unpaid bill, teaching at a school of nursing, or serving as president of a state or national organization. My hope is that once nurse practitioners have this base of knowledge about the business of health care and the legal foundation upon which nurse practitioners function, they can hasten the advancement of their careers.

Some of the medical practitioners asking these questions became clients, allowing me to research the answers and complete the appropriate legal documents for them to further their careers. Now, others will benefit from this extensive legal research.

CHAPTER 1

What Is a Nurse Practitioner?

Individuals who have never experienced the care of a nurse practitioner (NP)—whether they are physicians, reporters, lawmakers, bureaucrats, lobbyists, or new patients—often request clarification of just who NPs are and what they do.

It is the combination of skills of physician and nurse that seems to confuse people. Yet it is that combination of skills that makes an NP unique.

DEFINITION OF NURSE PRACTITIONER

The term *nurse practitioner* has been given a variety of definitions.

- According to a state NP organization, "Nurse practitioners are registered nurses with one to two years of additional education, which prepares them to provide many of the same services doctors provide. Nurse practitioners work with other health care professionals such as nurses, doctors, therapists, and counselors. Nurse practitioners provide health and wellness care to persons of all ages. Nurse practitioners are legally authorized to diagnose, order laboratory work and X-rays, and prescribe medication."[1]
- According to a national NP organization, "A nurse practitioner is a registered nurse with advanced academic and clinical experience, which enables him or her to diagnose and manage most common and many chronic illnesses. The nurse practitioner works either independently or as a part of a health care team."[2]
- A board of nursing defines NP as "a registered nurse who has obtained additional advanced specialized education."[3]
- According to federal law, "Nurse practitioner means a nurse practitioner who performs such services as such individual is legally authorized to perform (in the state in which the individual performs such services) in accordance with state laws and who meets such training, education and experience required as the Secretary has prescribed in regulations" [42 U.S.C.A. § 1395x(aa)(5)].

- In California state law, "nurse practitioner means a registered nurse who possesses additional preparation and skills in physical diagnosis, psych-social assessment and management of health-illness needs in primary health care and who has been prepared in a program conforming to board standards as specified in section 1484"[CA. CODE REGS. tit. 16, § 1480(a)].

For state-by-state definitions of the term *nurse practitioner,* see Appendix 1-A.

A NURSE PRACTITIONER, BY ANY OTHER NAME . . .

Other designations sometimes given NPs include *physician extender, mid-level practitioner,* and *advanced-practice nurse.* For a state-by-state listing of states' official terms for NPs, see Appendix 1-B.

Physician Extenders

The term *physician extender* is used by physicians' associations and publications aimed at the physician market, and usually is used to refer collectively to nurse practitioners, clinical nurse specialists, nurse anesthetists, nurse midwives, and physician assistants (PAs).

Mid-Level Practitioners

The term *mid-level practitioner* is used by some physician groups, some states, and the federal government in the Code of Federal Regulation sections dealing with Drug Enforcement Administration (DEA) registration. The DEA defines a mid-level practitioner as follows:

> The term *mid-level practitioner* means an individual practitioner other than a physician, dentist, veterinarian, or podiatrist, who is licensed, registered, or otherwise permitted by the United States or the jurisdiction in which he/she practices to dispense controlled dangerous substances in the course of professional practice. Examples of mid-level practitioners include, but are not limited to health care providers such as nurse practitioners, nurse midwives, nurse anesthetists, clinical nurse specialists, and physician assistants who are authorized to dispense controlled substances by the state in which they practice.
>
> *Citation:* 21 C.F.R. § 1300.01(28).

Some state laws provide a definition of *mid-level practitioner.* For example, in Minnesota, "'Midlevel practitioner' means a nurse practitioner, nurse midwife, nurse anesthetist, advanced clinical nurse specialist, or physician assistant" [MINN. STAT. § 144.1495(b)].

Advanced Practice Nurses

Advanced practice nurse is an umbrella term used by some states and some nursing associations to cover, collectively, NPs, clinical nurse specialists (CNSs), nurse midwives, and nurse anesthetists. NPs differ from other advanced practice nurses in that they offer a wider range of services to a wider portion of the population. Other advanced practice nurses compare with NPs in the following ways:

- *Nurse anesthetist:* Narrow range of services (preoperative assessment, administration of anesthesia, management of postanesthesia recovery) to a narrow base of patients (people having anesthesia)
- *Clinical nurse specialist:* Medium range of services (consultation, research, education, administration, coordination of care, case management, direct care within definition of registered nurse) to a narrow patient base (people under the care of a medical specialist)
- *Certified nurse midwife:* Narrow range of services (well-women gynecologic care; management of pregnancy and childbirth; antepartum and postpartum care) to a medium-sized base of patients (childbearing women)
- *Nurse practitioner:* Wide range of services (evaluation, diagnosis, treatment, education, risk assessment, health promotion, case management, coordination of care, counseling) to a wide base of patients, depending upon area of certification; a family nurse practitioner can have a patient base of any age, gender, or problem

SERVICES PROVIDED BY NPS

NPs may perform any service authorized by a state nurse practice act. Some nurse practice acts are so broad as to allow any service agreed upon by an NP and collaborating physician. Generally, NP services include:

- Obtaining medical histories and performing physical examinations
- Diagnosing and treating health problems
- Ordering and interpreting laboratory tests and X-rays
- Prescribing medications and other treatments
- Providing prenatal care and family planning services
- Providing well-child care and immunizations
- Providing gynecologic examinations and Pap smears
- Providing education about health risks, illness prevention, and health maintenance
- Case management and coordination of care

Typically, NPs have the following duties and responsibilities:

1. Conducts comprehensive medical and social history of individuals, including those who are healthy and those with acute illnesses and chronic diseases
2. Conducts physical examination of individuals, either comprehensive or problem focused
3. Orders, performs, and interprets laboratory tests for screening and for diagnosing
4. Prescribes medications
5. Performs therapeutic or corrective measures, including urgent care
6. Refers individuals to appropriate specialist nurses or physicians or other health care providers
7. Makes independent decisions regarding management and treatment of medical problems identified
8. Performs various invasive/clinical procedures such as suturing, biopsy of skin lesions, and endometrial biopsy, depending upon education, training, patient needs, and written agreement with physician collaborator
9. Prescribes and orders appropriate diet and other forms of treatment such as physical therapy
10. Provides information, instruction, and counseling on health maintenance, health promotion, social problems, illness prevention, illness management, and medication use
11. Evaluates the effectiveness of instruction and counseling and provides additional instruction and counseling as necessary
12. Initiates and participates in research studies and projects
13. Teaches groups of clients about health-related topics
14. Provides outreach health education services in the community
15. Serves as preceptor for medical, nursing, NP, or physician assistant (PA) students
16. Accepts after-hours calls and handles after-hours problems on a rotating schedule
17. Participates in development of pertinent health education materials
18. Participates in development of clinical practice guidelines
19. Initiates and maintains follow-up of noncompliant patients
20. Makes client home visits and provides care in the home as necessary
21. Makes hospital visits and follows hospital care of established patients
22. Consults with other health care providers about established clients who have been admitted to hospital, home care, rehabilitation, or nursing homes
23. Corresponds with insurers, employers, government agencies, and other health care providers about established clients as necessary
24. Manages care of clients; develops plan of treatment and/or follow-up and monitors progress, determines when referral to another provider is necessary, makes necessary arrangements for further care, determines when hospital admission or emergency room visit is necessary, and determines when illness is resolved

25. Assesses social/economic factors for each client, and tailors care to those factors
26. Manages care of clients in a way that balances quality and cost
27. Tracks outcome of interventions and alters interventions to achieve optimum results
28. Obtains informed consent from clients as appropriate and necessary
29. Maintains familiarity with community resources and connects clients with appropriate resources
30. Contracts with clients regarding provider responsibilities and client responsibilities
31. Supervises and teaches registered nurses (RNs) and nonlicensed health care workers
32. Participates in community programs and health fairs, school programs, and workplace programs
33. Represents the practice or the profession as an NP before local and state governing bodies, agencies, and private businesses as needed

PREPARATION AND LICENSE REQUIREMENTS

All NPs are RNs with education beyond the basic requirements for RN licensure. Many NPs have master's degrees, and some have doctorates. Master's degrees for NPs are required by law in 24 states. Three additional states will require a master's degree as of 2008. NPs without master's degrees have completed a program that meets requirements of state law.

State-required qualifications vary widely. For example, in Alaska, NPs must have completed a one-year academic course, have an RN license, be certified by a national certifying agency, and have 30 hours of continuing education every 2 years. In Pennsylvania, NPs must have an RN license, a master's degree, certification by a national organization, must provide evidence of continuing competence in medical diagnosis and therapeutics, and must have 30 hours of continuing education per year and 45 hours of advanced pharmacology. Federal law defers to state law regarding NP qualifications (42 C.F.T. 440.116).

In 35 states, NPs are required by state law to take and pass a national certification exam. A state requirement that an NP be nationally certified leads to a requirement of master's education because the certifying agencies of adult and pediatric NPs—the American Nurses Credentialling Center, the American Academy of Nurse Practitioners, and the National Certification Board of Pediatric Nurse Practitioners and Nurses—require a master's degree to sit for the certification examination. The National Certification Corporation, which certifies OB-GYN and neonatal nurse practitioners, does not require master's degrees, but will require master's degrees by 2007.

INITIALS

Among the initials used to designate NPs are CRNP (certified registered nurse practitioner); CANP (certified advanced nurse practitioner); ANP-C (advanced nurse practitioner–certified); CPNP (certified pediatric nurse practitioner); CANP (certified adult nurse practitioner); CGNP (certified geriatric nurse practitioner); RN, CS (registered nurse, certified specialist); ARNP (advanced registered nurse practitioner); and APRN (advanced practice registered nurse).

AREAS OF PRACTICE

NPs may be certified in the following areas:

- Adult primary care
- Family primary care
- Geriatric primary care
- Neonatal care
- Obstetrics and gynecology
- Pediatric primary care
- Acute care
- Primary care of school-aged children
- Family planning
- Emergency health care
- Maternal child health
- Mental health/psychiatric care
- Critical care
- Oncology
- Rehabilitation
- Community health
- Occupational health

Not all categories are recognized in all states.

LEGAL HISTORY OF NPS

Before the emergence of advanced practice nurses, the legal scope of practice of nurses excluded diagnosis and treatment of medical problems. Nurses carried out physicians' orders. In the mid-1970s, some state nurse practice acts were amended to include "nursing diagnoses" in the scope of nursing practice. A nursing diagnosis "limits the diagnostic process to those diagnoses that represent human responses to actual or potential health problems that are within the legal scope of nursing practice."[4]

When a physician shortage arose in the 1960s, it became evident that the shortage and the limitations on nurses' making medical diagnoses were limiting access to health care for people in medically underserved areas. Certain nurses and physicians joined forces to solve the problem. One answer was the NP.

The first NP educational program was a joint effort between Henry K. Silver, a pediatrician, and Loretta C. Ford, a nursing professor, at the University of Colorado in 1965. Their project was one of many efforts to deal with a physician shortage. The first NPs began practicing in the late 1960s.

As the concept was envisioned, NPs would make not only nursing diagnoses but also medical diagnoses. Further, they would treat patients with medical therapeutics, ordering pharmacotherapeutics and other treatments. It became necessary to broaden the legal scope of nursing practice.

As soon as NPs began to emerge from the training programs, a body of law emerged governing NP licensure and scope of practice. Idaho was the first state to revise its regulations to allow diagnosis and treatment by nurses.

By the mid-1970s, state legislators began to consider proposed laws regarding prescriptive authority for NPs. In some states, the prescriptive authority was granted through the regulatory process; in others, it was granted through the legislative process. By 2003, NPs had achieved some degree of prescriptive privileges in 49 states and the District of Columbia. The main legal goal of NPs for 30 years was achieved. The next legal hurdle became evident with the enrollment of a large percentage of the population into managed-care plans. NPs now need the legal authority to handle the primary care of panels of managed-care patients. In some states, NPs have that legal authority. In others, the law is unclear or does not address the issue.

DEMOGRAPHICS

There are approximately 103,000 NPs in the United States, according to statistics kept by Health Resources Services Administration (2001), as reported on the Web site of the American College of Nurse Practitioners.[2]

NPS IN PRIMARY CARE

The concept of the NP emerged from a need for more primary care providers in underserved areas of the nation. While some NPs work in specialty and acute care settings, the majority provide primary care.

As more and more health plans designate certain generalist physicians—pediatricians, internists, and family practitioners—as primary care providers (PCPs) for groups of patients, it is important for NPs to be included in the definition of PCP.

Definition of Primary Care

The following are definitions of primary care.

According to a national health policy think tank, the National Academy of Sciences' Institute of Medicine,

- "Primary care is the provision of integrated, accessible health care services by clinicians who are accountable for addressing a large majority of personal health care needs, developing a sustained partnership with patients, and practicing in the context of family and community."[5]

Two nurse practice acts written by state agencies define primary health care as:

- "that which occurs when a consumer makes contact with a health care provider who assumes responsibility and accountability for the continuity of health care regardless of the presence or absence of disease" [CA. CODE REGS. tit. 16, § 1480(b)] and as:
- "the prevention of disease, promotion and maintenance of health, assessment of needs, long-term nursing management of chronic illness and referrals of clients to other resources. The contact between advanced registered nurse practitioner and client may be for an episode of illness or it may be for continuous health care monitoring. The physical presence of the physician is not necessarily implied when care is given by the registered nurse practitioner." (KAN. ADMIN. REGS. 60-11-101)

A state legislature's definition is:

- "the health care which clients receive at the first point of contact with the health care system and [which] is continuous and comprehensive. Primary health care includes health promotion, prevention of disease and disability, health maintenance, rehabilitation, identification of health problems, management of health problems, and referral" (CODE ME. R. § 02 380 008).

Finally, here is a definition provided by the American Academy of Family Physicians:

- Primary care is that care provided by physicians specifically trained for and skilled in comprehensive first contact and continuing care for persons with any undiagnosed sign, symptom, or health concern (the "undifferentiated" patient) not limited by problem origin (biological, behavioral, or social), organ system, gender, or diagnosis. Primary care includes health promotion, disease prevention, health maintenance, counseling, patient education, diagnosis and treatment of acute and chronic illnesses in a variety of health care settings (e.g., office, inpatient, critical care, long-term care, home care, day care, etc.). Primary care is performed and managed by a personal physician, utilizing other health professionals, consultation and/or referral as appropriate."[6]

Primary care is not controversial in itself. Who performs primary care is somewhat controversial. Who receives reimbursement for primary care is very controversial.

The American Academy of Family Physicians (AAFP) is a professional group that has an interest in defining primary care as a physician-generated service.

Physicians want to limit reimbursement to physicians. Physicians are competing not only with NPs but also with other groups of physicians for the designation *primary care provider.* Professional groups representing NPs likewise could define primary care in NP-specific terms.

The Institute of Medicine definition of primary care given above is notably inclusive rather than restrictive regarding which professional might provide the care. That is because the committee developing the Institute of Medicine definition included several nurses and NPs as well as physicians. The Institute of Medicine definition can be cited by NPs as a definition written by a consensus group, not subject to bias by any one professional group.

NPS' LEGAL AUTHORITY TO BE PRIMARY CARE PROVIDERS

Some state's laws specifically authorize nurse practitioners to be *primary care providers* (PCPs); i.e., be designated as the individual responsible for the primary care of a patient enrolled in a managed care plan.

An example of one such law is Maryland's, which provides that ". . . each member [of a health maintenance organization] shall have an opportunity to select a primary physician or a certified nurse practitioner from among those available to the health maintenance organization. . . ."

The law continues:

> "A member may select a certified nurse practitioner as the member's primary care provider if:
>
> (I) The certified nurse practitioner provides services at the same location as the certified nurse practitioner's collaborating physician; and
>
> (II) The collaborating physician provides the continuing medical management required under subsections (B)(5) of this section.
>
> (III) A member who selects a certified nurse practitioner as a primary care provider shall be provided the name and contact information of the certified nurse practitioner's collaborating physician.
>
> (IV) This subsection may not be construed to require that a health maintenance organization include certified nurse practitioners on the health maintenance organization's provider panel as primary care providers." (MARYLAND HEALTH-GENERAL CODE ANNOTATED § 19-705.1)

In Maryland, a clause in the state law governing health maintenance organizations had been construed as prohibiting anyone other than a physician from being a PCP. Maryland NPs went to the legislature asking for a change in that law. In 2003, the change was made, and the language provided above was enacted.

In some states, no law prohibits a nurse practitioner from being designated as a PCP.

Nurse Practitioners as Team Members in Secondary and Tertiary Care

Whereas the role of nurse practitioners was originally contemplated to be in primary care, more and more nurse practitioners are working for specialists and in hospitals. For those nurse practitioners, state law on scope of practice and reimbursement and Federal law on reimbursement is most relevant.

NP VERSUS PA: WHAT'S THE DIFFERENCE?

While NPs and PAs may function very similarly and may, in some states, be interchangeable in terms of job description, there are differences between NPs and PAs in legal definition, scope of practice, licensure, and independence of practice. PAs practice medicine under the license of a physician, never independently. NPs practice under their own licenses. PAs are true physician extenders because they never practice under their own licenses. NPs may be physician extenders or practice independently, depending upon state law. The Institute of Medicine definition of primary care provider is misleading because, legally, it is a PA's physician employer who is practicing primary care. A PA has a job description, not a scope of practice.

Definition and Scope of Practice of PAs, Compared with NPs

By definition, a PA is a health care provider who practices medicine with physician supervision. Nurse practitioners define themselves as nurses with a broadened scope of practice and do not define themselves as physician supervised professionals.

PAs include in descriptions of their duties taking medical histories, performing physical examinations, ordering and interpreting laboratory tests, diagnosing and treating illnesses, assisting in surgery, prescribing and/or dispensing medication, and counseling patients.[7] NPs would include all of the above activities in their scope of practice, with the exception of assisting in surgery. While some NPs assist in surgery under practice agreements with physicians, it is not so common an activity that it is universally included in the scope of practice of NPs. NPs usually include special attention to health care maintenance and illness prevention in their statements of scope of practice. The nurse practice act of at least one state—Oregon—includes hospital admission in the scope of NP practice.

The scope of a PA's practice corresponds with a supervising physician's practice, with the understanding that the supervising physician will handle the more complicated medical cases. PAs are authorized to prescribe medications in 47 states, the District of Columbia, and Guam.[7]

Physician Involvement with PA Practice

PAs acknowledge their status as physician extenders. According to the American Academy of Physician Assistants, "The physician assistant is a representative of the physician, treating the patient in the style and manner developed and directed by the supervising physician."[7]

The Guidelines for Physician/Physician Assistant Practice, adopted by the American Medical Association House of Delegates in 1995, state the following:

1. Health care services delivered by physicians and PAs must be within the scope of each practitioner's authorized practice as defined by state law.
2. The physician is ultimately responsible for coordinating and managing the care of patients and, with the appropriate input of the PA, ensuring the quality of health care provided to patients.
3. The physician is responsible for the supervision of the PA in all settings.
4. The role of the PA in the delivery of health care should be defined through mutually agreed-upon guidelines that are developed by the physician and the PA and based on the physician's delegatory style.
5. The physician must be available for consultation with the PA at all times either in person or through telecommunication system or other means.
6. The extent of the involvement by the PA in the assessment and implementation of treatment will depend on the complexity and acuity of the patient's condition and the training and experience and preparation of the PA as adjudged by the physician.
7. Patients should be made clearly aware at all times whether they are being cared for by a physician or a PA.
8. The physician and PA together should review all delegated patient services on a regular basis, as well as the mutually agreed-upon guidelines for practice.
9. The physician is responsible for clarifying and familiarizing the PA with his or her supervising methods and style of delegating patient care.[7]

Demographics

As of January 2003, there were approximately 46,200 people in clinical practice as PAs.[7]

Education

PAs are educated in programs that use the medical model and are designed to complement physician training. The American Academy of Physician Assistants differentiates PA education from physician education in the following way:

> One of the main differences between PA education and physician education is not the core content of the curriculum, but the amount of time

> spent in formal education. . . . [P]hysicians are required to do an internship, and the majority also complete a residency in a specialty afterwards. PAs do not have to undertake an internship or residency.[7]

Licensure Requirements

According to the American Academy of Physician Assistants, "PAs are licensed in 44 jurisdictions, certified in four, and registered in three."[7] For licensure, PAs must graduate from an accredited PA program and pass a national certifying examination.

Certification Requirements

To maintain certification, PAs must log 100 hours of continuing medical education every two years and sit for recertification every six years. See Table 1-1 for a comparison of PAs, NPs, and physicians according to basic and continuing education.

History of PAs

As with NPs, the birth of the concept of PAs came after a physician shortage was recognized in the mid-1960s. Dr. Eugene Stead of Duke University Medical Center established the first PA program, using already trained Navy corpsmen. He based his program on a fast-track training program for physicians during World War II.

NP VERSUS PHYSICIAN: WHAT'S THE DIFFERENCE?

NPs differ from physicians in definition, scope of practice, and education.

Definition and Scope of Practice of Physicians

A physician is a provider of medical care according to the laws of the individual states. An example of state law defining the practice of medicine is New Jersey's statute:

> The phrase "the practice of medicine or surgery" and the phrase "the practice of medicine and surgery" shall include the practice of any branch of medicine and/or surgery and any method of treatment of human ailment, disease, pain, injury, deformity, mental or physical condition, and the term "physician and surgeon" or "physician or surgeon" shall be deemed to include practitioners in any branch of medicine and/or surgery or method of treatment of human ailment, disease, pain, injury, deformity, mental or physical condition.
>
> *Citation:* N.J. STAT. ANN. § 45:9-5.1.

TABLE 1–1

Nurse Practitioners' Education, License, and Certification Contrasted with That of Other Primary Care Providers

Health Professional	*Years of College*	*Undergraduate Degree or Other Education*	*Graduate Degree*	*License*	*Continuing Education (Minimum)*	*Certification (Renewal)*
Nurse practitioner	2–4	AA, BS, or RN diploma	Master's degree required in 24 states	Yes (RN plus specific area of NP certification)	75 hours/5 years	Yes, every 5 years
Physician assistant	2–4	BS or certificate	Not required	Not required	100 hours/2 years	Yes, every 6 years
Primary care physician	4	BA/BS	Doctor of medicine or osteopathy required in all states	Yes (MD or DO)	50 hours/year	Optional

Source: Data from the American Nurses Credentialling Center, American Academy of Physician Assistants and American Academy of Family Physicians.

Educational Requirements of Physicians

Physicians have four years of medical education. See Table 1-1 for a comparison of NPs, physicians, and PAs on requirements for basic education, continuing education, licensure, and certification.

NP VERSUS RN: WHAT'S THE DIFFERENCE?

NPs and RNs differ in definition, scope of practice, education, and physician supervision.

Definition of RN

The legal definition of *registered nurse* is provided by the laws of the states. Michigan, for example, defines *nursing* and *registered nurse* as follows:

> The "practice of nursing" means the systematic application of substantial specialized knowledge and skill derived from the biological, physical and behavioral sciences, to the care, treatment, counsel, and health teaching of individuals who are experiencing changes in the normal health processes or who require assistance in the maintenance of health and the prevention or management of illness, injury, or disability.
>
> "Registered nurse" means an individual licensed under this article to engage in the practice of nursing which scope of practice includes the teaching, direction and supervision of less skilled personnel in the performance of delegated nursing activities.

Citation: MICH. COMP. LAWS § 333.17201.

RNs' Scope of Practice

Nursing typically includes a variety of acts, described under state law. The nursing acts described below are taken from the law of North Dakota:

a. The maintenance of health and prevention of illness.
b. Diagnosing human responses to actual or potential health problems.
c. Providing supportive and restorative care and nursing treatment, medication administration, health counseling and teaching, case finding and referral of persons who are ill, injured, or experiencing changes in the normal health processes.
d. Administration, teaching, supervision, delegation, and evaluation of health and nursing practices.
e. Collaboration with other health care professionals in the implementation of the total health care regimen and execution of the health care regimen prescribed by a health care practitioner licensed to order health care regimens.

Citation: N.D. CENT. CODE § 43-12.1-02.

RNs' Education

An RN has two to four years of college education and may have a master's degree, a doctorate degree, or other advanced training over and above the basic education.

Supervision of RNs

Supervision is generally not mandated by law for those activities within the scope of nursing practice. To provide medical care, such as administering prescription medication, an RN needs an order from a health care provider authorized by law to give orders or prescribe medication.

NP VERSUS CNS: WHAT'S THE DIFFERENCE?

Definition and Scope of Practice of CNSs

Definition and scope of practice of a *clinical nurse specialist* (CNS) are specified by state law. For example, Maine law defines CNS as follows:

> The certified clinical nurse specialist applies research-based knowledge, skills and experience to intervene in human responses to complex health and illness problems. The certified clinical nurse specialist (1) provides case management skills to coordinate comprehensive health services and ensure continuity of care, (2) evaluates client progress in attaining expected outcomes, (3) consults with other health care providers to influence care of clients, effect change in symptoms, and enhance the ability of others to provide health care, (4) performs additional functions specific to the specialty areas. In addition to the above, the certified psychiatric clinical nurse specialist may independently assess, diagnose, and therapeutically intervene in complex mental health problems using psychotherapy and other interventions.
>
> *Citation:* CODE ME. R. § 0 2 380 CH 8.1.3.D.

Education of the CNS

CNSs have, at minimum, a master's degree in nursing and may have a doctorate degree.

Physician Supervision of CNSs

CNSs have no requirement for physician supervision unless they have prescriptive authority, in which case there often are collaboration or supervision requirements specified by state law. See Table 1-2 for a comparison of NPs, CNSs, and other types of advanced practice nurses in terms of education and licensure.

TABLE 1–2

Nurse Practitioners' Educational and Professional Credentials Contrasted with Those of Other Advanced Practice Nurses (APNs)

Type of APN	*Years of College*	*Years of Training*	*Undergraduate Degree*	*Graduate Degree*	*License*	*Continuing Education*	*Renewal of Certification*
Nurse Anesthetist	4	2	BA/BS	Not required	Yes, RN plus nurse anesthetist	40 hours/2 years	Yes, as CRNA by AANA Council on Accreditation of Nurse Anesthetists
Nurse midwife	2–4	1–2	BA/BS or RN diploma	Not required	Yes, RN plus nurse midwife	50 hours/5 years, with other recertification options available	Yes, as nurse midwife by ACNM Certification Council
Nurse psychotherapist	2–4	2, plus 100 hours of supervised practice	BA/BS	Master's	Yes, RN plus nurse psychotherapist	75 hours/ 5 years	Yes, as CNS by ANCC
Nurse practitioner	2–4	1–2	BA/BS or RN diploma	Master's degree required in 24 states	Yes, RN plus nurse practitioner	Varies with certifying body; 75 hours/ 5 years (ANCC)	Yes, as NP by ANCC, PNCB, or NCC

Note: ANCC, American Nurses Credentialling Center; CRNA, certified registered nurse anesthetist; AANA, American Association of Nurse Anesthetists; ACNM, American College of Nurse Midwives; NCC, National Certification Corporation; PNCB, Pediatric Nursing Certification Board.

Source: Data from the American Nurses Credentialling Center, American Association of Nurse Anesthetists, and American College of Nurse Midwives Web sites.

WHERE DO NURSE PRACTITIONERS PRACTICE?

NPs practice in health maintenance organizations, independent or collaborative private practices, hospitals and affiliated clinics, emergency departments, family planning clinics, college health services, school clinics, employee health clinics, long-term care facilities, homeless shelters, hospices, and home-based care services.

NOTES

1. Nurse Practitioner Association of Maryland. A Nurse Practitioner Is Your Partner in Health Care. Parkville, MD; 1995. (brochure)

2. Web site of the American College of Nurse Practitioners. Available at: http://www.nurse.org/acnp. Accessed July 2003.

3. Maryland Board of Nursing. Fact Sheet on Nurse Practitioners. Baltimore, MD; 1994.

4. C. Smith and F. Maurer. Community Health Nursing. Philadelphia: W.B. Saunders; 1995: 348.

5. Institute of Medicine. Primary Care: American's Health in a New Era. Washington, DC: IOM; 1996.

6. Web site of the American Academy of Family Physicians (AAFP). Available at: http://www.aafp.org. Accessed July 2003.

7. Web site of the American Academy of Physician Assistants. Available at: http://www.aapa.org. Accessed July 2003.

APPENDIX 1-A

State-by-State What is a Nurse Practitioner?

State-by-state definitions of nurse practitioner, including citation of code section:

ALABAMA

Practice as certified registered nurse practitioner means the performance of nursing skills by a registered nurse who has demonstrated by certification that he/she has advanced knowledge and skills in the delivery of nursing services within a health care system that provides for consultation, collaborative management, or referral as indicated by the health status of the client.

Citation: ALA. CODE § 32-21-81(4)a.

Advanced nurse practitioner. A registered nurse who has gained additional knowledge and skills through successful completion of an organized program of nursing education that prepares nurses for advanced practice rules and has been certified by the Board of Nursing to engage in the practice of advanced practice nursing.

Citation: ALA. ADMIN. CODE § r. 610-X-9-.07(3).

ALASKA

"Advanced nurse practitioner" means a registered nurse authorized to practice in the state who, because of specialized education and experience, is certified to perform acts of medical diagnosis and the prescription and dispensing of medical, therapeutic, or corrective measures under regulations adopted by the Board of Nursing.

Citation: ALAS. STAT. § 08.68.410.(1).

ARIZONA

"Registered nurse practitioner" means a professional nurse who is certified by the board in those areas authorized by the board through its rules for extended nursing practice and who has completed a nurse practitioner education program approved or recognized by the board.

Citation: ARIZ. REV. STAT. ANN. § 32-1601.12.

ARKANSAS

Practice of advanced nurse practitioner nursing means the performance for compensation of nursing skills by a registered nurse, who, as demonstrated by national certification, has advanced knowledge and practice skills in the delivery of nursing services.

Citation: ARK. CODE ANN. § 17-87-102(3).

CALIFORNIA

The Legislature finds that various and conflicting definitions of nurse practitioner are being created by state agencies and private organizations within California. The Legislature also finds that the public is harmed by conflicting usage of the title of nurse practitioner and lack of correspondence between use of the title and qualifications of the registered nurse using the title. Therefore, the Legislature finds the public interest served by the determination of the legitimate use of the title "nurse practitioner" by registered nurses.

Citation: CAL. BUS. & PROF. CODE § 2834.

Nurse practitioner means a registered nurse who possesses additional preparation and skills in physical diagnosis, psych-social assessment and management of health-illness needs in primary health care, and who has been prepared in a program conforming to board standards as specified in section 1484.

Citation: CAL. CODE REGS. tit. 16 § 1480(a).

COLORADO

"Advanced practice nurse" means a professional nurse who is licensed to practice pursuant to this article, who obtains specialized education and training as provided in this section and who applies to and is accepted by the board for inclusion in the advanced practice registry.

Citation: COLO. REV. STAT. ANN. § 12-38-111.5.(2).

"Advanced practice nurse" is the umbrella term for certified nurse midwife, clinical nurse specialist, certified registered nurse anesthetist, and nurse practitioner and these nurses may use APN in lieu of any of these designations.

Citation: 3 COLO. CODE REGS. § 716-1.

CONNECTICUT

Advanced nursing practice is defined as the performance of advanced level nursing practice activities which, by virtue of post-basic specialized education and experience, are appropriate to and may be performed by an advanced practice registered nurse.

Citation: CONN. GEN. STAT. § 20-87a(b).

DELAWARE

"Advanced practice nurse" means an individual whose education and certification meet criteria established by the Board of Nursing who is currently licensed as a registered nurse and has a master's degree or a post-basic program certified in a clinical nursing specialty with national certification. "Advanced practice nurses" (APNs) shall include, but not be limited to, nurse practitioners, certified registered nurse anesthetists, certified nurse midwives, or clinical nurse specialists. Advanced practice nursing is the application of nursing principles . . . at an advanced level and includes:

a. For those advanced practice nurses who do not perform independent acts of diagnosis or prescription, the authority as granted within the scope of practice rules and regulations promulgated by the Board of Nursing, and
b. For those advanced practice nurses performing independent acts of diagnosis and/or prescription with the collaboration of a licensed physician, dentist, podiatrist, or licensed Delaware health care delivery system without written guidelines or protocols and within the scope of practice as defined in the rules and regulations promulgated by the Joint Practice Committee and approved by the Board of Medical Practice.

Citation: DEL. CODE ANN. tit. 24, § 1902(d)(1).

DISTRICT OF COLUMBIA

"Practice of advanced registered nursing" means the performance of advanced-level nursing action by an advanced practice registered nurse certified pursuant to this chapter which, by virtue of post-basic specialized education, training, and experience, are proper to be performed. The advanced practice registered nurse may perform actions of nursing diagnosis and nursing treatment of alteration in health care status. The advanced registered nurse may also perform actions of medical diagnosis and treatment, prescription, and other functions which are identified in subchapter VI of this chapter and carried out in accordance with procedures required by this chapter.

Citation: D.C. CODE ANN. § 3-1201.02.

FLORIDA

"Advanced registered nurse practitioner" means any person licensed in this state to practice professional nursing and certified in advanced or specialized nursing practice.

Citation: FLA. STAT. ANN. § 464.003(6).

GEORGIA

"Advanced nursing practice" means practice by a registered professional nurse who meets those educational, practice, certification requirements, or any combination of such requirements, as specified by the board and includes certified nurse midwives, nurse practitioners, certified registered nurse anesthetists, clinical nurse specialists in psychiatry/mental health, and others recognized by the board.

Citation: GA. CODE ANN. § 43-26-3 (1).

An advanced practice registered nurse (APRN) is a registered professional nurse who has successfully completed/graduated from a post-basic educational program for nurse practitioners, at least nine months in length, which includes theoretical and practical components and evidence of advanced pharmacology within the curriculum or as a separate course.

Citation: GA. COMP. R. & REGS. § r. 410-12.03.

HAWAII

"Advanced Practice Registered Nurse" means a registered nurse who has met the qualifications for APRN set forth in this chapter and through rules of the board, which shall include educational requirements.

Citation: HAW. REV. STAT. § 457-2.

"Advanced practice registered nurse (APRN)" means a registered nurse licensed to practice in this State who has met the qualifications set forth in chapter 457, HRS, and this subchapter, who, because of advanced education, prevention, and the utilization of medical, therapeutic, or corrective measures.

Citation: HAW. ADMIN. § R. 16-89-77.

IDAHO

"Nurse practitioner" means a licensed professional nurse who has graduated from a nationally accredited nurse practitioner program, passed a qualifying examination recognized by the board, and has current initial certification or current recertification from a national group recognized by the board.

Citation: IDAHO CODE § 54-1402(1)(c).

ILLINOIS

"Advanced practice nurse" or "APN" means a person who: (1) is licensed as a registered professional nurse under this Act; (2) meets the requirements for licensure as an advanced practice nurse under Section 15-10; (3) except as provided in Section 15-25, has a written collaborative agreement with a collaborating physician in the diagnosis of illness and management of wellness and other conditions as appropriate to the level and area of his or her practice in accordance with Section 15-15; and (4) cares for patients (A) by using advanced diagnostic skills, the results of diagnostic tests and procedures ordered by the advanced practice nurse, a physician assistant, a dentist, a podiatrist, or a physician, and professional judgment to initiate and coordinate the care of patients; (B) by ordering diagnostic tests, prescribing medications and drugs in accordance with Section 15-20, and administering medications and drugs; and (C) by using medical, therapeutic, and corrective measures to treat illness and improve health status.

Citation: 225 ILL. COMP. STAT. § 65/15-5 and
ILL. ADMIN. CODE tit. 68 § 1305.10.

INDIANA

"Advanced practice nurse" means (1) a nurse practitioner, (2) a nurse midwife, (3) a clinical nurse specialist, who is a registered nurse qualified to practice nursing in a specialty role based upon the additional knowledge and skill gained through a formal organized program of study and clinical expertise, or the equivalent as determined by the board, which does not limit but extends or expands the function of the nurse.

Citation: IND. CODE ANN. § 25-23-1-1(b).

IOWA

"Advanced registered nurse practitioner" means a nurse with current licensure as a registered nurse in Iowa who is registered in Iowa to practice in the advanced role.

Citation: IOWA ADMIN. CODE § r. 655-7.1(152).

"Certified nurse practitioner" means an ARNP educated in the discipline of nursing who has advanced knowledge of nursing, physical and psychosocial assessment, appropriate interventions and management of health care, and who possesses evidence of current certification by a national professional association approved by the board.

Citation: IOWA ADMIN. CODE § r. 655-7.1(152).

KANSAS

"Advanced registered nurse practitioner" or "ARNP" means a professional nurse who holds a certificate of qualification from the board to function as a professional nurse in an expanded role, and this expanded role shall be defined by rules and regulations adopted by the board in accordance with the KSA 65-1130.

Citation: KAN. STAT. ANN. § 65-1113(g).

KENTUCKY

"Advanced registered nurse practitioner" shall mean one who is registered and designated to engage in advanced registered nursing practice, including, but not limited to, the nurse anesthetist, nurse midwife, and nurse practitioner pursuant to KRS 314.042.

Citation: KY. REV. STAT. ANN. § 314.011(7).

LOUISIANA

Nurse practitioner or "NP" is an advanced practice registered nurse educated in a specified area of care and certified according to the requirements of a nationally recognized accrediting agency such as the American Nurses Association Credentialling Center, National Certification Corporation for the Obstetric, Gynecologic and Neonatal Nursing Specialties, or the National Certification Board of Pediatric Nurse Practitioners and Nurses, or as approved by the board and who is authorized to provide primary, acute, or chronic care as an advanced nurse practitioner acting within his scope of practice to individuals, families, and other groups in a variety of settings including, but not limited to, homes, institutions, offices, industry, schools, and other community agencies.

Citation: LA. REV. STAT. ANN. § 37:913d.

MAINE

"Certified nurse practitioner" means a registered professional nurse who has received post-graduate education designed to prepare the nurse for advanced practice registered nursing in a specialty area in nursing that has a defined scope of practice and has been certified in the clinical specialty by a national certifying organization acceptable to the Board.

Citation: CODE ME. R. § 02 380 008.

MARYLAND

Nurse practitioner means a registered nurse who by means of certification may engage in the activities authorized by regulation.

Citation: MD. REGS. CODE § 10.27.07.01.B(4).

MASSACHUSETTS

Practice in the expanded role means professional nursing activity engaged in by a registered nurse in accordance with 244 CMR 4.00 and involving the employment of advanced skills including the evaluation, diagnosis, and treatment of patients with diseases and adverse health conditions. It also means the management of therapeutic regimens for acute and chronic problems associated with such diseases and conditions. It does not mean activity which the Board recognizes as the generic practice of registered nurses.

Citation: MASS. REGS. CODE tit. 244, § 4.05.

The definition of "Nurse Practitioner is found in Massachusetts law relating to "Controlled Substances":

"Nurse practitioner," a nurse with advanced training who is authorized to practice by the board of registration in nursing as a nurse practitioner, as provided for in section 80B of Chapter 112."
Section 80B of Chapter 112 describes the information which nurse practitioners must furnish to the board of registration in nursing in order to become licensed.

MICHIGAN

The board of nursing may issue a specialty certification to a registered professional nurse who has advanced training beyond that required for initial licensure and who has demonstrated competency through examination or other evaluative processes and who practices in 1 of the following health profession specialty fields: nurse midwifery, nurse anesthetist, or nurse practitioner.

Citation: MICH. COMP. LAWS § 333.17210.

"Certified nurse practitioner" means an individual licensed as a registered professional nurse under part 172 who has been issued a specialty certification as a nurse practitioner by the board of nursing.

Citation: MICH. COMP. LAWS § 333.2701(c).

MINNESOTA

"Advanced practice registered nurse" means an individual licensed as a registered nurse by the board and certified by a national nurse certification organization acceptable to the board to practice as a clinical nurse specialist, nurse anesthetist, nurse midwife, or nurse practitioner.

Citation: MINN. STAT. § 148.171.

MISSISSIPPI

Certified Nurse Practitioner: A registered nurse who has met all requirements for certification, as stated in the Nursing Practice Law, Rules and Regulations, and who has been certified as a nurse practitioner by the Board.

Citation: MISS. NURSING REGS., CH. V, § 1.

MISSOURI

"Advanced practice nurse" is a nurse who has education beyond the basic nursing education and is certified by a nationally recognized professional organization as having a nursing specialty, or who meets criteria for advanced practice nurses established by the board of nursing.

Citation: MO. CODE REGS. ANN. § 335.016 (2).

"Advanced practice nurse" is a registered professional nurse as defined in section 335.016(2) RSM and who is a nurse anesthetist, nurse midwife, nurse practitioner, or clinical nurse specialist.

Citation: MO. CODE REGS. ANN. tit. 4, § 200-4.100.

MONTANA

Advanced practice registered nurses are nurses who must have additional professional education beyond the basic nursing degree required of a registered nurse. Additional education must be obtained in courses offered in a university setting or its equivalent. The applicant must be certified or in the process of being certified by a certifying body for advanced practice registered nurses. Advanced practice registered nurses include nurse practitioners, nurse-midwives, nurse-anesthetists, and clinical nurse specialists.

Citation: MONT. CODE ANN. § 37-8-202(5)(a).

NEBRASKA

Advanced practice registered nurse shall mean a registered nurse who meets the requirements established in section 71-1722 and who holds a current license as an advanced practice registered nurse issued by the department.

Citation: NEB. REV. STAT. § 71-1707.

NEVADA

"Advanced practitioner of nursing" means a registered professional nurse who has specialized skill, knowledge, and experience obtained from an organized formal program of training and who is authorized in special conditions as defined by NAC 632.255 to 632.295, inclusive, to provide designated services in addition to those which a registered nurse is authorized to perform.

Citation: NEV. ADMIN. CODE § 632.020.

NEW HAMPSHIRE

"Advanced Registered Nurse Practitioner" or "A.R.N.P." means a registered nurse who is licensed as having specialized clinical qualifications as provided by RSA 326-B:10.

Citation: N.H. REV. STAT. ANN. § 326-B:2.II.

NEW JERSEY

"Nurse practitioner/clinical nurse specialist" means a person who holds a certification in accordance with section 8 or 9 of P.L. 1991, c.377(C.45:11-47 or 45.11-48).

Citation: N.J. STAT. ANN. § 45:11-23.d.

NEW MEXICO

"Certified nurse practitioner" means a registered nurse who is licensed by the board for advanced practice as a certified registered nurse anesthetist and whose name and pertinent information are entered on the list of certified registered nurse practitioners maintained by the board.

Citation: N.M. STAT. ANN. § 61-3-3.C.

NEW YORK

The practice of registered nursing by a nurse practitioner, certified under section six thousand nine hundred ten of this article, may include the diagnosis of illness and physical conditions and the performance of therapeutic and corrective measures within a specialty area of practice, in collaboration with a licensed physician qualified to collaborate in the specialty involved, provided such services are performed in accordance with a written practice agreement and written practice protocols.

Citation: N.Y. EDUC. LAW § 6902.3(a).

NORTH CAROLINA

"Nurse Practitioner" means a currently licensed registered nurse approved to perform medical acts under an agreement with a licensed physician for ongoing supervision, consultation, collaboration, and evaluation of the medical acts performed. Only a registered nurse approved by the Medical Board and the Board of Nursing may legally identify oneself as a nurse practitioner. It is understood that the nurse practitioner, by virtue of registered nurse licensure, is independently accountable for those nursing acts which he or she may perform.

Citation: N.C. ADMIN. CODE tit. 21, § r. 36.0227(a)(4).

NORTH DAKOTA

"Advanced practice registered nurse" means a person who holds current license to practice in this state as an advanced practice registered nurse and either has a graduate degree with a nursing focus or has completed the educational requirements in effect when the person was initially licensed.

Citation: N.D. CENT. CODE § 43-12.1-02.1.

OHIO

"Certified nurse practitioner" means a registered nurse who holds a valid certificate of authority issued under this chapter that authorizes the practice of nursing as a certified nurse practitioner in accordance with section 4723.43 of the Revised Code and rules adopted by the Board of Nursing.

Citation: OHIO REV. CODE ANN. § 4723.01(5).

OKLAHOMA

"Advanced practice nurse" means a licensed registered nurse who has successfully completed a formal program of study approved by the Board which is designed to prepare registered nurses to perform in an expanded role in the delivery of health care, is nationally certified by an appropriate certifying body, recognized by the Board, and has received a certificate of recognition from the Board. The term advanced practice nurse shall include Advanced Registered Nurse Practitioners, Clinical Nurse Specialists, Nurse Midwives, and Certified Registered Nurse Anesthetists.

Citation: OKLA. STAT. ANN., tit. 59, § 567.3a(5).

"Advanced registered nurse practitioner" means a licensed registered nurse who has met the requirements of paragraph 5 of this section. The advanced registered nurse practitioner performs an expanded role in the delivery of health care that is:

a. Consistent with advanced educational preparation as an advanced practice nurse in the area of specialty,
b. Functions within the advanced registered nurse practitioner scope of practice denoted for the area of specialization, and
c. Is in accord with the standards for advanced practice nurses as identified by the certifying body and approved by the Board.

Citation: OKLA. STAT. ANN. tit. 59, § 567.3a(6).

OREGON

"Nurse practitioner" (NP) means a registered nurse who provides health care in an expanded specialty role. The title nurse practitioner and specialty category of practice shall not be used unless the individual is certified by the Board.

Citation: OR. ADMIN. § R. 851-050-0000.

PENNSYLVANIA

"Certified registered nurse practitioner" is a registered nurse licensed in this Commonwealth who is certified by the Board in a particular clinical specialty area and who , while functioning in the expanded rule as a registered nurse, performs acts of medical diagnosis or prescription of medical therapeutic or corrective measures in collaboration with and under the direction of a physician licensed to practice medicine in this Commonwealth. Nothing in this subchapter is to be deemed to limit or prohibit a nurse from engaging in those activities which normally constitute the practice of nursing as defined in section 2 of the Professional Nursing law.

Citation: 49 PA. CODE § 21.251.

RHODE ISLAND

"Certified registered nurse practitioner" is an advanced role utilizing independent knowledge of physical assessment and management of health care and illnesses. The practice includes prescriptive privileges. The practice includes collaboration with other licensed health care professionals including but not limited to physicians, pharmacists, podiatrists, dentists, and nurses.

Citation: R.I. GEN. LAWS § 5-34-3.(b).

"Certified Registered Nurse Practitioner" means a registered nurse who practices in an advanced role utilizing independent knowledge of physical assessment and management of health care and illnesses.

Citation: R.I. CODE R. 14 140 022-5.

The practice includes prescriptive privileges, and collaboration with other licensed health care professionals, including, but not limited to, physicians, pharmacists, podiatrists, dentists, and nurses.

Citation: R.I. R. R5-34-NUR/ED 1.8.

SOUTH CAROLINA

"Nurse practitioner" means a registered nurse who has completed a post-basic or advanced formal education program acceptable to the board and who demonstrates advanced knowledge and skill in assessment and management of physical and psychosocial health-illness status of individuals and/or families, and/or groups.

Citation: 26 S.C. CODE ANN. REGS. § R91-2.d.

SOUTH DAKOTA

"Nurse practitioner" means a person duly authorized under this chapter to practice the specialty of nurse practitioner as defined in 36-9A-12.

Citation: S.D. CODIFIED LAWS § 36-9A-1.

South Dakota Codified Laws § 36-9A-12 defines the medical functions delegated to nurse practitioners. See Appendix 2-A for those functions.

TENNESSEE

"Advanced practice nurse" means a registered nurse with a master's degree or higher in a nursing specialty and national specialty certification as a nurse practitioner, nurse anesthetist, nurse midwife, or clinical nurse specialist.

Citation: TENN. CODE ANN. § 63-7-126(a)

TEXAS

Advanced practice nurse—A registered professional nurse approved by the board to practice as an advanced practice nurse based on completing an advanced educational program acceptable to the board. The term includes a nurse practitioner, nurse midwife, nurse anesthetist, and a clinical nurse specialist. The advanced practice nurse is prepared to practice in an expanded role to provide health care to individuals, families, and/or groups in a variety of settings including, but not limited to homes, hospitals, institutions, offices, industry, schools, community agencies, public and private clinics, and private practice. The advanced practice nurse acts independently and/or in collaboration with other health care professionals in the delivery of health care services.

Citation: TEX. ADMIN. CODE § 219.2(3).

UTAH

"Practice of advanced practice registered nursing" means the practice of nursing within the generally recognized scope and standards of advanced practice registered nursing as defined by rule and consistent with professionally recognized preparation and education standards of an advanced practice registered nurse by a person licensed under this chapter as an advanced practice registered nurse. Advanced practice nursing includes:

(a) Maintenance and promotion of health and prevention of disease;

(b) Diagnosis, treatment, correction, consultation, or referral for common health problems; and

(c) Prescription or administration of prescription drugs or devices, including local anesthesia; schedule IV-V controlled substances; and schedule II-III controlled substances in accordance with a consultation and referral plan.

Citation: UTAH CODE ANN. § 58-31b-102(16).

VERMONT

"Advanced practice registered nurse" means a licensed registered nurse authorized to practice in this state who, because of specialized education and experience is endorsed to perform acts of medical diagnosis and to prescribe medical, therapeutic, or corrective measures under administrative rules adopted by the board.

Citation: VT. STAT. ANN. tit. 26, § 1572(4).

VIRGINIA

"Licensed nurse practitioner" means a registered nurse who has met the requirements for licensure as stated in Part II of this chapter and has been licensed by the boards [of medicine and nursing].

Citation: 18 VA. CODE ANN. § 90-30-60.

"Nurse practitioner" means a registered nurse who has met the additional requirements of education and examination for licensure as a nurse practitioner in the Commonwealth.

Citation: 18 VA. CODE ANN. § 90-40-10.

WASHINGTON

An advanced practice registered nurse is a registered nurse prepared in a formal education program to assume primary responsibility for continuous and comprehensive management of a broad range of patient care, concerns, and problems.

Citation: WASH. ADMIN. CODE § 246-840-300.

WEST VIRGINIA

"Nurse practitioner" means a registered nurse qualified by virtue of his or her education and credentials and approved by the West Virginia board of examiners for registered professional nurses to practice as an advanced practice nurse independently or in a collaborative relationship with a physician.

Citation: W. VA. CODE § 9-4B-1(c).

"Advanced nurse practitioner" means a registered nurse with substantial theoretical knowledge in a specialized area of nursing practice and proficient clinical utilization of the knowledge in implementing the nursing process, and who has met the further requirements of title 19, legislative rules for West Virginia board of examiners for registered professional nurses, series 7, who has mutually agreed upon association in writing with a physician and has been selected by or assigned to the person and has primary responsibility for treatment and care of the person.

Citation: W. VA. CODE § 16-30-3(c).

WISCONSIN

"Nurse practitioner" means a registered nurse licensed under ch. 441 or in a party state, as defined in § 441.50(2)(j), whose practice of professional nursing under § 441.001(4) includes performance of delegated medical services under the supervision of a physician, dentist, or podiatrist.

Citation: WIS. STAT. § 225.06(d).

WYOMING

"Advanced practitioner of nursing" means a registered professional nurse who performs advanced nursing acts and who may perform medical acts including prescribing or providing prepackaged medications, except schedule I and schedule II drugs as defined in W.S. 35-7-1013 through 35-7-1016, in collaboration with a licensed or otherwise legally authorized physician or dentist, in such manner to assure quality and appropriateness of services rendered. The advanced practitioner of nursing performs such acts by reason of postgraduate education and additional nursing preparation which provides for the knowledge, judgement, and skill beyond that required of a registered professional nurse in paragraph (ix) of this subsection and who has completed a nationally accredited educational program for preparation as an advanced practitioner of nursing or who has passed a national certification examination of a nationally recognized accrediting agency accepted by the board.

Citation: WYO. STAT. ANN. § 33-21-120(a)(i).

State-by-State Titles for Nurse Practitioners

ALABAMA: Certified Registered Nurse Practitioner (CRNP)

ALASKA: Advanced Nurse Practitioner (ANP)

ARIZONA: Registered Nurse Practitioner (RNP)

ARKANSAS: Registered Nurse Practitioner (RNP)

CALIFORNIA: Nurse Practitioner (NP)

COLORADO: Nurse Practitioner (NP) or Advanced Practice Nurse (APN)

CONNECTICUT: Advanced Practice Registered Nurse (APRN) or Certified Nurse Practitioner (CNP)

DELAWARE: Advanced Practice Nurse (APN) or Nurse Practitioner (NP)

DISTRICT OF COLUMBIA: Nurse-Practitioner, Certified Nurse-Practitioner, or C.N.P.

FLORIDA: Advanced Registered Nurse Practitioner (ARNP)

GEORGIA: Advanced Practice Registered Nurse (APRN) or Nurse Practitioner (NP)

HAWAII: Advanced Practice Registered Nurse (APRN)

IDAHO: Nurse Practitioner (NP) or Advanced Practice Professional Nurse

ILLINOIS: Certified Nurse Practitioner (CNP)

INDIANA: Advanced Practice Nurse (APN) or Nurse Practitioner (NP)

IOWA: Advanced Registered Nurse Practitioner (ARNP)

KANSAS: Advanced Registered Nurse Practitioner (ARNP)

KENTUCKY: Advanced Registered Nurse Practitioner (ARNP)

LOUISIANA: Advanced Practice Registered Nurse (APRN) or Nurse Practitioner (NP)

MAINE: Advanced Practice Registered Nurse (APRN) or Certified Nurse Practitioner (CNP)

MARYLAND: Certified Registered Nurse Practitioner (CRNP)

MASSACHUSETTS: Nurse Practitioner (NP)

MICHIGAN: Nurse Practitioner (NP)

MINNESOTA: Nurse Practitioner (NP)

MISSISSIPPI: Advanced Practice Registered Nurse (APRN) or Certified Nurse Practitioner (CNP)

MISSOURI: Advanced Practice Nurse (APN) or Nurse Practitioner (NP)

MONTANA: Advanced Practice Registered Nurse (APRN) or Nurse Practitioner (NP)

NEBRASKA: Advanced Practice Registered Nurse

NEVADA: Advanced Practice Nurse (APN)

NEW HAMPSHIRE: Advanced Registered Nurse Practitioner (ARNP)

NEW JERSEY: Registered Nurse, Nurse Practitioner, Certified (RN, NP, C)

NEW MEXICO: Certified Nurse Practitioner (CNP)

NEW YORK: Nurse Practitioner (NP)

NORTH CAROLINA: Nurse Practitioner (NP)

NORTH DAKOTA: Advanced Practice Registered Nurse (APRN) or Nurse Practitioner (NP)

OHIO: Certified Nurse Practitioner (CNP)

OKLAHOMA: Advanced Registered Nurse Practitioner (ARNP)

OREGON: Nurse Practitioner (NP)

PENNSYLVANIA: Certified Registered Nurse Practitioner (CRNP)

RHODE ISLAND: Certified Registered Nurse Practitioner (RNP)

SOUTH CAROLINA: Nurse Practitioner (NP)

SOUTH DAKOTA: Certified Nurse Practitioner (CNP)

TENNESSEE: Certified Nurse Practitioner (CNP)

TEXAS: Advanced Practice Nurse (APN) or Nurse Practitioner (NP)

UTAH: Advanced Practice Registered Nurse (APRN)

VERMONT: Advanced Practice Registered Nurse (APRN) is used to describe all the categories of RNs in advanced nursing practice.

VIRGINIA: Advanced Practice Nurse (APN) or Nurse Practitioner (NP)

WASHINGTON: Advanced Practice Registered Nurse Practitioner (APRN)

WEST VIRGINIA: Advanced Practice Nurse (APN) or Nurse Practitioner (NP)

WISCONSIN: Advanced Practice Nurse (APN) or Nurse Practitioner (NP)

WYOMING: Advanced Practitioner of Nursing (APN)

CHAPTER 2

Legal Scope of Nurse Practitioner Practice

Having an adequate legal description of NPs' scope of practice in state law is important for the following reasons:

1. To allow NPs to perform at their level of education and training
2. To avoid any charges of practicing medicine without a license
3. To avoid imputation of liability for medical malpractice to someone other than the NP, usually a physician
4. To place accountability for benefits to patients and harm to patients squarely on the NP
5. To provide a basis for inclusion of NPs in the legal definition of primary care providers, which is necessary for admission to provider panels
6. To establish that the NP is a professional entity, not just a "nonphysician," a "physician extender," or whatever an agency, employer, or delegating physician decides an NP is
7. To get reimbursement for physician services, when provided by an NP.

State law is the most powerful source of authority for professional practice. However, federal agencies and private businesses may have policies on NP scope of practice, and professional societies may have accepted certain tasks, functions, and decisions as part of NP scope of practice.

PROFESSIONAL ASSOCIATION DEFINITION OF SCOPE OF PRACTICE

Some associations define the scope of practice for NPs in general or for individual NPs. For example, the American Academy of Nurse Practitioners' statement on scope of practice says:

> Nurse practitioners are primary care providers who practice in ambulatory, acute, and long-term care settings. According to their practice specialty these primary care providers provide nursing and medical services to individuals, families and groups. In addition to diagnosing

> and managing acute episodic and chronic illnesses, NPs emphasize health promotion and disease prevention. Services include but are not limited to ordering, conducting and interpreting diagnostic and laboratory tests, prescription of pharmacologic agents and treatments and nonpharmacologic therapies. Teaching and counseling individuals, families and groups are a major part of nurse practitioners' practice. Nurse practitioners practice autonomously and in collaboration with health care professionals and other individuals to diagnose, treat and manage the patient's health problems. They serve as health care resources, interdisciplinary consultants and patient advocates.[1]

STATUTORY VERSUS REGULATORY SCOPE OF NP PRACTICE

Some states define scope of practice in statutes enacted by the state legislature. In other states, the legislature gives the board of nursing the authority to define the scope of NP practice. Either way is enforceable, and regulations carry the same force of law as statutes.

Some states describe scope of practice specifically, and some define it generally. State statutes describing NP scope of practice fall into six categories:

1. Scope of practice is clearly defined by statute.
2. Scope of practice is clearly defined by regulation.
3. Scope of practice is vaguely defined by statute.
4. Scope of practice is not defined.
5. Scope of practice is defined by exception from a state law prohibiting practice of medicine without a license.
6. Scope of practice is defined by the individual physician, who may delegate to an NP by law.

The first category is most secure for the NP.

At a time when NPs are viewed by physicians as competitors, the first response to competitive pressures will be for physicians to point to state law and ask for strict interpretation. For example, physicians may counter NP efforts to be designated as primary care providers (PCPs) for managed-care organizations by claiming that state law does not explicitly authorize NPs to perform the functions necessary for primary care. Then, only NPs in states where the NP scope of practice is clearly defined as including medical diagnosis and treatment, prescription of medication, and oversight of comprehensive health care services for patients will have legal grounds for arguing that NPs should be admitted to provider panels as PCPs.

On the other hand, a vaguely worded nurse practice act that states, for example, that the scope of NP practice includes "acts of advanced nursing practice" will not provide sound legal basis for arguments that NPs should be admitted to managed care provider panels or get fees for providing physician services. It is difficult to argue to managed-care executives, state administrators, and legislators that "acts of nursing practice" are the acts necessary to perform physician services.

PHYSICIAN CHALLENGES TO NPs' SCOPE OF PRACTICE

An example of a physician challenge to NPs' scope of practice is a 1984 Missouri court case, *Sermchief v. Gonzales* [660 S.W.2d 683 (Mo. 1984)]. It remains the only example of an NP being prosecuted for practicing medicine without a license. That case, which the NPs won only after it went to the state's supreme court, could be repeated in other states today where state law is not specific enough about the authority of NPs to diagnose and treat.

In *Sermchief,* two obstetrical-gynecologic NPs were working in a family planning clinic under written protocols with the clinic's physicians. The NPs were taking histories, performing physical examinations, treating minor illnesses, and prescribing contraceptives. There was no charge of malpractice. The Missouri Board of Medicine charged that the NPs were practicing medicine without a license.

The lower court found that the NPs were practicing medicine without a license. However, the Missouri Supreme Court, on analyzing the nurse practice act, noted that the legislature had deleted a requirement that a physician directly supervise nursing functions and decided that by that deletion the legislature had intended to broaden the scope of nursing.

The NPs eventually prevailed in the *Sermchief* case, but that will not necessarily help NPs in other states if there is no express statutory authority for NPs' medical functions. NPs need clear statutory definition of a scope of practice that includes medical diagnoses and treatment and prescriptive authority.

NEED FOR CLARITY OF SCOPE OF PRACTICE

Some state laws describe scope of practice succinctly, and others go into great detail. Longer is not necessarily better, and vague language should be avoided. Consider Oklahoma's statute on nurse practitioner scope of practice.[1]

> An advanced registered NP in accordance with the scope of practice of the advanced registered nurse practitioner shall be eligible to obtain recognition as authorized by the Board to prescribe, as defined by rules and subject to the medical direction of a supervising physician.
>
> *Citation:* OKLA. STAT. ANN. tit. 59, § 567.3a.(6).

Under Oklahoma's statutory definition of NP scope of practice, an NP can prescribe, but it is unclear what else an NP can do.*

An example of a general and succinct description of scope of practice is Pennsylvania's. A CRNP, while functioning in the expanded role as a registered nurse, performs acts of medical diagnosis or prescription of medical therapeutics or corrective measures in collaboration with and under the direction of a physician (49 PA code § 21.251). In one short sentence, Pennsylvania lawmakers give

---

*Oklahoma regulations give NPs "responsibility" for diagnosing and managing illness, referring, consulting, and counseling.

NPs authority to diagnose and treat medical conditions, including the writing of prescriptions.

The succinct Pennsylvania law actually provides more professional safety than the longer Oklahoma law. In Pennsylvania, it is clear that NPs are authorized to diagnose and treat. In Oklahoma, NPs may have an "expanded role," but it is not clear what that role is, other than to prescribe, which is authorized in the adjacent paragraph.

See Exhibit 2-1 for a breakdown of elements of NP practice found in various state laws. See Appendix 2-A for the law of each of the states regarding NP scope of practice.

NP SCOPE OF PRACTICE COMPARED WITH RN SCOPE OF PRACTICE

NP scope of practice usually includes medical diagnosis and treatment, while RN scope of practice usually includes "nursing diagnosis" and "nursing interventions" or "nursing treatments."

Compare Oregon's scope of practice for an RN to Oregon's scope of practice for an NP. Oregon's law on scope of practice of an RN states:

> The registered nurse shall:
>
> - Conduct and document nursing assessments of the health status of individuals and groups by collecting objective and subjective data from observations, examinations, interviews, and written records in an accurate and timely manner as appropriate to the client's health care needs.
> - Establish and document nursing diagnoses which serve as a basis for the plan of care.
> - Develop and modify the plan of care based on assessment and nursing diagnosis. This includes: identifying priorities in the plan of care; setting realistic and measurable goals to implement the plan of care; identifying nursing intervention(s) based on the nursing diagnosis; prescribing nursing orders based on the nursing diagnosis; identifying measures to maintain comfort, to support human functions and responses, to maintain an environment conducive to well being, and to provide health teaching and health counseling.
> - Implement the plan of care by initiating nursing interventions through giving direct care; assisting with care; following nursing orders; assigning, delegating, and supervising care; teaching clients, family members, or significant others; referring to appropriate resources. . . .
> - Evaluate the responses of individuals or groups to nursing interventions. Evaluation should involve the client, family, significant others, and health team members.
>
> *Citation:* OR. ADMIN. § R. 851-45-010.

Exhibit 2-1 Specific Functions Included in States' Definitions of NP Scope of Practice

Diagnose	**Treat**	**Prescribe**	**Admit to**	KS
AL	AL	AL	**Hospital**	LA
AZ	AZ	AZ	AZ	ME
CO	CO	CO	OR	MT
CT	CT	CT	WA	NV
DE	DE	DE		NC
DC	DC	DC	**Refer**	NH
GA	FL	FL	AL	OK
ID	GA	ID	AZ	OR
IL	ID	IL	DC	SD
IN	IL	KS	DE	
LA	LA	LA	IN	**Order Tests**
ME	ME	MD	LA	AL
MD	MD	MA	ME	AZ
MA	MA	MN	MD	DE
MN	MN	NC	MT	FL
NC	NE	NE	NC	HI
NE	NV	NH	NE	ID
NH	NH	NJ	NH	IL
NY	NY	NM	NV	KY
OK	NC	NY	OK	LA
OR	OK	OH	OR	MA
PA	OR	OK	SD	NE
SC	PA	OR	WA	NH
SD	SC	PA		NJ
UT	SD	RI	**Repair**	NV
VT	UT	SC	**Laceration**	NC
WA	VT	SD	NV	WA
WV	WA	TX		
	WV	UT	**Teach**	
		VT	AL	
		WA	DE	
		WI	HI	
		WY	IN	

Oregon's board of nursing has elegantly defined scope of NP practice as follows:

> The nurse practitioner is independently responsible and accountable for the continuous and comprehensive management of a broad range of health care, which may include:
> - Promotion and maintenance of health
> - Prevention of illness and disability
> - Assessment of clients, synthesis and analysis of data, and application of nursing principles and therapeutic modalities

- Management of health care during acute and chronic phases of illness
- Admission of his/her clients to hospitals and long term care facilities and management of client care in these facilities
- Counseling
- Consultation and/or collaboration with other care providers and community resources
- Referral to other health care providers and community resources
- Management and coordination of care
- Use of research skills
- Diagnosis of health/illness status
- Prescription and/or administration of therapeutic devices and measures including legend drugs and controlled substances . . . consistent with the definition of the practitioner's specialty category and scope of practice.

The nurse practitioner is responsible for recognizing limits of knowledge and experience, and for resolving situations beyond his/her nurse practitioner expertise by consulting with or referring clients to other health care providers.

Citation: OR. ADMIN. § R. 851-050-0005.

In some states, the scope of practice of an NP is defined only marginally differently from the scope of practice of an RN. For example, compare North Dakota's scope of practice for NPs with its scope of practice for RNs. North Dakota's regulations on NP scope of practice states:

> The scope of practice for a registered nurse with advanced licensure is based upon understanding that a broad range of health care services can be appropriately and competently provided by a registered nurse with validated knowledge, skills, and abilities in specific practice areas. The health care needs of the citizens of North Dakota require that nurses in advanced practice roles provide care to the fullest extent of their scope of practice. The advanced practice registered nurse retains the responsibility for that scope of practice and is ultimately accountable to the patient within the Nurse Practice Act.
>
> *Citation:* N.D. ADMIN. CODE § 54-05-03.1-01.

In North Dakota, an RN's practice includes:

- Maintenance of health and prevention of illness
- Diagnosing human responses to actual or potential health problems
- Providing supportive and restorative care and nursing treatment, medication administration, health counseling and teaching, case finding, and referral of persons who are ill, injured, or experiencing changes in the normal health processes

- Administration, teaching, supervision, delegation, and evaluation of health and nursing practices
- Collaboration with other health care professionals in the implementation of the total health care regimen and execution of the health care regimen prescribed by a health care practitioner under title 43.

Citation: N.D. CENT. CODE § 43-12.1-02.6.

A non-nurse might have trouble distinguishing between the legal scope of practice of an RN and NP based on these definitions, but the distinction is clear to nurses: RNs may not step over the line from nursing into medical diagnosis and treatment, while NPs may. Although the difference between NP and RN practice in Oregon is clear when laws regarding NP and RN scope of practice are compared, the distinction is not so clear in North Dakota. What is not clear from reading North Dakota's definition of scope of practice for NPs is that NPs have prescriptive authority in North Dakota. The legal authority for prescription writing is not found in the definition of scope of practice, but is found elsewhere in North Dakota law.

NP AND MD SCOPE OF PRACTICE COMPARED

When NP scope of practice is defined to include diagnosis, treatment, prescriptive authority, and admission of patients to hospitals, as in Oregon law, there is little legal difference between NP and physician scope of practice. However in other states, attempts by physician associations to differentiate medical scope of practice from that of any other type of clinician is more pronounced. Consider Mississippi's definition of the practice of medicine:

> The practice of medicine shall mean to suggest, recommend, prescribe, or direct for the use of any person, any drug, medicine, appliance, or other agency, whether material or not material, for the cure, relief, or palliation of any ailment or disease of the mind or body, or for the cure or relief of any wound or fracture or other bodily injury or deformity, or the practice of obstetrics or midwifery, after having received, or with the intent of receiving therefor, either directly or indirectly, any bonus, gift, profit, or compensation; provided, that nothing in this section shall apply to females engaged solely in the practice of midwifery.

Citation: MISS. CODE ANN. § 73-25-33.

The liberal use of the word *any* differentiates physician scope of practice from NP scope of practice. There are no laws that authorize as wide a scope of practice for NPs as the Mississippi law authorizes for physician practice.

MANDATED PHYSICIAN INVOLVEMENT WITH NP PRACTICE

In some states, there is no legal requirement for physician involvement in NP practice. However, in the majority of states, there is some legal requirement for physician involvement. That involvement may be "supervision," "collaboration," or some other form of involvement. It may be limited to situations where the NP is prescribing medications, or it may be required for all advanced practice.

See Exhibit 2-2 for a chart listing requirements of physician involvement by state. For text of state laws regarding physician involvement, see Appendix 2-B.

Some states require that NPs practice using written protocols. Some states require a written agreement between the NP and the physician that states how the physician will participate in NP practice, what medications the NP may prescribe, what procedures an NP may perform, how often a physician will review NP documentation, and under what circumstances an NP must contact a physi-

Exhibit 2-2 Physician Involvement Required for NP Practice

Collaborate
AL
AZ
AR
CA
CO
CT
DE
DC
ID
IL
IN
IA
KE
LA
MA
MD
MS
MO
MN
NE
NJ
NY
ND
RI
SD
TX
VT
WV
WI
WY

Supervise
CA
FL
ID
ME*
NE
NC
OK
TN
TX
VA

Direct
CT
MA
OK
PA
VA

Protocols
AL
AR
CA
CT
DC
FL
GA
ID
KS
KY
LA
MA
MS
MO
NC
NV
NJ
NY
PA
SC
TX
VT
VA
WV

Collegial Relationship
HI

Referral Process
MT

Standard Care Arrangement
OH

Consultation/ Referral Plan
UT

None
AK
ME**
NH
NM
OR
WA

None, but No Scope of Practice in State Law
MI

*First 24 months of practice only.
**After 24 months.

cian. A protocol is a written instrument that guides the NP in collecting data from the patient and recommends specific action based upon the collected data. It consists of mutually agreed-upon medical guidelines between the physician and the NP that define the individual and shared responsibilities of the physician and NP. The protocol is considered a standard because it provides a guideline for a minimum level of safe practice in specific situations.[2]

Here is an example of a protocol:

Exhibit 2-3 Protocol

PROTOCOL

1. Definition
   Knee injury is an acute traumatic incident which can contuse, fracture, or tear various knee structures.
2. Data base
   a. Subjective data
      The following history is suggested:
      Description of injury or work activities surrounding the onset of symptoms. History of valgus, varus and/or associated rotary stress injury
      Audible "pop" at moment of injury
      Other subjective data as appropriate
   b. Objective Data
      The following assessment is suggested, and any or all of these findings may be noted:
      Knee:
      Examine for swelling, effusion, redness, ecchyymosis, decreased range of motion, tenderness, or any combination of these.
      Assessment:
      Knee injury
      Diagnostic Plan
      Treatment Plan
      - Supportive therapy:
        Encourage rest
        Apply ice
        Apply compression wrap for swelling
        Elevate affected extremity
      - Recommended drug therapy for severe pain
        Acetaminophen with Codeine 1–2 tablets every 4 hours to a maximum of 12 tablets/24 hours.
        Hydrocodone and Acetaminophen 1–2 tablets every 4–6 hours; maximum dosage of Acetaminophen, 4 g/day.
        Limit the number of tablets to 20, 30, or 50 with no refills.

Source: California Board of Registered Nursing. Available at: www.rn.ca.gov. Accessed July 2003.

NOTES

1. Web site of the American Academy of Nurse Practitioners. Available at http://www.aanp.org. Accessed July 2003.

2. R.S. Phillips. Nurse Practitioners: Their Scope of Practice and Theories of Liability. *Journal of Legal Medicine* 1985; 6:391-414.

APPENDIX 2-A

State-by-State Law Nurse Practitioner Scope of Practice

In some states scope of practice is specified by statute; in other states it is specified by regulation. Both statutes and regulations carry the same legal weight. Statutes are legislature-made law and are changed by a vote of the legislature. Regulations are executive agency made law, and can be changed by the agency, or overridden by statute.

The following are excerpts from state law. For the complete language, see the state's Nurse Practice Act, usually available online through the state's Board of Nursing Web site.

ALABAMA

> Practice as a certified registered nurse practitioner means the performance of nursing skills by a registered nurse who has demonstrated by certification advanced knowledge and skills in the delivery of nursing services within a health care system that provides for consultation, collaborative management, or referral as indicated by the health status of the client.
>
> *Citation:* ALA. ADMIN. CODE r. 610-X-9-.07(4).
>
> Functions and activities. CRNP is responsible for continuous and comprehensive management of a broad range of health services for which the CRNP is educationally prepared and for which competency is maintained. These services could include:
>
> a. Evaluate current health status and risk factors based on comprehensive health history and physical examination and assessment,
> b. Formulate a working diagnosis, develop and implement a treatment plan, and evaluate/modify therapeutic regimens to promote positive patient outcomes,
> c. Prescribe, administer and provide therapeutic measures, tests, procedures, and drugs,

d. Counsel, teach, and assist individuals/families to assume responsibility for self-care in prevention of illness, health maintenance, and health restoration,

e. Consult with and refer to other health care providers as appropriate.

A CRNP can request that additional functions be added to the protocol.

Citation: ALA. ADMIN. CODE r. 610-X-9-.16.

ALASKA

The board recognizes advanced and specialized acts of nursing practice as those described in the scope of practice statements for nurse practitioners certified by national certifying bodies recognized by the board.

Citation: ALAS. ADMIN. CODE tit. 12, § 44.430.

ARIZONA

Nurse practitioners

- Examine patients and establish medical diagnoses by client history, physical exam and other criteria
- Admit patients to health care facilities
- Order, perform, and interpret laboratory, radiographic, and other diagnostic tests
- Identify, develop, implement, and evaluate a plan of care for a patient to promote, maintain, and restore health
- Prescribe and dispense medications when granted authority under section R4-19-507
- Refer to and consult with appropriate health care providers.

Citation: ARIZ. ADMIN. CODE R4-19-505.

ARKANSAS

"Practice of advanced nurse practitioner nursing" means the performance for compensation of nursing skill by a registered nurse who, as demonstrated by national certification, has advanced knowledge and practice skills in the delivery of nursing services.

Citation: ARK. CODE ANN. § 17-87-102.(3)(A).

CALIFORNIA

The nurse practitioner shall function within the scope of practice as specified in the Nurse Practice Act and as it applies to all registered nurses.

Citation: CAL. CODE REG. tit.16 § 1485.

COLORADO

"Practice of professional nursing" means the performance of both independent nursing functions and delegated medical functions in accordance with accepted practice standards. Such functions include initiation and performance of nursing care through health promotion, supportive and restorative care, disease prevention, diagnosis and treatment of human disease, ailment, pain, injury, deformity, and physical or mental conditions using specialized knowledge, judgment, and skill.

Citation: COLO. REV. STAT. ANN. § 12-38-103(10).

An advanced practice nurse who is listed in the advanced practice registry, has license in good standing without disciplinary sanctions issued pursuant to section 12-38-11, and has fulfilled requirements established by the board pursuant to this section may be authorized by the board to prescribe controlled substances or prescription drugs as defined in article 22 of this title.

Citation: COLO. REV. STAT. ANN. § 12-38-111.5.

The scope of practice for an advanced practice nurse may be determined by the Board in accordance with this article.

Citation: COLO. REV. STAT. ANN. § 12-38-111.6(8)(a).

CONNECTICUT

Advanced nursing practice is defined as the performance of advanced level nursing practice activities, which by virtue of post-basic specialized education and experience are appropriate to and may be performed by an Advanced Practice Registered Nurse, and include acts of diagnosis and treatment of alteration in health status as described in subsection (a) of this section.

The advanced practice registered nurse may, under the direction of a physician licensed to practice medicine in this state and in accordance with written protocols, and if practicing in (1) an institution licensed pursuant to subsection (a) of section 19a-491 as a hospital, home for the aged, health care facility for the handicapped, nursing home, rest home, mental health facility, substance abuse treatment facility, infirmary operated by an educational institution for the care of students enrolled in, or the faculty and staff of, such institution, or facility operated and maintained by any state agency and providing services for the prevention, diagnosis and treatment or care of human health conditions, or (2) an industrial health facility licensed pursuant to subsection (h) of section 31-374 which serves at least two thousand employees, or

(3) a clinic operated by a state agency, municipality, or private non-profit corporation, or (4) a clinic operated by any educational institution prescribed by regulations adopted pursuant to section 10-99a, prescribe, dispense, or administer medical therapeutics and corrective measures, except that [an advanced practice nurse certified as a nurse anesthetist and administering therapeutics in surgery may do so only if a physician is present in the institution.] In all other settings, the advanced practice nurse may, under the direction of a physician licensed to practice medicine in the state and in accordance with written protocol, prescribe and administer medical therapeutics and corrective measures and may dispense drugs in the form of professional samples in accordance with section 20-14c to 20-14e, inclusive.

Citation: CONN. GEN. STAT. ANN § 20-87a.

DELAWARE

Advanced practice nursing is the application of nursing principles, including those in subsection (b) of this section, at an advanced level and includes:

a. For those advanced practice nurses who do not perform independent acts of diagnosis or prescription, the authority is granted within the scope of practice rules and regulations promulgated by the Board of Nursing; and
b. For those advanced practice nurses performing independent acts of diagnosis and prescriptions with the collaboration of a licensed physician, dentist, podiatrist, or licensed Delaware health care delivery system without written guidelines or protocols and within the scope of practice as defined in rules and regulations promulgated by the Joint Practice Committee and approved by the Board of Medical Practice.

Citation: DEL. CODE ANN. tit. 24, § 1902(d)(1).

Generic functions of the advanced registered nurse practitioner within the specialized scope of practice, include but are not limited to:

- Eliciting detailed health history(s)
- Defining nursing problem(s)
- Performing physical examination(s)
- Collecting and performing laboratory tests
- Interpreting laboratory data
- Initiating requests for essential laboratory procedures
- Initiating requests for essential X-rays
- Screening patients to identify abnormal problems
- Initiating referrals to appropriate resources and services as necessary

- Initiating or modifying treatment(s) within established guidelines
- Assessing and reporting changes in the health of individuals, families, and communities
- Providing health education through teaching and counseling
- Planning and/or instituting health care programs in the community with other health care professionals and the public
- Prescribing medications and treatments independently pursuant to Rules and Regulations. . . .

Citation: DEL. NURSING REGS. ART. VIII, § 7.

DISTRICT OF COLUMBIA

An advanced practice registered nurse may:

1. Initiate, monitor, and alter drug therapies
2. Initiate appropriate therapies or treatments
3. Make referrals for appropriate therapies or treatments
4. Perform additional functions within his or her specialty determined in accordance with rules and regulations promulgated by the Board.

Citation: D.C. CODE ANN. § 3-1206.04.

The advanced practice registered nurse may perform actions of medical diagnosis, treatment, prescription, and other functions authorized by this subchapter.

Citation: D.C. CODE ANN. § 3-1206.01.

FLORIDA

An ARNP shall perform those functions authorized in this section within the framework of an established protocol. Within the established framework, an ARNP may:

a. Monitor and alter drug therapies
b. Initiate appropriate therapies for certain conditions
c. Perform additional functions as may be determined by rule . . .
d. Order diagnostic tests and physical and occupational therapy.

Citation: FLA. STAT. CH. 464.012.

The nurse practitioner may perform any or all of the following acts within the framework of an established protocol:

1. Manage selected medical problems
2. Order physical and occupational therapy
3. Initiate, monitor, or alter therapies for certain uncomplicated acute illnesses

4. Monitor and manage patients with stable chronic diseases
5. Establish behavioral problems and diagnose and make treatment recommendations.

Citation: FLA. STAT. CH. 064.012.

GEORGIA

A certified nurse practitioner is an advanced registered nurse who provides primary nursing and medical services to individuals, families and groups, emphasizing health promotion and disease prevention as well as the diagnosis and management of acute and chronic disease.

Citation: GA. COMP. R. & REGS. § r. 410-12.03(2).

A physician may delegate to a nurse or physician's assistant the authority to order dangerous drugs, medical treatments, or diagnostic studies and a nurse or physician's assistant is authorized to dispense dangerous drugs, in accordance with dispensing procedure and under the authority of an order issued in conformity with a nurse protocol or job description, if that nurse or physician's assistant orders or dispenses those dangerous drugs, medical treatments, or diagnostic studies. [The law lists possible job settings where the delegation may occur; i.e. employee of public health department, any 501(c)(3) organization, the public health service, outpatient department of a hospital.]

Citation: GA. CODE ANN. § 43-34-26.1.

HAWAII

In addition to those functions specified for the registered nurse, the advanced practice registered nurse may perform the following generic acts which include, but are not limited to:

1. Provide direct nursing care by utilizing advanced practice scientific knowledge, nursing theory and skills to assess, plan, and implement appropriate health and nursing care to patients;
2. Provide indirect nursing care. Plan, guide, evaluate, and direct the nursing care given by other personnel associated with the health care team;
3. Teach and counsel individuals or groups. Utilize theories and skills to increase communication and knowledge among all members of the health care team;
4. Serve as a consultant and resource of advanced nursing knowledge and skills to those involved directly or indirectly in patient care; and
5. Participate in joint and periodic evaluation of services rendered.

Citation: HAW. ADMIN. R. 16-89-81(b).

Nurse practitioner scope of practice:

A. Evaluate the physical and psychosocial health status of the patient through a comprehensive health history and physical examination, using skills of observation, inspection, palpation, percussion, and auscultation, and using or ordering diagnostic instruments or procedures that are basic to the nursing evaluation of physical signs and symptoms;
B. Assess the normal and abnormal findings from the history, physical examination, and diagnostic reports;
C. Plan, implement, and evaluate care;
D. Consult with the patient, support systems, and members of the health care team to provide for acute and ongoing health care or referral of the patient;
E. Manage the plan of care prescribed for the patient;
F. Initiate and maintain accurate records, appropriate legal documents, and other health and nursing care reports;
G. Develop individualized teaching plans with the patient based on overt and covert health needs;
H. Counsel individuals, families, and groups about health and illness and promotion of health maintenance;
I. Recognize, develop, and implement professional and community educational programs related to health care;
J. Participate in periodic and joint evaluation of services rendered;
K. Conduct research and analyze the health needs of individuals and populations and design programs which target at-risk groups and cultural and environmental factors which foster health and prevent illness;
L. Participate in policy analysis and development of new policy initiatives in the area of practice specialty; and
M. Contribute to the development, maintenance, and change of health care delivery systems to improve quality of health care services and consumer access to services.

Citation: HAW. ADMIN. R. 16-89-81(c)(1).

IDAHO

Nurse practitioners . . . may perform comprehensive health assessments, diagnosis, health promotion, and the direct management of acute and chronic illness and disease which may include the prescribing of pharmacologic and non-pharmacologic treatments as defined by rules of the board.

Citation: IDAHO CODE § 54-1402(1)(c).

ILLINOIS

"Advanced practice nurse" or "APN" means a person who has a written collaborative agreement with a collaborating physician in the diagnosis of illness and management of wellness and other conditions as appropriate to the level and area of his or her practice in accordance with Section 15-15; and cares for patients (A) by using advanced diagnostic skills, the results of diagnostic tests and procedures ordered by the advanced practice nurse, a physician assistant, a dentist, a podiatrist, or a physician, and professional judgment to initiate and coordinate the care of patients; (B) by ordering diagnostic tests, prescribing medications and drugs in accordance with Section 15-20, and administering medications and drugs; and (C) by using medical, therapeutic, and corrective measures to treat illness and improve health status.

Citation: 225 ILL. COMP. STAT. 65/15-5.

INDIANA

An NP shall perform as an independent and interdependent member of the health team as defined in 848 IAC 2-1-3. "Health team" means a group of health care providers which may, in addition to health care practitioners, include the patient/client, family, and any significant others.

Citation: IND. ADMIN. CODE tit. 848, r. 2-1-3.

Nurse practitioner means an advance practice nurse who provides advanced levels of nursing client care in a specialty role, who meets the requirements of the advanced practice nurse as outlined in section 3 of these rules.

Citation: IND. ADMIN. CODE tit. 848, r. 4-1-4.

[Indiana law does not use the words "scope of practice," but describes "standards for each nurse practitioner" as follows:]

1. Assess clients by using advanced knowledge and skills to:
   A. identify abnormal conditions;
   B. diagnose health problems;
   C. develop and implement nursing treatment plans;
   D. evaluate patient outcomes; and
   E. collaborate with or refer to a practitioner, as defined in IC 25-23-1-19.4, in managing the plan of care.
2. Use advanced knowledge and skills in teaching and guiding clients and other health team members.
3. Use appropriate critical thinking skills to make independent decisions, commensurate with the autonomy, authority, and responsibility of a nurse practitioner.

4. Function within the legal boundaries of their advanced practice area and shall have and utilize knowledge of the statutes and rules governing their advanced practice area; including the following:
   A. State and federal drug laws and regulations.
   B. State and federal confidentiality laws and regulations.
   C. State and federal medical records access laws.
5. Consult and collaborate with other members of the health team as appropriate to provide reasonable client care, both acute and ongoing.
6. Recognize the limits of individual knowledge and experience, and consult with or refer clients to other health care providers as appropriate.
7. Retain professional accountability for any delegated intervention, and delegate interventions only as authorized by IC 25-23-1 and this title.
8. Maintain current knowledge and skills in the nurse practitioner area.
9. Conduct an assessment of clients and families which may include health history, family history, physical examination, and evaluation of health risk factors.
10. Assess normal and abnormal findings obtained from the history, physical examination, and laboratory results.
11. Evaluate clients and families regarding development, coping ability, and emotional and social well-being.
12. Plan, implement, and evaluate care.
13. Develop individualized teaching plans with each client based on health records.
14. Counsel individuals, families, and groups about health and illness and promote attention to wellness.
15. Participate in periodic or joint evaluations of service rendered, including, but not limited to, the following:
    A. Chart reviews.
    B. Client evaluations
    C. Outcome statistics.
16. Conduct and apply research findings appropriate to the area of practice.
17. Participate, when appropriate, in the joint review of the plan of care.

Citation: IND. ADMIN. CODE tit. 848, r. 4-2-1.

IOWA

In the advanced role, the nurse practices nursing assessment, intervention, and management within the boundaries of the nurse-client relationship. Advanced nursing practice occurs in a variety of settings within an interdisciplinary health care team, which provides for consultation, collaborative management, and referral. The ARNP may perform selected medically designated functions when a collaborative practice agreement exists.

Citation: IOWA ADMIN. CODE r. 655-6.1.

KANSAS

An advanced registered nurse practitioner functions in an expanded role to provide primary health care to individuals, families or groups, or some combination of these groups of clients, in a variety of settings, including homes, institutions, offices, industries, schools, community agencies, and private practice. ARNPs function in a collegial relationship with physicians and other health care professionals in the delivery of primary health care services. ARNPs make independent decisions about nursing needs of families and clients, and interdependent decisions with physicians in carrying out health regimes for families and clients. ARNPs are directly accountable and responsible to the consumer.

Citation: KANS. ADMIN. REGS. 60-11-101(a).

A nurse practitioner is authorized to:

- Evaluate the physical and psychosocial health status of the client through a comprehensive health history and physical examination using skills of observation, inspection, palpation, percussion, and consultation and using diagnostic instruments or laboratory procedures that are basic to the screening of physical signs and symptoms.
- Assess normal and abnormal findings from the history, physical examination, and laboratory reports.
- Plan, implement, and evaluate care.
- Consult with the client and members of the health care team to provide for acute and ongoing health care or referral of the client.
- Manage the medical plan of care prescribed for the client, based on protocols or guidelines adopted jointly by the nurse practitioner and the attending physician.
- Institute and maintain accurate records, appropriate legal documents and other health and nursing care reports.
- Develop individualized teaching plans with the client based on overt and covert health needs.
- Counsel individuals, families, and groups about health and illness and promote health maintenance.
- Recognize, develop, and implement professional and combined education programs related to health care.

- Participate in periodic and joint evaluation of services rendered, including but not limited to chart review, patient evaluations, and outcome of case statements.
- Participate, when appropriate, in the joint review and revision of adopted protocols or guidelines when the ARNP is involved in the medical plan of care.

Citation: KANS. ADMIN. REGS. 60-11-104.

A nurse practitioner may prescribe drugs pursuant to a written protocol as authorized by a responsible physician.

Citation: KANS. STAT. ANN. § 65-1130(d).

KENTUCKY

Practice of an advanced registered nurse practitioner shall be in accordance with standards and functions defined by each specialty area professional organization; such as American Nurses Association or Association of Women's Health, Obstetrical and Neonatal Nurses and [others listed].

Citation: 201 KY. ADMIN. REGS. 20:057.2.

Practice shall include prescribing treatments, drugs and devices, and ordering diagnostic tests which are consistent with the scope and standard of practice of the ARNP.

Citation: 201 KY. ADMIN. REGS. 20:057.4.

LOUISIANA

The advanced practice registered nurse shall practice as set forth in R.S. 37:913(3)(a) and the standards set forth in these administrative rules. The patient services provided by an APRN shall be in accord with the educational preparation of that APRN. . . .

Standards of practice are essential for safe practice by the APRN and shall be in accordance with the published professional standards for each recognized specialty and/or functional role. The core standards for all categories of advanced practice registered nurses include, but are not limited to:

1. An APRN shall meet the standards of practice for registered nurses as defined in LAC 46:XLVII3901-3915;
2. An APRN shall assess patients at an advanced level, identify abnormal conditions, analyze and synthesize data to establish a diagnosis, develop and implement treatment plans, and evaluate patient outcomes;

3. The APRN shall use advanced knowledge and skills in providing patients and health team members with guidance and teaching;
4. An APRN shall use critical thinking and independent decision-making at an advanced level commensurate with the autonomy, authority, and responsibility of the practice role and/or specialty while working with patients and their families in meeting health care needs;
5. An APRN shall demonstrate knowledge of the statutes and rules governing advanced registered nursing practice and function within the legal boundaries of the appropriate advanced registered nursing practice role;
6. An APRN shall demonstrate knowledge of and apply current nursing research findings relevant to the advanced nursing practice role and specialty;
7. An APRN shall make decisions to solve patient care problems and select medical treatment regimens in collaboration with a licensed physician or dentist;
8. An APRN shall retain professional accountability for his/her actions and/or interventions.

Citation: LA. ADMIN. CODE tit. 46 § XLVII-4513.

(3) (a) "Advanced practice registered nursing" means nursing by a certified registered nurse anesthetist, certified nurse midwife, clinical nurse specialist, or nurse practitioner which is based on knowledge and skills acquired in a basic nursing education program, licensure as a registered nurse, and a minimum of a master's degree with a concentration in the respective advanced practice nursing specialty which includes both didactic and clinical components, advanced knowledge in nursing theory, physical and psychosocial assessment, nursing interventions, and management of health care.

Advanced practice registered nursing includes:

i. Assessing patients, analyzing and synthesizing data, and knowledge of and applying nursing principles at an advanced level.
ii. Providing guidance and teaching.
iii. Working with patients and families in meeting health care needs.
iv. Collaborating with other health care providers.
v. Managing patients' physical and psychosocial health-illness status with regard to nursing care.
vi. Utilizing research skills.
vii. Analyzing multiple sources of data and identifying alternative possibilities as to the nature of a health care problem.

viii. Making decisions in solving patient care problems and selecting treatment regimens in collaboration with a licensed physician, or dentist.

ix. Consulting with or referring patients to licensed physicians, dentists, and other health care providers in accordance with a collaborative practice agreement.

(b) (i) Subject to the provision of subparagraph ii of this subparagraph, advanced practice registered nursing may include certain acts of medical diagnosis, in accordance with R.S. 37:913(8) and (9), or medical prescriptions of therapeutic or corrective nature, prescribing assessment studies, drugs, therapeutic regimens and distributing drugs for administration to and use by other individuals within the scope of practice and in accordance with R.S. 37:1031-1034.

(ii) Until such time as rules and regulations are promulgated under the provision of subparagraph (i) of this paragraph, the rules and regulations promulgated under the provisions of R.S. 37:1032 shall apply to advanced practice registered nursing. Other than limited prescriptive authority, nothing contained herein shall be construed to limit an advanced practice registered nurse's scope of practice as defined by the Nurse Practice Act.

Citation: LA. REV. STAT. 37:913(3)(a).

MAINE

The certified nurse practitioner shall provide only those health care services for which the certified nurse practitioner is educationally and clinically prepared, and for which competency has been maintained. The Board reserves the right to make exceptions. Such health care services, for which the certified nurse practitioner is independently responsible and accountable, includes:

1. Obtaining a complete health data base that includes a health history, physical examination, and screening and diagnostic evaluation
2. Interpreting health data by identifying wellness and risk factors and variations from norms
3. Diagnosing and treating common diseases and human responses to actual and potential health problems
4. Counseling individuals and families
5. Consulting and/or collaborating with other health care providers and community resources
6. Referring client to other health care providers and community resources.

Citation: CODE ME. R. § 02 380 008.

A certified nurse practitioner who is approved by the board as an advanced practice nurse may choose to perform medical diagnosis or practice therapeutic or corrective measures when the services are delegated by a licensed physician.

Citation: ME. REV. STAT. ANN. tit. 32, § 2205-B.

MARYLAND

A nurse practitioner may perform independently the following functions under the terms and conditions set forth in the written agreement:

1. Comprehensive physical assessment of patients,
2. Establishing medical diagnosis for common short-term or chronic stable health problems,
3. Ordering, performing, and interpreting laboratory tests,
4. Prescribing drugs,
5. Performing therapeutic or corrective measures,
6. Referring patients to appropriate licensed physicians or other health care providers,
7. Providing emergency care.

Citation: MD. REGS. CODE tit. 10 § 27.07.02.A.

MASSACHUSETTS

Nursing practice involves clinical decision making leading to the development and implementation of a strategy of care to accomplish defined goals, the administration of medication, therapeutics, and treatment prescribed by duly authorized nurses in advanced roles, including . . . nurse practitioners . . . and the evaluation of responses to care and treatment.

Advanced practice nurse regulations which govern the ordering of tests, therapeutics and prescribing of medications shall be promulgated by the board of nursing and in conjunction with the board of medicine.

Citation: MASS. ANN. LAWS CH. 112, § 80B.

The area of NP practice includes assessing the health status of individuals and families by obtaining health and medical history, performing physical examinations, diagnosing health and developmental problems, and caring for patients suffering from acute and chronic disease by managing therapeutic regimes according to guidelines appropriate and developed in compliance with 244 Code of Massachusetts Regulations 4.22, and such other additional professional activities as authorized by the guidelines under which a particular NP practices.

Citation: MASS. REGS. CODE tit. 224, § 4.26(2).

MICHIGAN

[There is no requirement for physician supervision or collaboration. However, there is no legal scope of practice for NPs. Physicians may delegate at their discretion (MICH. COMP. LAWS § 333.16215(1)).]

MINNESOTA

"Nurse practitioner practice" means, within the context of collaborative management:

1. Diagnosing, directly managing, and preventing acute and chronic illness and disease; and
2. Promoting wellness, including providing non-pharmacologic treatment.

Citation: MINN. STAT. ANN. § 148.171.

MISSISSIPPI

The nurse practitioner shall practice according to standards and guidelines of the national certification organization, and in a collaborative/consultative relationship with a licensed physician . . . according to a Nursing Board-approved protocol or practice guidelines. . . .

Citation: MISS. RULES, CH. IV. § 2.3.

MISSOURI

Advanced practice nurses shall function clinically within the professional scope and standards of their advanced practice nursing clinical specialty area and consistent with their formal advanced nursing education and national certification, if applicable, or within their education, training, knowledge, judgment, skill, and competence as registered professional nurses.

Citation: MO. CODE REGS. ANN. tit. 4 § 200-4.100.

MONTANA

NP practice means the management of primary health care of individuals, families, and communities including the ability to:

- Assess the health status of individuals and families using methods appropriate to the client population and area of practice such as health history taking, physical examination, and assessing developmental health problems;
- Institute and provide continuity of health care to clients, work with clients to insure their understanding of and compliance with therapeutic regimens;

- Promote wellness and disease prevention programs;
- Recognize when to refer clients to a physician or other health care provider;
- Provide instruction and counseling to individuals, families, and groups in the areas of health promotion and maintenance, including involving such persons in planning for their health care; and
- Work in collaboration with other health care providers and agencies to provide and, where appropriate, coordinate services to individuals and families.

Citation: MONT. ADMIN. R. 8.32.301.

NEBRASKA

An advanced practice registered nurse practitioner may provide health care services within specialty areas.

An advanced practice registered nurse shall function by establishing collaborative, consultative, and referral networks as appropriate with other health care professionals.

Patients who require care beyond the scope of practice of an advanced practice registered nurse shall be referred to an appropriate health care provider.

Advanced practice registered nurse practice shall mean health promotion, health supervision, illness prevention and diagnosis, and treatment and management of common health problems and chronic conditions, including:

1. Assessing patients, ordering diagnostic tests and therapeutic treatments, synthesizing and analyzing data, and applying advanced nursing principles;
2. Dispensing, incident to practice only, sample medication which are provided by the manufacturer and are provided at no charge to the patient; and
3. Prescribing therapeutic measures and medications, except controlled substances listed in Schedule II of section 28-405 not otherwise provided for in this section, related to health conditions within the scope of practice. An advanced practice registered nurse may prescribe controlled substances listed in Schedule II of section 28-405 used for pain control for a maximum of seventy-two hours supply if any subsequent renewal of such prescription is by a licensed physician.

Citation: NEB. REV. STAT. § 71-1721.

NEVADA

An advanced practitioner of nursing may perform the following acts in addition to the ordinary functions of a registered nurse if he is properly prepared and the acts are currently within the standard of medical practice for his specialty and appear in his protocols:

1. Systematically assess the health status of persons and families by
   a. Taking, recording, and interpreting medical history and performing physical examinations and
   b. Performing or initiating selected diagnostic procedures.
2. Based on information obtained in the assessment of a person's health, manage the care of selected persons and families with common, acute, recurrent, or long-term health problems.
   a. Initiation of a program of treatment.
   b. Evaluation of response to health problems and programs of treatment.
   c. Informing a person or family of the status of the patient's health and alternatives for care.
   d. Evaluation of compliance with a program of treatment agreed upon by the person or family and the advanced practice nurse.
   e. Modification of programs to treat, based on the response of the person or family to treatment.
   f. Referral to appropriate provider of health care.
   g. Treatment of minor lacerations which do not involve damage to a nerve, tendon, or major blood vessel.
   h. Commencement of care required to stabilize a patient's condition in an emergency until a physician can be consulted.
   i. Any other act for which an advanced practitioner of nursing is certified to perform by an organization recognized by the board, taught in a comprehensive program which included clinical experience, or is within the scope of practice of an advanced practitioner of nursing as determined by the board.

Citation: NEV. ADMIN. CODE § 632.255.

NEW HAMPSHIRE

The ARNP shall have the ability to:

- Elicit and record physical and mental health status, psychosocial history, including review of bodily systems
- Perform physical examination
- Initiate appropriate diagnostic tests to screen or evaluate the care-recipient's current health status
- Assess findings of history, review of systems, physical examination and diagnostic tests, and formulate a diagnosis prior to implementing a treatment regimen
- Identify health problems and learning needs of the care recipient
- Plan, teach, promote, and manage physical and mental health-care in a continuous program

- Implement and manage treatment regiments and administer, prescribe, dispense, and procure pharmacological agents
- Arrange appropriate referrals
- Initiate appropriate emergency treatment in life-threatening or unusual situations in order to stabilize the care-recipient; and
- Provide other functions common to the nurse practitioner for which the ARNP is educationally and experientially prepared.

Citation: N.H. CODE ADMIN. R. ANN. [NUR] 304.05.

NEW JERSEY

a. In addition to all other tasks which a registered professional nurse may, by law, perform, a nurse practitioner/clinical nurse specialist may manage specific common deviations from wellness and stabilized long-term illnesses by:
   1. initiating laboratory and other diagnostic tests; and
   2. prescribing or ordering medications and devices, as authorized by subsections b. and c. of this section.

Citation: N.J. STAT. ANN. § 45:11-49.a.

NEW MEXICO

Certified nurse practitioners who have fulfilled requirements for prescriptive authority may prescribe in accordance with the rules, regulations, guidelines, and formularies for individual certified nurse practitioners promulgated by the board.

Citation: N.M. STAT. ANN. § 61-3-23.2.C.

Certified nurse practitioners may:

1. Perform an expanded practice that is beyond the scope of practice of professional registered nursing; and
2. Practice independently and make independent decisions regarding health care needs of the individual, family, or community and carry out health regimens, including the prescription and dispensing of dangerous drugs, including controlled dangerous substances included in Schedule II-V of the Controlled Dangerous Substances Act.
3. Serve as a primary acute, chronic long-term, and end of life health care provider and as necessary collaborate with licensed medical doctors, osteopathic physicians, or podiatrists.

Citation: N.M. STAT. ANN. § 61-3-23.2.B.

NEW YORK

Nurse practitioner practice may include diagnosis of illness and physical conditions and the performance of therapeutic and corrective measures within a specialty area of practice, in collaboration with a licensed physician qualified to collaborate in the specialty involved, provided such services are performed in accordance with a written practice agreement and written practice protocols. The written practice agreement shall include explicit provisions for the resolution of any disagreement between the collaborating physician and the nurse practitioner regarding a matter of diagnosis or treatment that is within the scope of practice of both. To the extent the practice agreement does not so provide, then the collaborating physician's diagnosis or treatment shall prevail.

Citation: N.Y. EDUC. LAW, Art. 139 § 6902.3(a).

Prescriptions for drugs, devices, and immunizing agents may be issued in accordance with the practice agreement and practice protocols.

Citation: N.Y. EDUC. LAW Art. 139 § 6902.3(b).

NORTH CAROLINA

The NP shall be responsible and accountable for the continuous and comprehensive management of a broad range of personal health services for which the NP shall be educationally prepared and for which competency has been maintained, with physician supervision as described in paragraph (i) of this Rule. These services include but are not restricted to:

1. Promotion and maintenance of health;
2. Prevention of illness and disability;
3. Diagnosis, treating, and managing acute and chronic illnesses;
4. Guidance and counseling of both individuals and families;
5. Prescribing, administering, and dispensing therapeutic measures, tests, procedures, and drugs;
6. Planning for situations beyond the NP's expertise and consulting with and referring to other health care providers as appropriate; and
7. Evaluating health outcomes.

Citation: N.C. ADMIN CODE tit. 21 § r. 36.0227(b).

NORTH DAKOTA

The scope of practice for a registered nurse with advanced licensure is based upon understanding that a broad range of health care services can be appropriately and competently provided by a registered nurse with validated knowledge, skills, and abilities in specific practice areas. The health care needs of the citizens in North Dakota require that nurses in advanced practice roles provide care to the fullest extent of their scope of practice. The advanced practice registered nurse retains the responsibility and accountability for that scope of practice and is ultimately accountable to the patient within the Nurse Practice Act.

Citation: N.D. ADMIN. CODE § 54-05-03.1-01.

OHIO

[A] certified nurse practitioner, in collaboration with one or more physicians or podiatrists, may provide preventive and primary care services and evaluate and promote patient wellness within the nurse's nursing specialty, consistent with the nurse's education and certification, and in accordance with rules adopted by the Board. A certified nurse practitioner who holds a certificate to prescribe . . . may, in collaboration with one or more physicians or podiatrists, prescribe drugs and therapeutic devices in accordance with section 4723.481 of the Revised Code. When a certified nurse practitioner is collaborating with a podiatrist, the nurse's scope of practice is limited to the procedures that the podiatrist has the authority to perform.

Citation: OHIO REV. CODE ANN. § 4723.43(C).

OKLAHOMA

An advanced registered NP in accordance with the scope of practice of the advanced registered nurse practitioner shall be eligible to obtain recognition as authorized by the Board to prescribe, as defined by rules and subject to the medical direction of a supervising physician. This authorization shall not include dispensing drugs, but shall not preclude, subject to federal regulations, the receipt of, the signing for, or the dispensing of professional samples to patients.

The ARNP accepts responsibility, accountability, and obligation to practice in accordance with usual and customary advanced practice nursing standards and functions as defined by the scope of practice/role definition statements for the advanced registered nurse practitioner.

Citation: OKLA. STAT. ANN. tit. 59, § 567.3a (6).

The advanced practice registered nurse is responsible and accountable for the continuous and comprehensive management of a broad range of health services, which include, but are not limited to:

A. Promotion and maintenance of health;

B. Prevention of illness and disability;

C. Diagnosis and prescription of medications, treatments and devices;
D. Management of health care during acute and chronic phases of illness;
E. Guidance and counseling services;
F. Consultation and/or collaboration with other health care providers and community resources;
G. Referral to other care providers and community resources.

Citation: OKLA. ADMIN. CODE § 485:10-15-6(c).

OREGON

1. The nurse practitioner provides holistic health care to individuals, families, and groups across the life span in a variety of settings, including hospitals, long term care facilities and community-based settings.
2. Within his or her specialty, the nurse practitioner is responsible for managing health problems encountered by the client and is accountable for health outcomes. This process includes:
   (a) Assessment;
   (b) Diagnosis;
   (c) Development of a plan;
   (d) Intervention;
   (e) Evaluation.
3. The nurse practitioner is independently responsible and accountable for the continuous and comprehensive management of a broad range of health care, which may include:
   (a) Promotion and maintenance of health;
   (b) Prevention of illness and disability;
   (c) Assessment of clients, synthesis and analysis of data, and application of nursing principles and therapeutic modalities;
   (d) Management of health care during acute and chronic phases of illness;
   (e) Admission of his/her clients to hospitals and long term care facilities and management of client care in these facilities;
   (f) Counseling;
   (g) Consultation and/or collaboration with other care providers and community resources;
   (h) Referral to other health care providers and community resources;
   (i) Management and coordination of care;
   (j) Use of research skills;
   (k) Diagnosis of health/illness status;

(l) Prescription and/or administration of therapeutic devices and measures including legend drugs and controlled substances as provided in OAR 851-050-0131 and dispensing drugs as provided in OAR 851-050-0133, 0134, and 0145, consistent with the definition of the practitioner's specialty category and scope of practice.

4. The nurse practitioner is responsible for recognizing limits of knowledge and experience, and for resolving situations beyond his/her nurse practitioner expertise by consulting with or referring clients to other health care providers.
5. The nurse practitioner will only provide health care services within the nurse practitioner's scope of practice for which he/she is educationally prepared and for which competency has been established and maintained. Educational preparation includes academic course work, workshops or seminars, provided both theory and clinical experience are included.

Citation: OR. ADMIN. R. 851-050-0005.

PENNSYLVANIA

A CRNP, while functioning in the expanded role as a registered nurse, performs acts of medical diagnosis or prescription of medical therapeutics or corrective measures in collaboration with and under the direction of a physician.

Citation: 49 PA. CODE § 21.251.

A certified registered nurse practitioner . . . shall practice within the scope of practice of the particular clinical specialty area in which the nurse is certified by the Board.

Citation: ACT 206 OF 2002, § 8.2.

RHODE ISLAND

[A certified registered nurse practitioner] practices in an advanced role utilizing independent knowledge of physical assessment and management of health care and illnesses. The practice includes prescriptive privileges. . . .

Citation: R.I. R-5-34-NUR/ED 1.8.

SOUTH CAROLINA

The Nurse Practitioner, Clinical Nurse Specialist functioning in the extended role, or Certified Registered Nurse Anesthetist is subject, at all times, to the scope and standards or practice established by the nationally recognized credentialing organization representing the specialty area of practice, and must function within the scope of practice of the South Carolina Nurse Practice Act and shall not be in violation of the South Carolina Medical Practice Act.

The scope and standards of practice for each specialty area of nursing practice shall be on file in the Board office and available upon request.

Citation: 26 S.C. CODE ANN. REGS. 91-6f.

"Extended Role" means a collaborative process whereby a nurse with advanced education and training is recognized by the Board to assume additional acts. The extended role of the Registered Nurse includes performing delegated medical acts under the general supervision of a licensed physician who is readily available for consultation. This does not authorize violation of the Medical Practice Laws of South Carolina (Section 40-47-10 1976 Code of Laws, as amended), or the Pharmacy Practice Laws of South Carolina (Section 40-43-140, 1976 Code of Laws, as amended).

Citation: 26 S.C. CODE ANN. REGS. 91-2a.

"Delegated Medical Acts" means those additional acts delegated by the physician that include formulating a medical diagnosis and initiating, continuing, and modifying therapies, including prescribing drug therapy, under approved written protocols.

Citation: 26. S.C. CODE ANN. REGS. 91-1.c.

SOUTH DAKOTA

A nurse practitioner may perform the following overlapping scope of advanced practice nursing and medical functions pursuant to § 36-9A-15, including:

1. The initial medical diagnosis and the institution of a plan of therapy or referral;
2. The prescription of medications and provision of drug samples or a limited supply of labeled medications, including controlled drugs or substances listed in Schedule II in Chapter 34-20B for one period of not more than forty-eight hours for treatment of causative factors and symptoms. Medications or sample drugs provided to patients shall be accompanied with written administration instructions and appropriate documentation shall be entered in the patient's medical record;
3. The writing of a chemical or physical restraint order when the patient may do personal harm or harm others;
4. The completion and signing of official documents such as death certificates, birth certificates, and similar documents required by law;

5. The performance of a physical examination for participation in athletics and the certification that the patient is healthy and able to participate in athletics.

Citation: S.D. CODIFIED LAWS § 36-9A-12.

The nurse practitioner or nurse midwife advanced practice nursing functions include:

1. Providing advanced nursing assessment, nursing intervention, and nursing case management;
2. Providing advanced health promotion and maintenance education and counseling to clients, families, and other members of the health care team;
3. Utilizing research findings to evaluate and implement changes in nursing practice, programs, and policies; and
4. Recognizing limits of knowledge and experience, planning for situations beyond expertise, and consulting with or referring clients to other health care providers as appropriate.

These advanced practice nursing functions are under the jurisdiction of the Board of Nursing.

Citation: S.D. CODIFIED LAWS § 36-9A-13.1.

TENNESSEE

There is no description of the scope of practice for a nurse practitioner in Tennessee law, other than the authority to write and sign prescriptions and/or issue drugs.

Citation: [for prescriptive authority]
TENN. CODE ANN. § 63-7-123(a) and (b)(2).

TEXAS

The advanced practice nurse provides a broad range of personal health services, the scope of which shall be based on educational preparation, continued experience, and the accepted scope of professional practice of the particular specialty area. Advanced practice nurses practice in a variety of settings and, according to their practice specialty and role, they provide a broad range of health care services to a variety of patient populations. The scope of practice of particular specialty areas shall be defined by national professional society organizations or advanced practice nursing organizations recognized by the Board. The advanced practice nurse may perform only those functions which are within that scope of practice and which are consistent with the Nursing Practice Act, Board rules, and other laws and regulations of the State of Texas.

The advance practice nurse's scope of practice shall be in addition to the scope of practice permitted a registered nurse and does not prohibit the advanced practice nurse from practicing in those areas deemed to be within the scope of practice of a registered nurse.

Citation: 21 TEXAS ADMIN. CODE 221.12.

UTAH

"Practice of an advanced practice registered nursing" means the practice of nursing within the generally recognized scope of advanced practice registered nursing as defined in division rule and consistent with professionally recognized preparation and education standards of an advanced practice registered nurse by a person licensed under this chapter as an advanced practice registered nurse. Advanced practice registered nursing includes:

a. Maintenance and promotion of health and prevention of disease;
b. Diagnosis, treatment, correction, consultation, or referral for common health problems; and
c. Prescription or administration of prescription drugs or devices, including local anesthesia, schedule IV-V controlled substances; and schedule II-II controlled substances in accordance with a consultation and referral plan.

Citation: UTAH CODE ANN. § 58-31b-102(16).

"Generally recognized scope and standards of practice of advanced practice registered nursing" means the scope and standards of practice set forth in the "Scope and Standards of Advanced Practice Registered Nursing," 1996, published by the American Nurses Association, which is hereby adopted and incorporated by reference, or as established by the professional community.

Citation: UTAH ADMIN. CODE R156-31-102(12).

An APRN who chooses to change or expand from a primary focus of practice must be able to document competency within that expanded practice based on education, experience, and certification. The burden to demonstrate competency rests upon the licensee.

Citation: UTAH ADMIN. CODE R156-31-702.

VERMONT

Advanced practice registered nurses are endorsed to perform acts of medical diagnosis and to prescribe medical, therapeutic, or corrective measures under administrative rules adopted by the board.

Citation: VT. STAT. ANN. tit. 26, § 1572.

The advanced practice registered nurse accepts the responsibility, accountability, and obligation to practice in accordance with current standards and functions as defined by the scope of practice statements for each specialty area and as developed by national professional nursing organizations.

Citation: VT. CODE R. CH. 4, RULE VIII.C.1.

The APRN performs medical acts independently within a collaborative practice with a licensed physician under practice guidelines which are mutually agreed upon between the APRN and collaborating physician and which are jointly acceptable to the medical and nursing professions.

Citation: VT. CODE R. CH. 4, RULE VIII.C.4.a.

VIRGINIA

A licensed nurse practitioner shall be authorized to engage in practices constituting the practice of medicine in collaboration with and under the medical direction and supervision of a licensed physician in accordance with 18 Virginia Administrative Code 90-30-130.

Citation: 18 VA. ADMIN. CODE 90-30-120B.

WASHINGTON

An advanced registered nurse practitioner under his or her license may perform for compensation nursing care, as that term is usually understood, of the ill, injured, or infirm and in the course thereof, she or he may do the following things that shall not be done by a person not so licensed, except as provided in RCS 18.79.260 and 18.79.270:

1. Perform specialized and advanced levels of nursing as recognized jointly by the medical and nursing professions, as defined by the commission;
2. Prescribe legend drugs and Schedule V controlled substances, as defined in the Uniform Controlled Substances Act, chapter 69.50 RCS, and Schedule II through IV subject to RCW 18.79.240(1)(r) or (s) within the scope of practice defined by the commission;
3. Perform all acts provided in RCS 18.79.260;
4. Hold herself or himself out to the public or designate herself or himself as an advanced registered nurse practitioner or as a nurse practitioner.

Citation: WASH. REV. CODE 18.79.250.

Advanced registered nurse practitioners function within the specialty scopes of practice and/or description of practice and/or standards of care developed by national professional organization and reviewed and approved by the commission.

Advanced registered nurse practitioners are prepared and qualified to assume primary responsibility and accountability for the care of their patients. This practice is grounded in nursing and incorporates the use of independent judgment as well as collaborative interaction with other health care professionals when indicated in the assessment and management of wellness and conditions as appropriate to the ARNP's area of specialization.

Within the scope of the advanced registered nurse practitioner's knowledge, experience, and specialty scope of practice statement(s), licensed advanced registered nurse practitioners may perform the following functions:

- Examine patients and establish medical diagnoses by client history, physical examination, and other assessment criteria;
- Admit patients to health care facilities;
- Order, collect, perform, and interpret laboratory tests;
- Initiate requests for radiographic and other testing measures;
- Identify, develop, implement, and evaluate a plan of care and treatment for patients to promote, maintain, and restore health;
- Prescribe medications when granted authority under this chapter;
- Refer clients to other health care professionals or facilities.

Citation: WASH. ADMIN. CODE § 246-840-300.

WEST VIRGINIA

Advanced nursing practice is the practice of nursing at a level that required substantial theoretical knowledge in a specialized area of nursing practice and proficient clinical utilization of the knowledge in implementing the nursing process. The competencies of specialists include but are not limited to the ability to assess, conceptualize, diagnose, analyze, plan, implement, and evaluate complex problems related to health.

Citation: W.V. CODE ST. R. tit. 19 § 19-7-2.1.

WISCONSIN

The intent of the board of nursing in adopting rules in this chapter is to specify education, training, or experience that a registered nurse must satisfy to call himself or herself an advanced practice nurse; to establish appropriate education, training, and examination requirements that an advanced practice nurse must satisfy to qualify for a certificate to issue prescription orders; to define the scope of practice within which an advanced practice nurse prescriber may issue prescription orders; to specify the classes of drugs, individual drugs, or devices that may not be prescribed by an advanced practice nurse prescriber; to specify the conditions to be met for a registered nurse to administer a drug prescribed or directed by an advanced practice nurse prescriber; to establish procedures for maintaining a certificate to issue prescription orders, including requirements for continuing education; and to establish the minimum amount of malpractice insurance required of an advanced practice nurse prescriber.

Citation: WIS. ADMIN. CODE § N 8.01.

There is no defined scope of practice for Wisconsin NPs, other than the above regulation which indicates that NPs may prescribe. Physicians may delegate medical functions to a nurse at the physician's discretion.

WYOMING

"Advanced practice of nursing" means a registered professional nurse who performs advanced nursing acts and who may perform medical acts including prescribing or providing prepackaged medications except Schedule I and Schedule II drugs as defined in Wyoming Statutes Annotated § 35-7-1013–35-7-1016.

Citation: WYO. STAT. ANN. § 33-21-120(a)(i).

APPENDIX 2-B

State-by-State Requirement, If Any, of Physician Collaboration

ALABAMA

The joint committee shall be the state authority designated to recommend rules and regulations to the State Board of Medical Examiners and the Board of Nursing for the purpose of regulating the collaborative practice of physicians and certified registered practitioners and certified nurse midwives. No person may practice as a certified registered nurse practitioner or a certified nurse midwife in this state unless that person possesses a certificate of qualification issued by the Board of Nursing and practices under written protocols approved by the State Board of Medical Examiners and the Board of Nursing and signed by a qualified collaborating physician or physicians and certified registered nurse practitioner or certified nurse midwife or is exempt from the requirement of a written protocol according to rules promulgated by the State Board of Medical Examiners and the Board of Nursing. The joint committee shall recommend to the State Board of Medical Examiners and the Board of Nursing rules and regulations designed to govern the collaborative relationship between physicians and certified registered nurse practitioners and certified nurse midwives certified by the Board of Nursing to engage in these areas of advanced practice nursing. These rules and regulations shall be finally adopted by July 1, 1996. These rules and regulations and any and all additions, deletions, corrections, or changes thereto shall be considered rules and regulations requiring publication under the Alabama Administrative Procedure Act; however, the following shall not be considered rules or regulations under the Administrative Procedure Act:

1. Protocols for use by certified registered nurse practitioners and certified nurse midwives certified to engage in these two areas of advanced practice nursing in collaboration with a physician; and
2. The formulary of legend drugs that may be prescribed by certified registered nurse practitioners and certified nurse midwives authorized to do so.

Citation: ALA. CODE § 34-21-85.

Requirements for Collaborative Practice:

1. Role of Collaborating Physician
   (a) The collaborating physician is responsible for providing professional oversight and direction to the certified registered nurse practitioner.
2. Availability of Collaborating Physician
   (a) The collaborating physician shall be available for direct communication or by radio, telephone, or telecommunications.
   (b) The collaborating physician shall be available for consultation or referrals of patients from the certified registered nurse practitioner.
   (c) In the event the collaborating physician is not available, provisions must be made for medical coverage by a physician who is pre-approved by the State Board of Medical Examiners and is familiar with these rules.
   (d) If the certified registered nurse practitioner is to perform duties at a site away from the collaborating physician, the application must clearly specify the circumstances and provide written verification of physician availability for consultation and/or referral, and direct medical intervention in emergencies and after hours, if indicated. The Joint Committee may, at its discretion, waive the requirements of written verification upon documentation of exceptional circumstances. Employees of state and county health departments are exempt from the requirements of written verification of physician availability.
3. Written Standard Protocol
   (a) A written standard protocol specific to the specialty practice area of the certified registered nurse practitioner, approved and signed by both the collaborating physician and the certified registered nurse practitioner shall be maintained at each practice site.
   (b) The written standard protocol shall include a formulary of drugs, devices, medical treatments, tests, and procedures that may be prescribed, ordered, and implemented by the certified registered nurse practitioner consistent with these rules and which are appropriate for the collaborative practice setting.

(c) The written standard protocol shall include a pre-determined plan for emergency services.
(d) The written standard protocol shall specify the process by which the certified registered nurse practitioner shall refer a patient to a physician other than the collaborating physician.

4. Mechanism for Quality Analysis
   (a) A written plan for review of medical records and patient outcomes shall be submitted with the application, with documentation of the reviews maintained.
   (b) Countersignature by physician must be pursuant to established policy and/or applicable legal regulations and accreditation standards.
5. Exemptions
   (a) Certified registered nurse practitioners practicing in settings in which they are solely performing in a nursing role may apply for an exemption from the collaborative practice requirements.

Citation: ALA. ADMIN. CODE 610-X-9-.15.

Collaboration. A formal relationship between one or more CRNPs and a physician under which these nurses may engage in advanced practice nursing as evidenced by written protocols. The term collaboration does not require direct, on-site supervision of the activities of a CRNP, by the collaborating physician. The term does require such professional oversight and direction as may be required by the rules and regulations of the Board of Nursing and the Board of Medical Examiners.

Citation: ALA. ADMIN. CODE r. 610-X-9-.07(5) and ALA. CODE § 32-21-81(5).

Protocol. A document establishing the permissible functions and activities to be performed by CRNP and signed by collaborating physician and by any NPs practicing with those physicians.

Citation: ALA. ADMIN. CODE r. 610-X-9-.07(11) and ALA. CODE § 32-21-81(11).

Protocol must include a formulary of drugs, treatments, tests, and procedures, a pre-determined plan for emergency services, a process for referral, a mechanism for quality analysis, and a written plan for review of medical records.

Citation: ALA. ADMIN. CODE r. 610-X-9-.15.

Collaborating physician must get an exemption to collaborate with more than three full-time equivalent NPs, unless MD and NPs are employed by the State Health Department.

Citation: ALA. ADMIN. CODE r. 610-X-9-.10, r. 610-X-9-.18.

ALASKA

There is no requirement for a written agreement with a physician.

There is a requirement for a written plan which outlines procedures for consultation with other health care providers and referral of clients to other health care providers as indicated by clients' needs.

Citation: ALAS. ADMIN. CODE tit. 12, § 44.400.

ARIZONA

In addition to the scope of practice permitted by a professional nurse, an RNP may perform the following acts in collaboration with a physician:

- Examine patients and establish medical diagnoses by client history, physical exam, and other criteria;
- Admit patients to health care facilities;
- Order, perform, and interpret laboratory, radiographic, and other diagnostic tests;
- Identify, develop, implement, and evaluate a plan of care for a patient to promote, maintain, and restore health;
- Prescribe and dispense medications when granted authority under section R4-19-507;
- Refer to and consult with appropriate health care providers.

Citation: ARIZ. ADMIN. CODE R4-19-505.

ARKANSAS

NPs must practice under a collaborative practice agreement, which must address physician availability for consultation or referral, protocols for prescriptive authority, coverage in the emergency absence of NP or physician, and quality assurance.

Citation: ARK. CODE ANN. § 17-87-310(C)(1).

CALIFORNIA

Neither this chapter nor any other provision of law shall be construed to prohibit a nurse practitioner from furnishing or ordering drugs or devices when all of the following apply:

(a) The drugs or devices are furnished or ordered by a nurse practitioner in accordance with standardized procedures or protocols developed by the nurse practitioner and his or her supervising physician and surgeon under any of the following circumstances:
   1. When furnished or ordered incidental to the provision of family planning services.

2. When furnished or ordered incidental to the provision of routine health care or prenatal care.
3. When rendered to essentially healthy persons.

(b) The nurse practitioner is functioning pursuant to standardized procedure, as defined by Section 2725, or protocol. The standardized procedure or protocol shall be developed and approved by the supervising physician and surgeon, the nurse practitioner, and the facility administrator or his or her designee.

(c) The standardized procedure or protocol covering the furnishing of drugs or devices shall specify which nurse practitioners may furnish or order drugs or devices, which drugs or devices may be furnished or ordered, under what circumstances, the extent of physician and surgeon supervision, the method of periodic review of the nurse practitioner's competence, including peer review, and review of the provisions of the standardized procedure.

(d) The furnishing or ordering of drugs or devices by a nurse practitioner occurs under physician and surgeon supervision. Physician and surgeon supervision shall not be construed to require the physical presence of the physician, but does include: (1) collaboration on the development of the standardized procedure, (2) approval of the standardized procedure, and (3) availability by telephonic contact at the time of patient examination by the nurse practitioner.

(e) For purposes of this section, no physician and surgeon shall supervise more than four nurse practitioners at one time.

(f) Drugs or devices furnished or ordered by a nurse practitioner may include Schedule III through Schedule V controlled substances under the California Uniform Controlled Substances Act [Division 10 (commencing with Section 11000) of the Health and Safety Code] and shall be further limited to those drugs agreed upon by the nurse practitioner and physician and surgeon and specified in the standardized procedure. When Schedule III controlled substances, as defined in Section 11056 of the Health and Safety Code, are furnished or ordered by a nurse practitioner, the controlled substances shall be furnished or ordered in accordance with a patient-specific protocol approved by the treating or supervising physician. A copy of the section of the nurse practitioner's standardized procedure relating to controlled substances shall be provided upon request, to any licensed pharmacist who dispenses drugs or devices, when there is uncertainty about the nurse practitioner furnishing the order.

(g) The board has certified in accordance with Section 2836.3 that the nurse practitioner has satisfactorily completed:

1. At least six month's physician and surgeon-supervised experience in the furnishing or ordering of drugs or devices, and
2. A course in pharmacology covering the drugs or devices to be furnished or ordered under this section. The board shall establish the requirements for satisfactory completion of this subdivision.

(h) Use of the term "furnishing" in this section, in health facilities defined in subdivisions (b), (c), (d), (e), and (i) of Section 1250 of the Health and Safety Code, shall include (1) the ordering of a drug or device in accordance with the standardized procedure and (2) transmitting an order of a supervising physician and surgeon.

(i) Nothing in this section, nor any other provision of law, shall be construed to authorize a nurse practitioner in solo practice to furnish drugs or devices, under any circumstances.

(j) "Drug order" or "order" for purposes of this section means an order for medication which is dispensed to or for an ultimate user, issued by a nurse practitioner as an individual practitioner, within the meaning of Section 1306.02 of Title 21 of the Code of Federal Regulations. Notwithstanding any other provision of law,

1. A drug order issued pursuant to this section shall be treated in the same manner as a prescription of the supervising physician;
2. All references to "prescription" in this code and the Health and Safety Code shall include drug orders issued by nurse practitioners; and
3. The signature of a nurse practitioner on a drug order issued in accordance with this section shall be deemed to be the signature of a prescriber for purposes of this code and the Health and Safety Code.

Citation: ANN. CAL. BUS. & PROF. CODE § 2836.1.

Furnishing or ordering of drugs or devices by nurse practitioners is defined to mean the act of making a pharmaceutical agent or agents available to the patient in strict accordance with a standardized procedure. All nurse practitioners who are authorized pursuant to Section 2831.1 to furnish or issue drug orders for controlled substances shall register with the United States Drug Enforcement Administration.

Citation: ANN. CAL. BUS. & PROF. CODE § 2836.1.

COLORADO

For prescriptive authority, NP must show evidence of execution of a written collaborative agreement with a physician licensed in Colorado whose medical education, training, experience, and active practice correspond with that of the APN.

Written agreement shall include the duties and responsibilities of each party, provisions regarding consultation and referral, a mechanism designed by the APN to assure appropriate prescriptive practice, and other provisions as established by the board. Nothing in this paragraph shall be construed to permit the independent practice of medicine, as defined in section 12-36-106(1) and (2), by an APN, limit the ability of an advanced practice nurse to make an independent judgment, require supervision by a physician or require the use of methods for prescribing medication that are codified and that do not allow the use of professional judgment or variation according to the needs of the patient.

Citation: COLO. REV. STAT. ANN. § 12-38-111.6(4)(d)(I)-(IV).

CONNECTICUT

The advanced practice registered nurse may, under the direction of a physician licensed to practice medicine in this state and in accordance with written protocols, and if practicing in: (1) an institution licensed pursuant to subsection (a) of section 19a-491 as a hospital, home for the aged, health care facility for the handicapped, nursing home, rest home, mental health facility, substance abuse treatment facility, infirmary operated by an educational institution for the care of students enrolled in, or the faculty and staff of, such institution, or facility operated and maintained by any state agency and providing services for the prevention, diagnosis, and treatment or care of human health conditions, or (2) an industrial health facility licensed pursuant to subsection (h) of section 31-374 which serves at least two thousand employees; or (3) a clinic operated by a state agency, municipality, or private non-profit corporation; or (4) a clinic operated by any educational institution prescribed by regulations adopted pursuant to section 10-99a, prescribe, dispense, or administer medical therapeutics and corrective measures, except that [an advanced practice nurse certified as a nurse anesthetist and administering therapeutics in surgery may do so only if the physician is present in the institution]. In all other settings, the advanced practice nurse may, under the direction of a physician licensed to practice medicine in the state and in accordance with written protocol, prescribe and administer medical therapeutics and corrective measures and may dispense drugs in the form of professional samples in accordance with section 20-14c to 20-14e, inclusive.

Citation: CONN. GEN. STAT. ANN. § 20-87a.

. . . "[C]ollaboration" means a mutually agreed upon relationship between an advanced practice registered nurse and a physician who is educated, trained, or has relevant experience that is related to the work of such advanced practice registered nurse. The collaboration shall address a reasonable and appropriate level of consultation and referral, coverage for the patient in the absence of the advanced practice registered nurse, a method to review patient outcomes, and a method of disclosure of the relationship to the patient. Relative to the exercise of prescriptive authority, the collaboration between an advanced practice registered nurse and a physician shall be in writing and shall address the level of schedule II and III controlled substances that the advanced practice registered nurse may prescribe and provide a method to review patient outcomes, including, but not limited to, the review of medical therapeutics, corrective measures, laboratory tests, and other diagnostic procedures that the advanced practice registered nurse may prescribe, dispense, and administer.

Citation: CONN. GEN. STAT. ANN. § 20-87a.

A clinical practice relationship shall exist between each Advanced Practice Registered Nurse performing advanced level nursing practice activities and a physician licensed to practice medicine in this state, and shall be based upon mutually agreed upon written protocols which shall be available upon request of the Department of Health Services or the Department of Consumer Protection. Such protocols shall include, but not be limited to:

(a) A list of categories of medical therapeutics, corrective measures, laboratory tests, and other diagnostic procedures which may be prescribed, dispensed, or administered by the Advanced Practice Registered Nurse in various circumstances;
(b) A list of appropriate laboratory tests and other diagnostic procedures which may be required and ordered by the Advanced Practice Registered Nurse before medical therapeutics or corrective measures may be prescribed, dispensed, or administered by the Advanced Practice Registered Nurse;
(c) Situations in which medical consultation or referral may be required before prescribing, dispensing, or administering shall occur;
(d) Follow-up evaluative procedures.

Citation: CONN. GEN. STAT. ANN. § 20-87a-4.

Policies shall be in place to insure that prescribing activities are reviewed by the physician directing the prescribing in a manner that is consistent with the type of setting in which care is rendered. Such policies shall provide for a periodic review consistent with the type of setting and the nature of patients' health care needs.

Citation: CONN. GEN. STAT. ANN. § 20-87a-5.

DELAWARE

Advanced practice nurses shall operate in collaboration with a licensed physician, dentist, podiatrist, or licensed health care delivery system to cooperate, coordinate, and consult with each other as appropriate pursuant to a collaborative agreement defined in the Rules and Regulations promulgated by the Board of Nursing, in the provision of health care to their patients.

Advanced practice nurses desiring to practice independently or to prescribe independently must do so pursuant to Title 24, § 1906(20) (1997).

Citation: DEL. CODE ANN. tit. 24 § 1902(d)(1).

The Joint Practice Committee with the approval of the Board of Medical Practice shall have the authority to grant, restrict, suspend, or revoke practice or independent practice authority and the Joint Practice Committee with the approval of the Board of Medical Practice shall be responsible for promulgating Rules and Regulations to implement the provisions of this chapter regarding "advanced practice nurses" who have been granted authority for independent practice and/or independent prescriptive authority.

Citation: DEL. CODE ANN. tit. 24, § 1906(20).

Those individuals who wish to engage in independent practice without written guidelines or protocols and/or wish to have independent prescriptive authority shall apply for such privilege or privileges to the Joint Practice Committee and do so only in collaboration with a licensed physician, dentist, podiatrist, or licensed health care delivery system. This does not include those individuals who have protocols and/or waivers approved by the Board of Medical Practice.

Citation: DEL. CODE ANN. tit. 24, § 1902(d)(2).

DISTRICT OF COLUMBIA

Generally, advanced practice registered nurses shall carry out acts of advanced registered nursing in collaboration with a licensed physician or osteopath.

Citation: D.C. CODE ANN. § 3-1206.03.

Functions shall be clearly delineated in a written protocol. The protocol requirement shall not apply to a NP who is directly employed by or practicing in a hospital, health maintenance organization, ambulatory surgical facility, or similar facility or agency . . . who practices in accordance with the protocols of that facility, which require at least general collaboration.

Citation: D.C. MUN. REGS. § 5907.

The protocol shall be reviewed biennially by the collaborating parties, and shall be initialed and dated by each party at the time of review.

Citation: D.C. MUN. REGS. § 5907.8

FLORIDA

A nurse practitioner shall only perform medical acts of diagnosis, treatment, and operation pursuant to a protocol between advanced registered nurse practitioner and a licensed medical doctor, osteopathic physician, or dentist. The degree and method of supervision, determined by the nurse practitioner and physician shall be specifically identified in the protocol and shall be appropriate for prudent health care providers under similar circumstances. General supervision is required, unless otherwise specified.

Citation: FLA. ADMIN. CODE CH. 64B9-4.010.

GEORGIA

The certified nurse practitioner collaborates as necessary with a variety of individuals to diagnose and manage clients' health care problems.

Citation: GA. COMP. R. & REGS, r. 410-12.03

A physician may delegate to a nurse recognized as a . . . certified nurse practitioner in accordance with a nurse protocol . . . the authority to order controlled substances selected from a formulary of such drugs established by the composite State Board of Medical Examiners and the authority to order dangerous drugs, medical treatments, and diagnostic studies.

"Nurse protocol" means a written document mutually agreed upon and signed by a nurse and licensed physician by which document the physician delegates to the nurse the authority to perform certain medical acts. . . .

Citation: GA. CODE ANN. § 43-34-26.1.

HAWAII

(a) Each relationship between a recognized APRN with prescriptive authority and a licensed physician shall be documented in an agreement, the form of which is provided by the department, which attests that:

1. The physician shall be actively engaged in the same or related specialty practice and affiliated with the same institution in which the recognized APRN is to practice;

2. The physician and the recognized APRN jointly acknowledge and accept the responsibility that the collegial working relationship is based upon written policies for the delivery of health care services that will have the interest and welfare of the patient foremost in mind;
3. The recognized APRN and the physician acknowledge and accept the responsibility that the recognized APRN's prescriptive authority is governed by the exclusionary formulary and that there shall be strict adherence to the exclusionary formulary; and
4. Details of the collegial working relationship between the recognized APRN with prescriptive authority and the physician shall, at minimum, include:
   (A) Name and area of practice specialty of the recognized APRN;
   (B) Name and area of practice of the physician or physicians;
   (C) Any limitation, agreed to by the parties, such as drugs not to be prescribed (although permitted by the exclusionary formulary) or the party to prevail when there is disagreement on the prescription for a patient;
   (D) Method of communication between the recognized APRN and the physician or physicians;
   (E) Name of the institution or institutions which employ or is affiliated with the recognized APRN and the physician; and
   (F) Name of interim physician or physicians who will act in place of the primary physician in the event unforeseen circumstances preclude the relationship with the primary physician. The interim physician shall comply with all conditions of the agreement.

(b) The collegial working relationship agreement shall be signed by the recognized APRN with prescriptive authority, the physician, and the interim physician, dated, notarized, and filed with the department for approval at least five weeks prior to the intended implementation of the relationship. Approval by the director of the department or designee is required, and in the case of disapproval of any relationship, the recognized APRN shall be provided the reason for disapproval and the right to a hearing pursuant to chapter 91, HRS.

(c) Any modifications, including, but not limited to, a change in the interim physician, institution, or changes in the specific conditions set forth in the collegial working relationship agreement previously filed, shall be submitted to the department in a written document by the recognized APRN at least ten working days prior to the intended implementation of the change. The modified relationship shall at minimum meet the requirements of subsections (a) and (b). Until the department has approved the modified relationship, modifications shall not be implemented.

(d) Either the recognized APRN or the physician may unilaterally terminate the physician and recognized APRN collegial working relationship at any time by notifying the other party. Either the recognized APRN or the physician shall notify the department of the termination in writing within three calendar days of the termination. At the time the collegial working relationship ceases, the recognized APRN shall not have prescriptive authority until such time as another collegial working relationship agreement has been reestablished and approved by the department.

(e) The director may assess a processing fee for the approval of, modifications to, termination, or reestablishment of, a collegial working relationship agreement.

(f) The director shall have the authority to summarily suspend a collegial working relationship agreement, and the prescriptive authority of a recognized APRN in accordance with section 436B-23, HRS.

(g) The collegial working relationship agreement shall be made available to licensed pharmacies.

Citation: HAW. ADMIN. R § 16-89C-10.

IDAHO

The nurse practitioner shall practice with physician supervision, consultation and collaborative management, and appropriate referral.

Citation: IDAHO CODE § 54-1402(1)(c).

ILLINOIS

(Section scheduled to be repealed on January 1, 2008)

(a) Except as provided in Section 15-25, no person shall engage in the practice of advanced practice nursing except when licensed under this Title and pursuant to a written collaborative agreement with a collaborating physician.

(b) A written collaborative agreement shall describe the working relationship of the advanced practice nurse with the collaborating physician and shall authorize the categories of care, treatment, or procedures to be performed by the advanced practice nurse. Collaboration does not require an employment relationship between the collaborating physician and advanced practice nurse. Collaboration means the relationship under which an advanced practice nurse works with a collaborating physician in an active clinical practice to deliver health care services in accordance with (i) the advanced practice nurse's training, education, and experience and (ii) medical direction as documented in a jointly developed written collaborative agreement. The agreement shall be defined to promote the exercise of professional judgment by the advanced practice nurse commensurate with his or her education and experience. The services to be provided by the advanced practice nurse shall be services that the collaborating physician generally provides to his or her patients in the normal course of his or her clinical medical practice. The agreement need not describe the exact steps that an advanced practice nurse must take with respect to each specific condition, disease, or symptom but must specify which authorized procedures require a physician's presence as the procedures are being performed. The collaborative relationship under an agreement shall not be construed to require the personal presence of a physician at all times at the place where services are rendered. Methods of communication shall be available for consultation with the collaborating physician in person or by telecommunications in accordance with established written guidelines as set forth in the written agreement.

(c) Physician medical direction under an agreement shall be adequate if a collaborating physician:
   1. Participates in the joint formulation and joint approval of orders or guidelines with the APN and he or she periodically reviews such orders and the services provided patients under such orders in accordance with accepted standards of medical practice and advanced practice nursing practice;
   2. Is on site at least once a month to provide medical direction and consultation; and
   3. Is available through telecommunications for consultation on medical problems, complications, or emergencies or patient referral.

(d) A copy of the signed, written collaborative agreement must be available to the Department upon request from both the advanced practice nurse and the collaborating physician and shall be annually updated. An advanced practice nurse shall inform each collaborating physician of all collaborative agreements he or she has signed and provide a copy of these to any collaborating physician, upon request.

Citation: 225 ILL. COMP. STAT. § 65/15-15.

INDIANA

An advanced practice nurse shall operate in collaboration with a licensed practitioner as evidenced by a practice agreement, or by privileges granted by the governing board of a hospital . . . with the advice of the medical staff of the hospital that sets forth the manner in which the advanced practice nurse and a licensed practitioner will cooperate, coordinate, and consult with each other in the provision of health care to their patients.

Citation: IND. CODE ANN. § 25-23-1-19.4(b).

"Practitioner" means [for the purpose of this section]:

- A licensed physician.
- A dentist.
- A podiatrist.
- An optometrist.

Citation: IND. CODE ANN. § 16-14-19-5.

NP must have a written practice agreement that sets forth the manner in which the APN and licensed practitioner will cooperate, coordinate, and consult with each other in the provision of health care to patients. [Written agreement has specific requirements for information included.]

Citation: IND. ADMIN. CODE tit. 848, r. 5-1-1(6).

IOWA

"Collaboration" is the process whereby an ARNP and physician jointly manage the care of a client.

"Collaborative practice agreement" means an ARNP and physician practicing together within the framework of their respective professional scopes of practice. This collaborative agreement reflects both independent and cooperative decision making and is based on the preparation and ability of each practitioner.

"Consultation" is the process whereby an ARNP seeks the advice or opinion of a physician, pharmacist, or another member of the health care team. ARNPs practicing in a noninstitutional setting as sole practitioners, or in small clinical practice groups, shall regularly consult with a licensed physician or pharmacist regarding the distribution, storage, and appropriate use of controlled substances.

Citation: IOWA ADMIN. CODE r. 655-7.1(152).

The ARNP may perform selected medically designated functions when a collaborative practice agreement exists.

Citation: IOWA ADMIN. CODE r. 655-6.1.

KANSAS

An advanced registered nurse practitioner may prescribe drugs pursuant to a written protocol as authorized by a responsible physician.

Each written protocol shall contain a precise and detailed medical plan of care for each classification of disease or injury for which the advanced registered nurse practitioner is authorized to prescribe and shall specify all drugs which may be prescribed by the advanced registered nurse practitioner. Any written prescription order shall include the name, address, and telephone number of the responsible physician.

Citation: KAN. STAT. ANN. § 65-1130(d).

Advanced registered nurse practitioners shall function in a collegial relationship with physician and other health professional in the delivery of primary health care services. Advanced registered nurse practitioners shall be authorized to make independent decisions about nursing needs of families and clients, and interdependent decisions with physician in carrying out health regimens for families and clients.

Citation: KAN. STAT. ANN. § 60-11-101(a).

KENTUCKY

In the performance of advanced registered nursing practice, the advanced registered nurse practitioner shall practice in accordance with the collaborative practice agreement, if applicable, and shall seek consultation or referral in those situations outside the advanced registered nurse practitioner's scope of practice.

Citation: 201 KY. ADMIN. REGS. 20:057.

LOUISIANA

"Collaboration" means a cooperative working relationship with another licensed physician, dentist, or other health care provider to jointly contribute to providing patient care, and may include, but not be limited to, discussion of a patient's diagnosis and cooperation in the management and delivery of health care with each provider performing those activities that he is legally authorized to perform.

"Collaborative practice" means the joint management of the health care of a patient by an advanced practice registered nurse performing advanced practice registered nursing and one or more consulting physicians or dentists. Except as otherwise provided in R.S. 37:930, acts of medical diagnosis and prescription by an advanced practice registered nurse shall be under the direction of a licensed physician or dentist and in accordance with a collaborative practice agreement.

"Collaborative practice agreement" means a formal written statement addressing the parameters of the collaborative practice which are mutually agreed upon by the advanced practice registered nurse and one or more licensed physicians or dentists which shall include, but not be limited to the following provisions:

(a) Availability of the collaborating physician or dentist for consultation or referral, or both.
(b) Methods of management of the collaborative practice which shall include clinical practice guidelines.
(c) Coverage of the health care needs of a patient during any absence of the advanced practice registered nurse, physician, or dentist.

Citation: LA. REV. STAT. ANN. § 37:913.

[A] collaborative practice agreement . . . shall include, but not be limited to:

(a) A plan of accountability among the parties that: (i) defines the limited prescriptive authority of the APRN and the responsibilities of the collaborating physician or physicians; (ii) delineates a plan for possible hospital admissions and privileges; (iii) delineates mechanisms and arrangements for diagnostic and laboratory requests for testing; (iv) delineates a plan for documentation of medical records and the frequency of collaborating physician review of patient charts; (v) delineates a plan to accommodate immediate consultation with the collaborating physician regarding complications or problems not addressed by clinical practice guidelines.
(b) Clinical practice guidelines . . . shall contain documentation of the types of categories or schedules of drugs available and generic substitution for prescription that complements the APRN's licensed category and area of specialization as delineated in the collaborative practice physician and be: (i) mutually agreed upon by the APRN and collaborating physician; (ii) specific to the practice setting; (iii) maintained on site; (iv) reviewed and signed at least annually by the APRN and physician to reflect current practice.
(c) Documentation of the availability of the collaborating physician when the physician is not physically present in the practice setting. . . .
(d) Documentation shall be shown that patients are informed about how to access care when both the APRN and collaborating physician are absent from the practice setting or otherwise unavailable.
(e) An acknowledgment of the mutual obligation and responsibility of the APRN and collaborating physician to insure that all acts of limited prescriptive authority of the APRN are properly documented in written form by the APRN and that each such entry is reviewed and countersigned by the collaborating physician within 24 hours with respect to inpatients in an acute care setting and patients in a hospital emergency department.

A physician may enter into collaborative practice agreements for the exercise of limited prescriptive authority with not more than two APRNs, except as may otherwise expressly approve by the Joint Administration Committee. . . .

Citation: LA. ADMIN. CODE tit. 46 § XLVII.4513.

MAINE

For temporary approval [to practice] for graduates of nurse practitioner programs, a nurse practitioner must practice for a minimum of 24 months under the supervision of a licensed physician, or be employed by a clinic or hospital that has a medical director who is a licensed physician.

Requirements for initial approval to practice . . . [I]f more than 5 years have elapsed since completion of an advanced practice registered nurse program and the applicant does not meet the practice requirement of 1500 hours, the applicant shall complete 500 hours of clinical practice supervised by a physician or nurse practitioner in the same speciality area of practice.

Citation: CODE ME. R. § 02 380 008.

MARYLAND

Before a nurse practitioner may practice he shall . . .

(2) Enter into a written agreement with a physician whereby the physician on a regularly-scheduled basis shall:
   (a) Accept referrals;
   (b) Establish and review drug and other medical guidelines with the nurse practitioner;
   (c) Participate with the nurse practitioner in periodically reviewing and discussing medical diagnosis and the therapeutic or corrective measures employed in the practice setting;
   (d) Jointly sign records if needed to document accountability of both the physician and nurse practitioner;
   (e) Be available for consultation in person, by telephone, or by some other form of telecommunication; and
   (f) Designate an alternate physician if the physician identified in the written agreement temporarily becomes unavailable.

Citation: MD. CODE REGS. tit. 20, § 27.07.02.B.

MASSACHUSETTS

1. All nurses practicing in an expanded role . . . shall practice in accordance with the written guidelines developed in collaboration with and mutually acceptable to the nurse and to:

a. A physician expert by virtue of training or experience in the nurse's area of practice . . . .

2. In all cases the written guidelines shall designate a physician who shall provide medical direction as is customarily accepted in the specialty area. Guidelines shall:
   a. Specifically describe the nature and scope of the nursing practice;
   b. Describe the circumstances in which physician consultation or referral is required;
   c. Describe the use of established procedures for the treatment of common medical conditions which the nurse may encounter; and
   d. Include provisions for managing emergencies.
3. The guidelines pertaining to prescriptive practice shall:
   a. Include a defined mechanism to monitor prescribing practices, including documentation of review with a supervising physician at least every three months;
   b. Include protocols for initiation of intravenous therapies and Schedule II drugs;
   c. Specify the frequency of review of initial prescription of controlled substances; the initial prescription of Schedule II drugs must be reviewed by the physician within 96 hours; and
   d. Conform to M.G.L. c.94C, the regulations of the Department of Public Health at 105 CMR 700.000 et seq., and M.G.L. c.112, § 80E or § 80G, as applicable.

Citation: CODE MASS. REGS. tit. 244 § 4.22.

MICHIGAN

[There is no requirement for physician supervision or collaboration. However, there is no legal scope of practice for NPs. Physicians may delegate at their discretion [MICH. COMP. LAWS § 333.16215(1)].]

MINNESOTA

"Collaborative management" is a mutually agreed upon plan between an advanced practice registered nurse and one or more physicians or surgeons licensed under chapter 147 that designates the scope of collaboration necessary to manage the care of patients.

Citation: MINN. STAT. ANN. § 148.171.

MISSISSIPPI

The nurse practitioner shall practice in a collaborative/consultative relationship with a licensed physician whose practice is compatible with that of the nurse practitioner. The nurse practitioner shall practice according to a Board-approved protocol which has been mutually agreed upon by the nurse practitioner and a Mississippi licensed physician whose practice or prescriptive authority is not limited as a result of a voluntary order or legal/regulatory order. The protocol must outline diagnostic and therapeutic procedures and categories or pharmacologic agents which may be ordered, administered, dispensed, and/or prescribed for patients with diagnoses identified by the nurse practitioner.

Citation: CODE OF MISSISSIPPI RULES, Ch. IV, § 2.3.b. & c.

MISSOURI

Collaborative practice arrangements refer to written agreements, jointly agreed upon protocols, or standing orders, all of which shall be in writing, for the delivery of health care services.

Citation: MO. CODE REGS. ANN. tit. 4, § 200-4.200 (1)(B).

The collaborating physician in a collaborative practice shall not be so geographically distanced from the collaborating registered professional nurse or advanced practice nurse as to create an impediment to effective collaboration in the delivery of health care services or the adequate review of those services.

Citation: MO. CODE REGS. ANN. tit. 4, § 200-4.200(2)(A).

The use of a collaborative practice arrangement by an advanced practice nurse who provides health care services that include the diagnosis and initiation of treatment for acutely or chronically ill or injured persons shall be limited to practice locations where the collaborating physician, or other physician designated in the collaborative practice arrangement, is no further than fifty (50) miles by road, using the most direct route available, from the collaborating advanced practice nurse if the advanced practice nurse is practicing in federally designated health professional shortage areas (HPSAs). Otherwise, in non-HPSAs, the collaborating physician and collaborating advanced practice nurse shall practice within thirty (30) miles by road of one another. The provision of the above specified health care services pursuant to a collaborative practice arrangement shall be limited to only an advanced practice nurse.

Citation: MO. CODE REGS. ANN. tit. 4, § 200-4.200(2)(B).

An advanced practice nurse who desires to enter into a collaborative practice arrangement to provide health care services that include the diagnosis and treatment of acutely or chronically ill or injured persons at a location where the collaborating physician is not continuously present shall practice at the same location with the collaborating physician for a period of at least one (1) calendar month before the collaborating physician is not present. The provision of the above specified health care services pursuant to a collaborative practice arrangement shall be limited to only an advanced practice nurse.

Citation: MO. CODE REGS. ANN. tit. 4, § 200-4.200(2)(C).

Guidelines for consultation and referral to the collaborating physician or designated health care facility for services or emergency care that is beyond the education, training, competence, or scope of practice of the collaborating registered professional nurse or advanced practice nurse shall be established in the collaborative practice arrangement.

Citation: MO. CODE REGS. ANN. tit. 4, § 200-4.200(3)(D).

The methods of treatment, including any authority to administer or dispense drugs, delegated in a collaborative practice arrangement between a collaborating physician and a collaborating advanced practice nurse shall be delivered only pursuant to a written agreement, jointly agreed-upon protocols, or standing orders that are specific to the clinical conditions treated by the collaborating physician and collaborating advanced practice nurse.

Citation: MO. CODE REGS. ANN. tit. 4, § 200-4.200(3)(G).

The collaborative practice arrangement between a collaborating physician and a collaborating registered professional nurse or advanced practice nurse shall be signed and dated by the collaborating physician and collaborating registered professional nurse or advanced practice nurse before it is implemented, signifying that both are aware of its content and agree to follow the terms of the collaborative practice arrangement. The collaborative practice arrangement and any subsequent notice of termination of the collaborative practice arrangement shall be in writing and shall be maintained by the collaborating professionals for a minimum of eight years after termination of the collaborative practice arrangement. The collaborative practice arrangement shall be reviewed and revised as needed by the collaborating physician and collaborating registered professional nurse or advanced practice nurse.

Citation: MO. CODE REGS. ANN. tit. 4, § 200-4.200(3)(H).

When a collaborative practice arrangement is utilized to provide health care services for conditions other than acute self-limited or well defined problems, the collaborating physician, or other physician designated in the collaborative practice arrangement, shall see the patient for evaluation and approve or formulate the plan of treatment for new or significantly changed conditions as soon as is practical, but in no case more than two (2) weeks after the patient has been seen by the collaborating advanced practice nurse. The provision of the above specified health care services pursuant to a collaborative practice arrangement shall be limited to only an advanced practice nurse.

Citation: Mo. Code Regs. Ann. tit. 4, § 200-4.200(3)(J).

In order to assure true collaborative practice and to foster effective communication and review of services, the collaborating physician, or other physician designated in the collaborative practice arrangement, shall be immediately available for consultation to the collaborating registered professional nurse or advanced practice nurse at all times, either personally or via telecommunications.

Citation: Mo. Code Regs. Ann. tit. 4, § 200-4.200(4)(A).

The collaborating physician shall review the work, records, and practice of the health care delivered pursuant to a collaborative practice arrangement at least once every two (2) weeks. This review shall be documented by the collaborating physician. This subsection shall not apply to the situation described in subsection (4)(E) below or during the time the collaborating physician and collaborating advanced practice nurse are practicing together as required in subsection (2)(C) above.

Citation: Mo. Code Regs. Ann. tit. 4, § 200-4.200(4)(B).

If a collaborative practice arrangement is used in clinical situations where a collaborating advanced practice nurse provides health care services that include the diagnosis and initiation of treatment for acutely or chronically ill or injured persons, then the collaborating physician shall be present for sufficient periods of time, at least once every two (2) weeks, except in extraordinary circumstances that shall be documented, to participate in such review and to provide necessary medical direction, medical services, consultations, and supervision of the health care staff. In such settings the use of a collaborative practice arrangement shall be limited to only an advanced practice nurse and the physician shall not enter into a collaborative practice arrangement with more than three (3) full-time equivalent advanced practice nurses.

Citation: Mo. Code Regs. Ann. tit. 4, § 200-4.200(4)(C).

The collaborating physician and collaborating registered professional nurse or advanced practice nurse shall determine an appropriate process of review and management of abnormal test results which shall be documented in the collaborative practice arrangement.

Citation: Mo. Code Regs. Ann. tit. 4, § 200-4.200(4)(D).

In the case of collaborating physicians and collaborating registered professional nurses or advanced practice nurses practicing in settings which provide care to well patients or to those with narrowly circumscribed conditions in public health clinics or community health settings that provide population-based health services limited to immunizations, well child care, human immunodeficiency virus (HIV) and sexually transmitted disease care, family planning, tuberculosis control, cancer and other chronic disease and wellness screenings, services related to epidemiologic investigations and prenatal care, review of services shall occur as needed and set forth in the collaborative practice arrangement. If the services provided in such settings include diagnosis and the initiation of treatment of any other disease or injury, then the provisions of subsection (4)(C) shall apply.

Citation: MO. CODE REGS. ANN. tit. 4, § 200-4.200(4)(E).

In the case of collaborating physicians and collaborating registered professional nurses or advanced practice nurses practicing in association with public health clinics that provide population-based health services limited to immunizations, well child care, HIV and sexually transmitted disease care, family planning, tuberculosis control, cancer and other chronic disease and wellness screenings, services related to epidemiologic investigations and related treatment, and prenatal care, the geographic areas, methods of treatment and review of services shall occur as set forth in the collaborative practice arrangement. If the services provided in such settings include diagnosis and initiation of treatment of disease or injury not related to population-based health services, then the provisions of sections (2), (3), and (4) above shall apply.

Citation: MO. CODE REGS. ANN. tit. 4, § 200-4.200(5)(A).

MONTANA

An APN with prescriptive privileges will have a referral process to a licensed physician and a method for documenting referral in client records.

Citation: MONT. ADMIN. R. 8.32.1507.

An advanced practice registered nurse with prescriptive authority will submit a method of quality assurance for evaluation of the advanced registered nurse practitioner's practice. The quality assurance method must be approved by the board of nursing prior to issuance of prescriptive authority.

The quality assurance method will include . . . 30 charts or 5% of all charts handled by the advanced practice nurse; whichever is less, must be reviewed quarterly. Review must be accomplished through the use of a mixture of peer review and review by a physician of the same specialty if appropriate.

Citation: MONT. ADMIN. R. 8.32.1508.

NEBRASKA

Integrated practice agreement shall mean a written agreement between an advanced practice registered nurse and a collaborating physician in which the advanced practice registered nurse and the collaborating physician provide for the delivery of health care through an integrated practice. The integrated practice agreement shall provide that the advanced practice registered nurse and the collaborating physician will practice collaboratively within the framework of their respective scopes of practice. Each provider shall be responsible for his or her individual decisions in managing the health care of patients. Integrated practice includes consultation, collaboration, and referral.

The advanced practice registered nurse and the collaborating physician shall have joint responsibility for patient care, based upon the scope of practice of each practitioner. The collaborating physician shall be responsible for supervision of the advanced practice registered nurse to ensure the quality of health care provided to patients.

Supervision shall mean the ready availability of the collaborating physician for consultation and direction of the activities of the advanced practice registered nurse within the advanced practice registered nurse's defined scope of practice.

Citation: REV. STAT. NEB. § 71-1716.03.

NEVADA

A protocol must reflect current practice of the advanced practitioner of nursing, reflect established national or customary standards for his medical specialty, be maintained at the place of his practice, and be available for review by the board. A comprehensive review and revision of the protocols by an advanced practitioner of nursing must be conducted and documented by the advanced practitioner and the collaborating physician at the time of renewal.

Citation: NEV. ADMIN. CODE CH. 632, § 632.2555.

An applicant for a certificate of recognition as an advanced registered practitioner of nursing will be authorized to issue written prescriptions for poisons, dangerous drugs and devices only if he:

a. Is authorized to do so by the board; and

b. Submits an application for authority to use written prescriptions for poisons, dangerous drugs, or devices to the board; and
c. Has successfully completed a program [specific requirements omitted].

In addition to the information contained in the application for a certificate of recognition as an advanced practitioner of nursing, the application for authority to write a prescription for poisons, dangerous drugs, and devices must include:

a. Documentation of 1,000 hours of active practice in the immediately preceding 2 years as an advanced practitioner of nursing under a collaborating physician. The documentation must consist of a signed statement from the collaborating physician indicating to the board that the applicant is competent to prescribe those drugs listed in his protocols.

Citation: NEV. ADMIN. CODE CH. 632, § 632.257.

NEW HAMPSHIRE

There is no requirement for physician collaboration for NP practice in New Hampshire.

NEW JERSEY

A nurse practitioner/clinical nurse specialist may order medications and devices in the inpatient setting, subject to the following conditions:

1. Controlled substances may be ordered;
2. The order is written in accordance with standing orders or joint protocols developed in agreement between a collaborating physician and the nurse practitioner/clinical nurse specialist, or pursuant to the specific direction of the physician;
3. The nurse practitioner/clinical nurse specialist authorizes the order by signing his own name, printing the name and certification number, and printing the collaborating physician's name;
4. The physician is present or readily available through electronic communications;
5. The charts and records of the patients treated by the nurse practitioner/clinical nurse specialist are reviewed by the collaborating physician and the nurse practitioner/clinical nurse specialist within the period of time specified by the rule adopted by the State Commissioner of Health pursuant to section 13 or P.O. 1991, c. 377 (c.45-11-52); and
6. The joint protocols developed by the collaborating physician and the nurse practitioner/clinical nurse specialist are reviewed, updated, and signed at least annually by both parties.

A nurse practitioner/clinical nurse specialist may prescribe medications and devices in all other medically appropriate settings subject to:

1. Controlled dangerous substances may be ordered;
2. The order is written in accordance with standing orders or joint protocols developed in agreement between a collaborating physician and the nurse practitioner/clinical nurse specialist, or pursuant to the specific direction of the physician;
3. The nurse practitioner/clinical nurse specialist writes the prescription on the prescription blank of the collaborating physician, signs his name to the prescription, and prints his name and certification number;
4. The prescription is dated and includes the name of the patient and the name, address, and telephone number of the collaborating physician;
5. The physician is present or readily available through electronic communications;
6. The charts and records of the patients treated by the nurse practitioner/clinical nurse specialist are periodically reviewed by the collaborating physician and nurse practitioner/clinical nurse specialist;
7. The joint protocols developed by the collaborating physician and the nurse practitioner/clinical nurse specialist are reviewed, updated, and signed at least annually by both parties.

Citation: N.J. STAT. ANN. § 45:11-49.

NEW MEXICO

[There is no legal requirement for physician collaboration for NP practice in New Mexico.]

The Certified Nurse Practitioner makes independent decisions regarding the health care needs of the client and also makes independent decisions on carrying out health care regimens.

Citation: N.M. ADMIN. CODE 16.12.2.13.P.

NEW YORK

[A practice agreement between NP and a physician is required.]

Each practice agreement shall provide for patient records review by the collaborating physician in a timely fashion but in no event less often than every three months. The names of the nurse practitioner and the collaborating physician shall be clearly posted in the practice setting of the nurse practitioner.

Citation: N.Y. EDUC. LAW § 6902.3(c).

No physician shall enter into practice agreements with more than four nurse practitioners who are not located on the same physical premises as the collaborating physician.

Citation: N.Y. EDUC. LAW § 6902.3(e).

The protocol shall reflect current accepted medical and nursing practice. The protocols shall be filed with the department within ninety days of the commencement of the practice and may be updated periodically. The commissioner shall make regulations establishing the procedure for the review of protocols and the disposition of any issues arising from such review.

Citation: N.Y. EDUC. LAW § 6902.3(d).

NORTH CAROLINA

The primary or back-up supervising physician(s) and the nurse practitioner shall be continuously available to each other for consultation and direct communication or telecommunication. Written protocols shall be agreed upon and signed by both the primary supervising physician and the nurse practitioner, and maintained in each practice site.

The written standing protocols shall include the drugs, devices, medical treatments, tests, and procedures that may be prescribed, ordered, and implemented by the nurse practitioner . . . and which are appropriate for the diagnosing and treatment of the most commonly encountered health problems in that practice setting.

The written standing protocols shall include predetermined plans for emergency services.

The nurse practitioner shall be prepared to demonstrate the ability to perform medical acts as outlined upon request by members or agents of either board.

[Other conditions omitted.]

Citation: N.C. ADMIN. CODE tit. 21, r. 36.0227(i).

NORTH DAKOTA

For prescriptive authority, APRN shall [submit] a scope of practice statement including . . .

- The nature and extent of the collaboration for prescriptive practices with a physician . . .;
- Methods and frequency of the collaboration for prescriptive practices, which must occur as client needs dictate, but no less than once every two months;
- Methods of documentation of the collaboration process regarding prescriptive practices;

- Alternative arrangements for collaboration regarding prescriptive practices in the temporary or extended absence of the physician; and submit an affidavit from the licensed physician who will be participating in the collaborative prescriptive agreement acknowledging the manner of review and approval of the planned prescriptive practices. Information in the affidavit must also indicate that the advanced practice registered nurse's scope of prescriptive practice is appropriately related to the collaborating physician's medical specialty or practice.

Citation: N.D. ADMIN. CODE § 54-05-03.1-09.

OHIO

. . . [A] certified nurse practitioner may practice only in accordance with a standard care arrangement entered into with each physician or podiatrist with whom the nurse collaborates . . . [additional conditions omitted].

Citation: OHIO REV. CODE ANN. § 4723.431.

OKLAHOMA

An advanced registered nurse practitioner in accordance with the scope of practice of the advanced registered nurse practitioner shall be eligible to obtain recognition as authorized by the Board to prescribe . . . subject to the medical direction of a supervising physician.

Citation: OKLA. STAT. ANN. tit. 59, § 567.3a(6).

OREGON

There is no requirement of physician collaboration.

PENNSYLVANIA

"Direction": The incorporation of physician supervision to the certified registered nurse practitioner's performance of medical acts in the following ways:

1. Immediate availability of a licensed physician through direct communication or by radio, telephone, or telecommunications.
2. A predetermined plan for emergency services which has been jointly developed by the supervising physician and the CRNP.
3. A physician available on a regularly scheduled basis for referrals, review of the standard of medical practice incorporating consultation and chart review establishing and updating standing orders, drug and other medication protocols within the practice setting,

periodic updating in medical diagnosis and therapeutics, and consigning records when necessary to document accountability by both parties.

Citation: 49 PA. CODE § 21.251.

In those health care facilities providing health services in which the practice of a certified registered nurse practitioner involves the acts of medical diagnosis, or prescription of medical therapeutics or corrective measures, there shall be a committee in each area of practice whose function is to establish standard policies and procedures, in writing, pertaining to the scope and circumstances of the practice of the nurse in the medical management of the patient. . . . The committee shall include equal representation from the medical staff, including a nurse practitioner and nursing administration.

Citation: 49 PA. CODE § 21.291.

If a certified registered nurse practitioner is associated with a physician or group of physicians, the committee may consist of, but need not be limited to, the nurse practitioners and the physician.

Citation: 49 PA. CODE § 21.294.

The committee shall review annually the effectiveness of the medical functions of the CRNP, through an evaluation of the care rendered to patients using the data sources of patient records, statistics, and patient follow-up.

Citation: 49 PA. CODE § 21.294.

The CRNP is responsible for his own professional judgements and is accountable to the individual consumer. He is also accountable to the physician and employing agency in the area of medical diagnosis and therapeutics.

Citation: 49 PA. CODE § 21.311.

A CRNP may perform acts of medical diagnosis in collaboration with a physician and in accordance with regulations promulgated by the Board.

Citation: ACT 206 OF 2002, SECTION 8.2.

RHODE ISLAND

A certified registered nurse practitioner is permitted to prescribe from a formulary . . . written in collaboration with the medical director or physician consultant of the individual establishments.

Citation: R.I. GEN. LAWS § 5-34-39.

SOUTH CAROLINA

"Approved written protocols" mean specific statements developed collaboratively by the physician or medical staff and the nurse that establish physician delegation for medical aspects of care, including the prescription of medications.

Citation: S.C. CODE ANN. § R91-2.g.

A nurse practitioner or clinical nurse specialist practicing in an extended role shall perform delegated medical acts pursuant to an approved written protocol between the nurse and physician.

An approved written protocol shall include the following information at a minimum:

- General Data:
  1. Name, address, and South Carolina license number of the registered nurse.
  2. Name, address, and South Carolina license number of the physician.
  3. Nature of practice and practice location(s) of the nurse and physician.
  4. Date developed and dates reviewed and amended.
  5. Description of how consultation with the physician is provided and provision for backup consultation in the physician's absence.
- Delegated Medical Acts:
  1. The medical conditions for which therapies may be initiated, continued, or modified.
  2. The treatments that may be initiated, continued, or modified.
  3. The drug therapies that may be prescribed.
  4. Situations that require direct evaluation by or referral to the physician.

The original protocol and any amendments to the protocol, dated and signed by the nurse and physician, shall be available to the Board for review within 72 hours of request. A random audit of approved written protocols will be conducted by the Board on an annual basis. Failure to produce protocols upon request of the Board shall be considered misconduct and subject the licensee to disciplinary action. Individuals who change practice settings or physician, shall notify the Board of such change within 15 days and provide verification of approved written protocols. Individuals who discontinue their practice shall notify the Board within 15 days.

Citation: S.C. CODE ANN. § 91-6.h.

SOUTH DAKOTA

"Collaborative agreement" defined. The term, collaborative agreement, as used in this chapter, means a written agreement authored and signed by the nurse practitioner or nurse midwife and the physician with whom the nurse practitioner or nurse midwife is collaborating. A collaborative agreement defines or describes the agreed upon overlapping scope of advanced practice nursing and medical functions that may be performed, consistent with § 36-9A-12 or 36-9A-13, and contains such other information as required by the boards. A copy of each collaborative agreement shall be maintained on file with and be approved by the boards prior to performing any of the acts contained in the agreement.

Citation: S.D. CODIFIED LAWS § 36-9A-15.

Advanced practice nursing and medical functions—Collaborative agreement required. A nurse practitioner or nurse midwife may perform the overlapping scope of advanced practice nursing and medical functions only under the terms of a collaborative agreement with a physician licensed under chapter 36-4. Any collaborative agreement shall be maintained on file with the boards. Collaboration may be by direct personal contact, or by a combination of direct personal contact and indirect contact via telecommunication, as may be required by the boards. If the collaborating physician named in a collaborative agreement becomes temporarily unavailable, the nurse practitioner or nurse midwife may perform the agreed upon overlapping scope of advanced practice nursing and medical functions in consultation with another licensed physician designated as a substitute.

Citation: S.D. CODIFIED LAWS § 36-9A-17.

Collaboration with a licensed physician or physicians. A nurse practitioner or nurse midwife may perform the overlapping scope of advanced practice nursing and medical functions defined in SDCL 36-9A-12 and 36-9A-13, in collaboration with a physician or physicians licensed under SDCL chapter 36-4. Collaboration by direct personal contact with each collaborating physician must occur no less than one-half day a week or a minimum of one hour per ten hours of practice. Collaboration with each collaborating physician shall occur at least once per month by direct personal contact.

Citation: S.D. ADMIN. R. 20:62:03:03.

Direct personal contact. For the purposes of this chapter, the term, direct personal contact, means that both the collaborating physician and the nurse practitioner or nurse midwife are physically present on site and available for the purposes of collaboration. When the collaborating physician is not in direct personal contact with the nurse practitioner or nurse midwife, the physician must be available by telecommunication. If the boards consider additional direct personal contact necessary for a nurse practitioner or nurse midwife, they shall set the terms of that additional collaboration and require inclusion of those terms in that nurse practitioner's or midwife's collaborative agreement as a condition for its approval.

Citation: S.D. ADMIN. R. 20:62:03:04.

TENNESSEE

A nurse who has been issued a certificate of fitness as a NP shall file a notice with the primary care advisory board containing the name of the NP, the name of the licensed physician having supervision, control and responsibility for prescriptive services rendered by the NP, and a copy of the formulary describing the categories of legend drugs to be prescribed and/or issued by the NP.

Upon joint adoption of physician supervisory rules concerning controlled substances, the NP who holds a certificate of fitness shall be authorized to prescribe and/or issue controlled substances listed in Schedules II, III, IV, and V.

Citation: TENN. CODE ANN. § 63-7-123(b)(1)(2).

TEXAS

The advanced practice nurse acts independently and/or in collaboration with the health team in the observation, assessment, diagnosis, intervention, evaluation, rehabilitation, care and counsel, and health teachings of persons who are ill, injured, or infirm or experiencing changes in normal health processes; and in the promotion and maintenance of health or prevention of illness.

Citation: 21 TEX. ADMIN. CODE § 221.13(c).

When providing medical aspects of care, advanced practice nurses shall utilize mechanisms that provide authority for that care. These mechanisms may include, but are not limited to, protocols or other written authorization. This shall not be construed as requiring authority for nursing aspects of care.

Protocols or other written authorization shall promote the exercise of professional judgment by the advanced practice nurse commensurate with his/her education and experience. The degree of detail within protocols/policies/practice guidelines/clinical practice privileges may vary in relation to the complexity of the situations covered by such protocols, the advanced specialty area of practice, the advanced educational preparation of the individual, and the experience level of the individual advanced practice nurse.

Protocols or other written authorization:
(A) Should be jointly developed by the advanced practice nurse and the appropriate physician(s);
(B) Shall be signed by both the advanced practice nurse and the physician(s);
(C) Shall be reviewed and re-signed at least annually;
(D) Shall be maintained in the practice setting of the advanced practice nurse; and
(E) Shall be made available as necessary to verify authority to provide medical aspects of care.

The advanced practice nurse shall retain professional accountability for advanced practice nursing care.

Citation: 21 TEX. ADMIN. CODE § 221.13(d).

The advanced practice nurse with a valid prescription authorization number shall carry out or sign prescription drug orders for only those drugs that are:
(A) Classified as dangerous drugs;
(B) Authorized by protocols or other written authorization for medical aspects of patient care; and
(C) Prescribed for patient populations within the accepted scope of professional practice for the advanced practice nurse's specialty area. . . .

Protocols or other written authorization shall be defined in a manner that promotes the exercise of professional judgement by the advanced practice nurse commensurate with the education and experience of that person. A protocol or other written authorization:
(A) Is not required to describe the exact steps that the advanced practice nurse must take with respect to each specific condition, disease, or symptom; and
(B) May state types or categories of medications that may be prescribed or contain the types or categories of medications that may not be prescribed.

Protocols or other written authorization:
(A) Shall be written, agreed upon and signed by the advanced practice nurse and the physician;
(B) Reviewed and signed at least annually; and
(C) Maintained in the practice setting of the advanced practice nurse.

Citation: 21 TEX. ADMIN. CODE § 222.4.

UTAH

"Practice of advanced practice registered nursing" means . . . prescription or administration of prescription drugs or devices, including:

(i) Local anesthesia;
(ii) Schedule IV-V controlled substances; and
(iii) Schedule II-III controlled substances in accordance with a consultation and referral plan.

Citation: UTAH CODE ANN. § 58-31b-102(16).

"Consultation and referral plan" means a written plan jointly developed by an advanced practice registered nurse and a consulting physician that permits the advanced practice registered nurse to prescribe schedules II-III controlled substances.

Citation: UTAH CODE ANN. § 58-31b-102(5).

VERMONT

APRN performs medical acts independently within a collaborative practice with a licensed physician under practice guidelines which are mutually agreed upon between the APRN and collaborating physician and which are jointly acceptable to the medical and nursing professions. Practice guidelines will be reviewed and approved by the Board of Nursing and kept on file in the workplace and made available to the Board of Nursing at any time upon request.

Practice guidelines shall include:

- A description of clinical practice, including practice site(s), focus of care, and general category of clients;
- An indexed copy of standards for clinical practice including method of data collection, assessment, plan of care and criteria for collaboration, consultation and referral, including emergency referral or delineation of clinical privileges;
- The name of at least one physician licensed in Vermont who practices in the same specialty area who will be routinely utilized for collaboration, consultation, and referral; and
- Method of quality assurance.

Citation: VT. CODE R. CH. 4, RULE VIII.C.4.

VIRGINIA

A licensed nurse practitioner shall be authorized to engage in practices constituting the practice of medicine in collaboration with and under the medical direction and supervision of a licensed physician.

Citation: 18 VA. ADMIN. CODE 90-30-120.A.

A nurse practitioner with prescriptive authority may prescribe only within the scope of a written practice agreement with a supervising physician.

Citation: 18 VA. ADMIN. CODE 90-40-90.

"Practice agreement" means a written agreement jointly developed by the supervising physician and the nurse practitioner that describes and directs the prescriptive authority of the nurse practitioner.

Citation: 18 VA. ADMIN. CODE 90-40-10.

"Supervision" means that the physician documents being readily available for medical consultation by the licensed nurse practitioner or the patient, with the physician maintaining ultimate responsibility for the agreed-upon course of treatment and medications prescribed.

Citation: 18 VA. ADMIN. CODE 90-40-10.

Physicians who enter into a practice agreement with a nurse practitioner for prescriptive authority shall:

1. Supervise and direct, at any one time, no more than four nurse practitioners with prescriptive authority.
2. Regularly practice in any location in which the licensed nurse practitioner exercises prescriptive authority. A separate practice setting may not be established for the nurse practitioner. Exceptions to this requirement are as follows:
   a. A separate office practice may be established for a certified nurse midwife or for a nurse practitioner employed by or under contract with local health department, federally funded comprehensive primary care clinics, or nonprofit health care clinics or programs.
   b. Physicians who do not regularly practice at the same location with the nurse practitioner and who provide supervisory services to such separate practices shall make regular site visits for consultation and direction for appropriate patient management. The site visits shall occur in accordance with the practice agreement, but no less frequently than once a quarter.
3. Conduct a monthly, random review of patient charts on which the nurse practitioner has entered a prescription for an approved drug or device.

Citation: VA. ADMIN. CODE 90-40-100.

WASHINGTON

No physician collaboration is required by law for nurse practitioner practice in Washington.

WEST VIRGINIA

For the purposes of prescriptive authority, an agreement to a collaborative relationship for prescriptive practice between a physician and an advanced nurse practitioner shall be set forth in writing.

Collaborative agreements shall include:

- Mutually agreed upon written guidelines or protocols for prescriptive authority as it applies the advanced nurse practitioner clinical practice.
- Statements describing the individual and shared responsibilities of the advanced nurse practitioner and the physician pursuant to the collaborative agreement between them.
- Periodic and joint evaluation of prescriptive practice.
- Periodic and joint review and updating of the written guidelines or protocols.

Citation: W.V. CODE § 30-7-15(b).

WISCONSIN

Advanced practice nurse prescribers shall facilitate collaboration with other health care professionals at least one of whom shall be a physician through the use of modern communication techniques.

Citation: WIS. ADMIN. CODE § N8.10(2).

WYOMING

"Advanced practitioner of nursing" means a registered professional nurse who performs advanced nursing acts and who may perform medical acts including prescribing or providing prepackaged medications . . . in collaboration with a licensed or otherwise legally authorized physician or dentist, in such a manner as to assure quality and appropriateness of services rendered.

Citation: WYO. STAT. ANN. § 33-21-120(a)(i).

A registered professional nurse who is applying for initial recognition as an advanced practitioner of nursing shall meet the following requirements: . . . . Submit a written plan of practice and collaboration. Such written plan shall conform to the following criteria:

(A) Specialty areas of advanced nursing practice;
  (1) Identify and describe the recognized specialty area(s) of advanced nursing practice.
(B) Scope of practice;
  (1) Describe the scope of practice for each recognized specialty area of advanced nursing practice, including recipients of care, in terms of:
    (1.) Education and experiential preparation; and
    (2.) Scope of practice statements from national professional nursing organizations and/or accrediting agencies representing that specialty area of advanced nursing practice.

(C) Standards of practice;
  (1) Describe the plan for practicing advanced nursing according to the standards of practice for recognized specialty areas, including but not limited to the following:
    (1.) Methods of quality assurance;
    (2.) Strategies for collaboration with licensed or otherwise legally authorized physician(s) or dentist(s); and
    (3.) Consultation and referral patterns.
(D) Advanced practitioner of nursing's signature; and
(E) Date.

Citation: WYO. BOARD OF NURSING RULES CH. IV.3.(a).

CHAPTER 3

State Regulation of Nurse Practitioner Practice

The law governing nurse practitioner (NP) definition, scope of practice, prescriptive authority, and requirement of physician collaboration, if any, may be enacted by a state legislature in great detail or in general terms. Alternatively, the state legislature may give authority to a licensing board to make the rules and regulations that will govern NPs.

The likely state board to make the rules regarding NPs is the board of nursing. In many states, the board of nursing makes the rules governing NP practice. In some states, however, the board of medicine has a role. Appendix 3-A lists, for each state, the agency that regulates NPs.

HOW LAWS ABOUT NP PRACTICE EVOLVE

State law takes two forms, statutes and regulations (regulations are sometimes referred to as *rules*). The legislature makes statutory law, and state agencies under the executive branch of government make regulations. Regulations cannot contradict statutes but often expand upon the statutes to include more detail of government administration.

When a member of the public wants to change a statute, the advocate must enlist the help of a state legislator, who can introduce a bill that will change the current statute. When a member of the public wants to change a regulation, the advocate must either convince the state agency that is responsible for the regulation to change the regulation or convince a legislator to introduce a bill that, if enacted, would override the regulation.

When an agency decides to change a regulation, the agency writes a new regulation, publishes the regulation in an official state publication, and invites comments from interested parties. The agency may or may not make changes to the proposed regulation based on comments received from interested parties. A proposed regulation becomes a final regulation—law—after it has been published in proposed form and comments have been reviewed. Final regulations are republished, in final form, in the state's "register," an official publication of the state.

WHAT IS REGULATED?

Much of the state law governing NPs appears in regulations; some law is statutory. The practice issues that come under state regulation are:

- Requirements for licensure
- Scope of practice
- Prescriptive authority
- Requirement of collaboration or supervision
- Basis for license suspension, revocation, or nonrenewal
- Reimbursement under Medicaid
- Reimbursement by indemnity insurers
- Requirements of educational programs
- Standards of practice

State law regarding definition of an NP is found in Chapter 1. State law regarding scope of practice of NPs and collaboration requirements is found in Chapter 2. State law regarding NP prescriptive privileges is found in Chapter 5.

Licensure Requirements

State law governs the requirements for holding a professional license in the state. All states require NPs to hold state licenses as RNs. Twenty-four states require NPs to have master's degrees. Three additional states will require master's degrees as of 2005, 2006, and 2008. Thirty-five states require NPs to have obtained national certification. Appendix 3-B lists, for each state, the requirements for holding and maintaining an NP license.

Bases for Loss of License

State law, usually a regulation, specifies the criteria under which an NP's license may be revoked, suspended, or not renewed. Examples of some state laws follow. North Carolina and Pennsylvania make continuation of practice contingent upon following the rules of physician supervision. Rhode Island law does not address physician collaboration or supervision, but is concerned about practice-related safety issues.

North Carolina's law is more specific than most about enforcing the requirement of a nurse practitioner to practice under physician supervision:

> The approval of NP may be restricted, denied, or terminated, after notice and hearing, if the appropriate Board finds:
> - That the NP held himself out as a licensed physician;
> - That the nurse practitioner has engaged or attempted to engage in the performance of medical acts other than according to the written protocols and collaborative practice agreement.
>
> *Citation:* N.C. ADMIN. CODE tit. 21 r. 36.0227.

In Pennsylvania, approval may be terminated by the board of nursing when, after notice and hearing, the board finds registrant has "engaged in performance of medical functions and tasks other than at the direction of a physician licensed by the state board of medicine" (with exceptions), or, "the registrant has performed a medical task or function which the registrant is not qualified by education to perform" (49 PA. CODE § 21.321).

In Rhode Island, grounds for revocation/suspension include:

- Guilty of fraud or deceit in procuring or attempting to procure a license to practice nursing.
- Guilty of crime of gross immorality.
- Unfit or incompetent by reason of negligence or habits.
- Habitually intemperate or . . . addicted to one of the habit-forming drugs.
- Mentally incompetent.
- Guilty of unprofessional conduct which includes:
  - Abandonment of a patient.
  - Willfully making and filing false reports or records in the practice of nursing.
  - Willful omission to file reports or record nursing records or reports as required by law.
  - Failure to furnish appropriate details of client's nursing needs to succeeding nurse legally qualified to provide continuing nursing services to a client.
  - Willful disregard of standards and failure to maintain standards of the nursing profession.
- Failure to comply with the provisions of section 5-34-40(c) of the General Laws, as a nurse practitioner.
- Guilty of willfully or repeatedly violating any of the provisions of the Act and/or the rules and regulations adopted thereunder.

Citation: R.I. NURSING RULES § 10.1.

APPENDIX 3-A

Agency That Regulates Nurse Practitioners, State by State[1]

ALABAMA: Joint Committee of Board of Medical Examiners and Board of Nursing

ALASKA: Board of Nursing

ARIZONA: Board of Nursing

ARKANSAS: Board of Nursing

CALIFORNIA: Board of Nursing

COLORADO: Board of Nursing

CONNECTICUT: Board of Nursing

DELAWARE: Board of Nursing and Board of Medical Practice

DISTRICT OF COLUMBIA: Board of Nursing

FLORIDA: Board of Nursing

GEORGIA: Board of Nursing

HAWAII: Board of Nursing

IDAHO: Board of Nursing

ILLINOIS: Advanced Practice Nursing Board

INDIANA: Board of Nursing

[1] *Source:* © Carolyn Buppert 2003.

IOWA: Board of Nursing

KANSAS: Board of Nursing

KENTUCKY: Board of Nursing

LOUISIANA: Board of Nursing

MAINE: Board of Nursing

MARYLAND: Board of Nursing

MASSACHUSETTS: Board of Nursing and Board of Medicine

MICHIGAN: Board of Nursing

MINNESOTA: Board of Nursing

MISSISSIPPI: Board of Nursing

MISSOURI: Board of Nursing

MONTANA: Board of Nursing

NEBRASKA: Board of Nursing

NEVADA: Board of Nursing

NEW HAMPSHIRE: Board of Nursing

NEW JERSEY: Board of Nursing

NEW MEXICO: Board of Nursing

NEW YORK: Board of Nursing

NORTH CAROLINA: Board of Nursing and Board of Medicine

NORTH DAKOTA: Board of Nursing

OHIO: Board of Nursing

OKLAHOMA: Board of Nursing

OREGON: Board of Nursing

PENNSYLVANIA: Board of Nursing

RHODE ISLAND: Board of Nursing regulates practice in general; Division of Professional Regulation, Board of Nursing, regulates prescription writing; Director of Health Department establishes formulary committee

SOUTH CAROLINA: Board of Nursing and Physician Consultant to Board of Nursing

SOUTH DAKOTA: Board of Nursing and Board of Medicine

TENNESSEE: Board of Nursing and Board of Medicine make rules on prescription writing

TEXAS: Board of Nursing

UTAH: Board of Nursing

VERMONT: Board of Nursing

VIRGINIA: Board of Nursing and Board of Medicine

WASHINGTON: Board of Nursing

WEST VIRGINIA: Board of Nursing

WISCONSIN: Board of Nursing

WYOMING: Board of Nursing

APPENDIX 3-B

State-by-State Nurse Practitioner Qualifications Required by Law

ALABAMA

- RN license
- Graduation from an organized program of study and clinical experience beyond basic educational preparation as a registered nurse, which is recognized by the Board of Nursing and/or the appropriate specialty certifying agency
- Master's degree in nursing
- Certification from a national certifying agency recognized by the Board of Nursing

Citation: ALA. ADMIN. CODE r. 610-X-9-.09.

ALASKA

Requirements for initial authority to practice:

- One-year academic course
- RN license
- Certification by a national certifying agency

Requirements to maintain authority to practice

- 30 hours of continuing education every 2 years

Citation: ALAS. ADMIN. CODE tit. 12, § 44.400.

ARIZONA

Board of nursing grants NP designation based on the following submission by candidate:

- RN license
- Application
- Description of educational background

- Specification of specialty area
- Specification of employer
- Statement of whether nationally certified [board specifies which certifying agencies it accepts]
- Statement of whether license has ever been denied
- Statement of whether ever subject to disciplinary action by board
- Transcript from educational institution
- As of January 1, 2001, master's degree

Citation: ARIZ. ADMIN. CODE R4-19-504.

ARKANSAS

- Evidence of education approved by board
- National certification approved by board

Citation: ARK. CODE ANN. § 17-87-302.

CALIFORNIA

- RN license
- Completion of a program of study which conforms to the board standards
- Certification by a national or state organization

Citation: CAL. CODE REGS. § 1482.

COLORADO

- RN license
- Completion of NP program accredited by nationally recognized accrediting agency and/or completion of an exam required by the national certifying agency
- On or after July 1, 2008, successful completion of a graduate degree in the appropriate specialty
- For prescriptive authority, a graduate degree in nursing, satisfactory completion of specific educational requirements in the use of controlled substances and prescription drugs . . . and post graduate experience as an APN in a relevant clinical setting . . . consisting of not less than 1800 hours completed within the preceding 5 years.

Citation: COLO. REV. CODE ANN. § 12-38-111.6(4).

CONNECTICUT

- RN license
- Certification as NP from a national certifying body
- 30 hours education in pharmacology for advanced nursing practice

- As of December 31, 1994, master's degree

Citation: CONN. GEN. STAT. ANN. § 20-94a.

DELAWARE

- RN license
- Master's or certificate with national certification
- If no national certificate is available in the specialty, master's degree will qualify

Citation: DEL. CODE ANN. tit. 24 § 1902(d)(1).

DISTRICT OF COLUMBIA

- RN license
- Good ethical standing within the profession
- Successful completion of a post-basic education program applicable to the area of practice that is acceptable to the Board or accredited by a national accrediting body that is relevant to the advanced practice registered nurse's area of practice
- Certification by a nationally recognized accrediting body

Citation: D.C. CODE ANN., § 3-1206.08.

FLORIDA

- RN license
- Malpractice insurance
- One of the following:
  1. Completion of a formal, post-basic educational program of at least one academic year, the purpose of which is to prepare nurses for advanced practice
  2. Certification by an appropriate specialty board
  3. Graduation from a program leading to a master's degree

Citation: FLA. STAT., CH. 464.012.

GEORGIA

- RN license
- Completion/graduation from a nurse practitioner education program greater than 9 months in length
- Certification by the certifying agent of the American Nurses Association, the National Association of Pediatric Nurse Associates and Practitioners, AWHONN, or AANP and authorization to practice by the board
- Master's degree as of January 1, 1999

Citation: GA. COMP. R. & REGS. § r.410-12.03.

HAWAII

- RN license
- Unencumbered licenses in all other states where licensed
- MSN or certification from a national certifying body recognized by the board

Citation: HAW. REV. STAT. ANN. § 457-8.5.

- Completed application
- Proof of unencumbered license as RN in other states
- Official complete transcript of master's degree in clinical nursing or nursing science or evidence of current certification in the nursing specialty sent from a recognized national certifying body
- Documentation relating to any disciplinary action ordered by or pending before any board of nursing
- Documentation regarding any criminal conviction within the past 20 years

Citation: HAW. ADMIN. R. § 16-89-83.

IDAHO

To practice:

- RN license
- Completion of NP program accredited by a national organization recognized by the board
- Passing results on the certification examination administered by an organization recognized by the board
- Current national certification as a nurse practitioner from an organization recognized by the board

Citation: IDAHO ADMIN. CODE 23.01.01.285.03.

To prescribe:

- 30 hours of pharmacology education

Citation: IDAHO ADMIN. CODE 23.01.01.315.01.

ILLINOIS

To practice:

- Current registered nurse licensure
- National certification from one of 5 accrediting bodies
- Master's degree or other advanced practice formal education program

Citation: ILL. ADMIN. CODE, tit. 68 § 1305.15.

INDIANA

To practice:

- Graduation from an accredited graduate or certificate program that prepares NPs

Citation: IND. ADMIN. CODE tit. 848, § r. 4-1-4.

To prescribe:

- Completion of a graduate-level course in pharmacology
- 30 hours of continuing education in the past two years
- Attestation to a lack of substance abuse or conviction of a felony
- A collaborative agreement

Citation: IND. ADMIN. CODE tit. 848, § r. 5-1-1.

IOWA

- Master's or completion of a formal advanced practice educational program of study in a nursing specialty area approved by the board
- Appropriate clinical experience as approved by Board of Nursing

Citation: IOWA ADMIN. CODE r. 655-7.2(3).

KANSAS

- Completion of a formal, post-basic nursing education program located or offered in Kansas, approved by the board, which prepares nurses to function in an expanded role for which application is made
- Completion of an out-of-state program approved by the board
- Possession of a certificate issued by another board of nursing that requires completion of a formal program
- 3 college hours in advanced pharmacology

Citation: KAN. ADMIN. REGS. § 60-11-103.

KENTUCKY

- RN licensure
- Completion of an organized post-basic program of study and clinical experience acceptable to the board
- Certification by a national organization recognized by the board
- Facility with English language

Citation: KY. REV. STAT. ANN. § 314.042.

LOUISIANA

To practice:

- RN license
- Master's degree in appropriate program

Citation: LA. ADMIN. CODE tit. 46 § XLVII.4507.

To prescribe:

- RN licensure
- APRN licensure
- Evidence of 500 hours of practice as a licensed ARNP within 6 months prior to applying for prescriptive authority
- 36 hours of education in pharmacotherapeutics
- 12 contact hours in physiology/pathophysiology
- Collaborative practice agreement
- Each year, six hours of continuing education in pharmacology or pharmacologic management

Citation: LA. ADMIN. CODE tit. 46 § XLVII.4513.

MAINE

- Transcript from NP program
- Evidence of current certification
- Evidence of a minimum of 1500 hours of practice in the expanded role within five years or completion of NP program within five years
- Evidence of satisfactory completion of 45 contact hours of pharmacology
- As of January 1, 2006, a master's degree

Citation: CODE ME. R. § 02 380 008.

For prescriptive and dispensing authority:

If the applicant has not prescribed drugs within the past two years, the applicant shall provide evidence of satisfactory completion of 15 contact hours of pharmacology within the two years prior to applying for approval to practice.

If the applicant has not prescribed drugs within the past five years, the applicant shall provide evidence of satisfactory completion of 45 contact hours (or three credits) of pharmacology within the two years prior to applying for approval to practice.

For certified nurse practitioners with prescriptive authority in other US jurisdictions:

1. Minimum of 200 hours of practice in an expanded specialty role within the preceding two years.
2. 45 contact hours (or three credits) of pharmacology equivalent to the requirements set forth in Section 64(3)(A) and (B).

If the applicant has not prescribed drugs within the past two years, the applicant shall provide evidence of satisfactory completion of 15 contact hours of pharmacology within the two years prior to applying for approval to practice.

If the applicant has not prescribed drugs within the past five years, the applicant shall provide evidence of satisfactory completion of 45 contact hours (or three credits) of pharmacology within the two years prior to applying for approval to practice.

Citation: CODE ME. R. § 02 380 008.

MARYLAND

- RN license
- Completion of a program for preparation of NPs approved by the board
- Passing of an examination as designated by the board

Citation: MD. REGS. CODE tit. 10 § 27.07.03.

MASSACHUSETTS

- RN license
- Advanced nursing knowledge and clinical skills acquired through an appropriate educational program
- Current certification in practice area

Citation: MASS. ANN. LAWS CH. 112 § 80B and CODE MASS. REGS tit. 244, § § 4.05 and 4.13(2).

MICHIGAN

- RN license
- Completion of formal advanced program for NPs
- Submission of an application for certification in a specialty area of nursing
- Meets standards of advanced practice certification agencies [5 agencies listed]

Citation: Mich. ADMIN. CODE R338.10404.

MINNESOTA

- RN license
- Graduation from NP program

- Certification as NP by national certifying agency
- To prescribe, a written agreement with a physician

Citation: MINN. STAT. ANN. §§ 148.235 and 148.284.

MISSISSIPPI

- RN license
- BS in nursing
- Applicants who graduated from a nurse practitioner program after December 31, 1998 are required to submit official evidence of graduation from a graduate program with a concentration in the applicant's respective advanced practice nursing specialty
- Graduation from a NP program and clinical experience that occurred following the bachelor's degree or as part of a master's degree program
- Certification by a national organization recognized by the board

Citation: MISS. Nursing REGS. CH. IV, § 2.

MISSOURI

- RN license
- Evidence of completion of advanced nursing education program
- Three graduate hours in pharmacology and evidence of 1500 hours of clinical practice in advanced practice, or
- Certification by a national organization

Citation: MO. CODE REGS. tit. 4, § 200-4.100.

MONTANA

- RN license
- National certification
- Completion of post-basic professional nursing program in APN area
- Master's degree or certificate from post-master's program

Citation: MONT. ADMIN. R. 8.32.305.

NEBRASKA

To practice:

- RN license
- Evidence of having successfully completed an approved advanced practice registered nurse program
- Evidence of having successfully completed 30 contact hours of education in pharmacotherapeutics

- Submission of proof of having passed an examination pertaining to the specific advanced practice registered nursing role in nursing adopted or approved by the boards

Citation: NEB. Rev. STAT. § 71-1722.

To prescribe:

- Master's or doctorate degree in nursing
- Completed an approved advanced practice registered nurse program
- Demonstration of separate course work in pharmacotherapeutics, advanced health assessment, and pathopsychology
- Completion of a minimum of 2000 hours of practice under the supervision of a physician

Citation: NEB Rev. STAT. § 71-1723.02

NEVADA

- Completion of a program for advanced practice, approved by the board
- Evidence of continuous practice (400 hours per year) in three of the five years immediately preceding application [exceptions omitted] or has maintained licensure in another state
- If completed an educational program after June 1, 2005, holds a master's degree in nursing or related field approved by the board

Citation: NEV. ADMIN CODE CH. 632, § 632.260.

NEW HAMPSHIRE

- Transcript of a nurse practitioner education program approved by the board, including 225 hours of theoretical nursing content and 480 hours of precepted practice
- 30 hours of continuing education in the past two years
- Documentation of competence
- National certification

Citation: N.H. CODE ADMIN. R. ANN. [NUR] 304.02.

NEW JERSEY

- Application with educational and experience data
- Proof of education–post-basic nursing certificate program accredited by or acceptable to the board
- Proof of current certification
- Graduation from master's program for NPs
- If five years have elapsed since completed graduate level pharmacology course, 30 continuing education units in pharmacology

- Passing of the highest level practice exam in the area of specialization approved by the board.

Citation: N.J. ADMIN. CODE tit. 13, § 37-7.1.

NEW MEXICO

- RN license
- Formal post-graduate program for the education and preparation of nurse practitioners; master's degree if applying after January 1, 2001 for initial licensure
- National certification

Citation: N.M. ADMIN. CODE § 16.12.2.13.A.

To prescribe:

- 400 hours of precepted work experience in past two years
- DEA registration
- Maintain a formulary

Citation: N.M. ADMIN. CODE § 16.12.2.13.P(5)(a).

NEW YORK

- Completion of an educational program approved by the Department of Education, or
- Certification as NP by a national certifying body, and
- Three semester hours in pharmacology

Citation: N.Y. COMP. Codes R. & REGS. tit. 8, § 64.4.

NORTH CAROLINA

To practice:

- RN license
- Successful completion of approved educational program
- Unrestricted license to practice as RN and unrestricted approval to practice as NP
- Submission of any information deemed necessary to evaluate the application
- A primary supervising physician agreement

To maintain license:

- 30 hours of continuing education every two years, including a course in medical and social effects of substance abuse

Citation: N.C. ADMIN. CODE tit. 21, § r36.0227.

NORTH DAKOTA

- RN license
- Appropriate education [completion of a graduate education program with nursing focus, with exceptions]
- Current certification by a national organization

Citation: N.D. CENT. CODE § 43-12.1-09 and N.D. ADMIN. CODE § 54-05-03.1-04.

To prescribe:

- A scope of practice statement [see N.D. ADMIN. CODE § 54-05-03.1-09(5)]
- Evidence of completion of 30 hours of education in pharmacotherapy
- An affidavit from a physician who will be participating in the collaborative prescriptive agreement. . . .

Citation: N.D. ADMIN. CODE § 54-05-03.1-09.

OHIO

For a certificate of authority:

- RN license
- Graduate degree in nursing specialty . . .
- Certification . . .
- Collaborating physician or podiatrist. . . .

Citation: OHIO REV. CODE ANN. § 4723.41.

OKLAHOMA

- Successful completion of a formal program of study approved by the Board
- Certification from program recognized by board of nursing
- Certificate of recognition from the Board

Citation: OKLA. STAT. ANN. tit. 59 § 567.3a(5).

For prescriptive authority:

- Submit a statement from a physician supervising prescriptive
- Submit documentation verifying completion of 45 contact hours in pharmeotherapeutics
- Master's degree in a clinical nurse speciality

Citation: OKLA. ADMIN. CODE § 485: 10-16-3.

OREGON

To practice:

- RN license
- Master's degree in nursing
- Satisfactory completion of an NP program specific to the expanded specialty/category for which application is made

Citation: OR. ADMIN. § R. 851-050-0002.

To prescribe:

- NP certificate in Oregon
- Completion of 30 hours of pharmacology instruction

Citation: OR. ADMIN. § R. 851-050-0120.

To renew certification:

- RN license
- 100 clock hours of continuing education obtained through independent learning activities, unstructured learning activities, and structured learning activities
- Minimum of 960 hours of practice in an expanded specialty role within the five-year period immediately preceding renewal or graduation from a nurse practitioner program within five years of renewal or completion of 400 hours of supervised practice in the two years preceding renewal

Citation: OR. ADMIN. § R. 851-050-0138.

PENNSYLVANIA

- RN license
- Master's degree and certification by a national certification organization
- Evidence of continuing competency in the area of medical diagnosis and therapeutics at the time of renewal of the applicant's certification
- 30 hours of continuing education per year

To prescribe:

- 45 hours of advanced pharmacology

Citation: 49 PA. CODE § 21.271 and ACT 206 OF 2002, § 8.3.

RHODE ISLAND

- RN license
- Completion of an accredited educational program resulting in a master's degree and/or an approved nurse practitioner course of study
- Passing of a national certifying examination recognized by the board

Citation: R.I. GEN. LAWS § 5-34-35.

To prescribe:

- Completion of 30 hours of education in pharmacology within three years prior to application

To maintain prescriptive privileges:

- Completion of 30 hours of CE in pharmacology every six years

Citation: R.I. GEN. LAWS § 5-34-39.

SOUTH CAROLINA

- RN license
- Certification by a national organization acceptable to the Board
- Master's degree in nursing

To prescribe:

- 45 contact hours of education in pharmacotherapeutics

Citation: 26 S.C. CODE ANN. § 91-6.

SOUTH DAKOTA

- RN license
- Completion of an approved program for the preparation of NPs
- Passing of any examination that the boards in their discretion may require
- Submission of a copy of proposed practice agreement and the practice agreement is approved by the boards

Citation: S.D. CODIFIED LAWS § 36-9A-4.

TENNESSEE

- RN license
- Graduation from a program conferring a master's or doctorate in nursing

- Preparation in specialized practitioner skills as the master's, post-master's, doctorate, or postdoctorate level
- Skills education shall include at least three quarter hours of pharmacology instruction
- Current national certification in the appropriate nursing specialty area

Citation: TENN. COMP. R. & REGS. tit. 11, CH. 1000-4-.03.

TEXAS

- Licensed as registered nurse and nurse practitioner in Texas
- Evidence of educational preparation
- Minimum 400 hours of current practice within preceding biennium unless graduated from appropriate program within the preceding biennium
- 20 contact hours of continuing education every two years

Citation: 21 TEXAS ADMIN. CODE § 221.4.

UTAH

- Physical and mental health that will allow the applicant to practice safely as an advanced practice registered nurse
- Current registered nurse license
- Graduate degree in nursing or a related area of specialized knowledge
- Successful completion of course work in patient assessment, diagnosis and treatment, and pharmacotherapeutics from an education program approved by the division in collaboration with the board
- Passing of examinations as required by division rule made in collaboration with the board
- Certification by a program approved by the division in collaboration with the board

Citation: UTAH CODE ANN. § 58-31b-302(3).

VERMONT

- RN license
- Completion of formal educational program approved by Board of Nursing
- Certification by national organization recognized by Board of Nursing

Citation: VT. CODE R. CH. 4, RULE VIII.B.

VIRGINIA

- RN license
- Completion of educational program designed to prepare nurse practitioners, approved by the board
- Evidence of professional certification by an agency accepted by the board

Citation: 18 VA. ADMIN. CODE 90-30-80A.

For prescriptive authority:

- Current license as a nurse practitioner
- Evidence of certification as a nurse practitioner
- Completion of a graduate level course in pharmacology as part of NP program within 5 years prior to submission of the application
- Practice as NP for no less than 1000 hours and 15 continuing education units related to the area of practice for each of the two years prior to submission of the application or 30 hours of education in pharmacology acceptable to the boards taken within 5 years prior to submission of the application
- Submit a practice agreement between NP and supervising physician
- Board approves practice agreement

Citation: 18 VA. ADMIN. CODE 90-40-40.

WASHINGTON

- RN license
- Completion of a formal advanced nursing education, meeting the requirements of Washington Administrative CODE 246-839-305
- Documentation of initial certification credential granted by a national certifying body recognized by the commission, approved ARNP specialty whose certification program is approved by the commission and subsequently maintain currency and competency as defined by the certifying body
- Accountability for practice based on and limited to the scope of his/her education, demonstrated competence, and advanced nursing experience
- Documentation of any additional formal education, skills training, or supervised clinical practice beyond the basic ARNP preparation . . . .

Citation: WASH. ADMIN. CODE § 246-839-300.

For prescriptive authority:

- RN license

- Advanced registered nurse practitioner license with authority for legend drugs and Schedule V drugs
- Joint practice arrangement that meets requirements of WAC 246-840-422 with a physician or physicians licensed under chapter 18.71 or 18.57 RCW who holds a license without restrictions related to prescribing scheduled drugs
- Submission of an application form for Schedule II-IV endorsement

Citation: WASH. ADMIN. CODE § 246-840-421.

WEST VIRGINIA

- RN license
- Current national certification in area recognized by West Virginia Board of Examiners for Registered Professional Nurses
- After December 31, 1998, a master's degree in nursing

Citation: W. VA. CODE ST. R. § 19-7-3.

For prescriptive authority

- Licensed as advanced nurse practitioner in West Virginia
- Baccalaureate degree
- Successful completion of 45 contact hours of education in pharmacology and clinical management of drug therapy under a program approved by the board, 15 hours of which shall be completed within the two-year period immediately before the date of application
- Evidence of good moral character and not addicted to alcohol or the use of controlled substances

Citation: W. VA. CODE ST. R. § 30-7-15b.

WISCONSIN

- RN license
- Certification by a national certifying body approved by the board as a nurse practitioner
- For applicants who receive certification after July 1, 1998, a master's degree in nursing or a related health field granted by a college or university accredited by a regional accrediting agency approved by the board of education in the state in which the college or university is located

Citation: WISC. ADMIN. CODE § N 8.02(1)(c).

WYOMING

- Post-graduate education and additional nursing preparation that provides for the knowledge, judgment, and skill beyond that required of a registered professional nurse

- Completion of a nationally accredited educational program for preparation as an advanced practitioner of nursing or national certification by a nationally recognized accrediting agency accepted by the board

Citation: Wyo. Stat. Ann. § 33-21-120(a)(1).

- RN license
- Completion of a nationally accredited educational program for advanced practitioners of nursing with a specific curriculum appropriate to the proposed specialty area of practice, accepted by the board
- Certification in a specific specialty area of advanced practice, accepted by the board, or master's degree in nursing, with specific curriculum preparation at the advanced practice/clinical specialist level, accepted by the board
- Submission of a written plan of practice and collaboration

Citation: Wyo. Board of Nursing Rules, ch. 4, § 3(a).

For prescriptive authority:

- Recognition as an advanced practitioner of nursing in Wyoming
- Documentation of completion of a minimum of two semester credit hours, three quarter credit hours, or 30 contact hours of course work approved by the board in pharmacology and clinical managment of drug therapy or pharmacotherapeutics within the five year period immediately before the date of application
- Documentation of completion of 400 hours of advanced nursing practice in recognized areas of specialty within the two year period immediately before the date of application
- Compliance with the standards of nursing practice, the rules and regulations, and the Act
- A written plan of practice and collaboration

Citation: Wyo. Board of Nursing Rules, ch. 4 § 8.c.

CHAPTER 4

Federal Regulation of the Nurse Practitioner Profession

The federal government regulates NP practice through statutes enacted by Congress, regulations written by federal agencies, and policies and guidelines written by federal agencies. Federal law may preempt state law, and when federal and state law conflict, the state law will not have effect. Where no federal law addresses an issue, or where Congress has expressly given the responsibility to the states to make law on an issue, state law controls.

Federal law addresses:

- Care of patients covered by Medicare
- Care of patients covered by Medicaid
- Care of hospitalized patients insofar as participation by hospitals in the Medicare program is contingent on a hospital's following certain regulations
- Care of residents of nursing homes
- In-office and hospital laboratories, under the Clinical Laboratories Improvement Act (CLIA)
- Self-referral by health care providers, under the Stark Acts
- Prescription of controlled substances, under the Drug Enforcement Administration (DEA)
- Reporting of successful malpractice lawsuits against NPs to the National Practitioner Data Bank (NPDB)
- Confidentiality of information about patients
- Discrimination in hiring and firing
- Facility access for disabled people

Federal law affects NPs by what it says and by what it does not say.

MEDICARE

Because much of the funding for hospitals and much of the reimbursement for office practice comes from Medicare, federal statutes and regulations and policies from the Center for Medicare and Medicaid Services (CMS), formerly the Health Care Financing Administration (HCFA), have great impact on the interest of hospitals and medical practices in having NP providers. For example, the Social Security Act, which governs Medicare and Medicaid, was written in 1965, before there were NPs. The act frequently uses the word *physician* as if there were no other health care provider. Other health care providers have had to get acts of Congress to be included in the laws governing Medicare. The act has been amended many times since the 1960s, but some relevant portions of the act remain that give permission to physicians and only physicians to provide care. Without specific legal authority in the Social Security Act for NPs to direct the care of patients covered by Medicare, CMS will not include NPs in its regulations. Without inclusion in law or regulations, NPs risk Medicare fraud if they take care of Medicare patients.

NPs made progress in 1997 when an act of Congress authorized NPs to be reimbursed directly for the care of Medicare patients. However, the Social Security Act still states that a physician must direct the care of hospitalized patients. In late 1997, HCFA proposed new regulations for hospital participation in Medicare (62 Fed. Reg. 66726-66763). The regulations state that every Medicare patient must be under the care of a physician, dentist, podiatrist, optometrist, chiropractor, or psychologist. The regulation is based on a section of the Social Security Act that states:

> "Hospital" means an institution which has a requirement that every patient with respect to whom payment may be made under this title must be under the care of a physician, except that a patient receiving qualified psychologist services . . . may be under the care of a clinical psychologist with respect to such services to the extent permitted under state law.
>
> *Citation:* 42 U.S.C.S. § 1395x(e)(4).

The regulation states that physicians, dentists, podiatrists, optometrists, chiropractors, or psychologists may delegate tasks to other qualified health care personnel to the extent recognized under state law or a state's regulatory mechanism [62 Fed. Reg. 42 C.F.R. § 482.20(a)(1)(i)]. Because the proposed regulation does not use the term *nurse practitioner,* it is not clear that the regulation contemplates NPs practicing in hospitals. However, it certainly is arguable that NPs are "other qualified health care personnel." Hospitals wishing to serve patients covered by Medicare will want NPs to give care only under delegation from a physician. This may be a limitation for NPs in states where physician collaboration is not required.

NPs may want to lobby Congress for statutory language that specifically authorizes NP participation in the care of Medicare patients in hospitals, at home, in nursing homes, or in offices. Being relegated to the "other qualified personnel" bin is suboptimal for the NP profession. Other providers, most recently psychologists, have successfully lobbied for greater inclusion in the Social Security Act.

With the passage of the Budget Reconciliation Bill of 1997, NPs were authorized to receive direct reimbursement for services to Medicare patients, regardless of the setting or location of the services.

Medicare Reimbursement

In 1997, direct reimbursement to NPs, regardless of geographic area of practice, was authorized by Congress. However, the specific procedures by which NPs are reimbursed are still being discussed as questions arise and answers are developed. For example, the Budget Reconciliation Act of 1997 (1) removed the provision of the prior law that restricted reimbursement of NPs to those practicing in rural areas and (2) set the amount paid to 80 percent of either the lesser of the actual charge or 85 percent of the fee schedule amount provided under section 1848. NPs who work for medical practices and who can fulfill the requirements of "incident to" relationships with physicians can submit their work under a physician's provider number and will receive full fee (not 85 percent of the physician fee). In general, however, NPs' work should be billed under the NP's provider number. Practitioners who are in doubt should seek an opinion from their Medicare payer or from an appropriate attorney.

What Is an "Incident to" Relationship?

The full term is *incident to a physician's professional service. Incident to* is a Medicare phrase meaning services furnished as an "integral, although incidental, part of the physician's personal professional services in the course of diagnosis or treatment of an injury or illness."[1] To qualify under this definition, the services of nonphysicians must be rendered under a physician's "direct personal supervision." Nonphysicians must be employees of a physician or physician group, leased employees, or have an independent contractor relationship with a physician or physician group. Services must be furnished during a course of treatment where a physician performs an initial service and subsequent services of a frequency that reflects the physician's active participation in and management of a course of treatment. Direct personal supervision in the office setting does not mean that a physician must be in the same room.

However, to bill an incident to a physician's service, the physician must be in the same suite as the nurse practitioner at the time the nurse practitioner is performing the service to be billed under the physician's provider number.

The 1997 law change that gave NPs direct Medicare reimbursement, while remaining the most significant national-level advance in years for NPs, changed the language in only a few of the ways needed if NPs are to practice without barriers.

Federal Definition of Collaboration

For example, in federal law the term *collaboration* means:

> A process in which a nurse practitioner works with a physician to deliver health care services within the scope of the practitioner's professional expertise, with medical direction and appropriate supervision as provided for in jointly developed guidelines or other mechanism as defined by the law of the State in which the services are performed.
>
> *Citation:* 42 U.S.C.S. § 1395x(aa)(6).

The emergence of an NP as a primary provider rather than a supervised helper is not reflected in the Social Security Act. In the act, an NP is someone to whom a physician may delegate certain tasks. Although state law either does not require collaboration or calls for "collaboration" and defines collaboration without using the term *supervision*, federal law requires, through its definition of collaboration, "supervision."

The enactment of the Budget Reconciliation Bill of 1997, which gave direct reimbursement to NPs for Medicare patients, does not change the law quoted above. That will take another act of Congress.

Medicare Fraud

CMS makes the rules that most affect NPs who care for Medicare patients. The US Justice Department enforces the rules. NPs who do not follow CMS's rules can expect to do poorly on audits and can possibly be charged with Medicare fraud and/or abuse.

In the past few years, CMS has reevaluated Medicare's payment system, upgrading the reimbursement for some evaluation and management functions and downgrading the reimbursement for other functions. At the same time, CMS has clarified how providers, hospitals, and medical groups should bill, based on the services provided. Of particular interest to NPs are the guidelines jointly developed by CMS and the American Medical Association for coding office visits. (See the Appendices to this chapter.)

NPs can expect that their Medicare billing choices will be audited and that they will be expected to know the rules for choosing appropriate evaluation and management codes that correlate with the type of visit performed and the documentation recorded. NPs also can expect that the rules for Medicare will soon be the rules for billing in general.

For the guidelines for coding office visits covered by Medicare, see Appendix 4-A. For more information on Medicare reimbursement in general, see Chapter 9. For more information on how to avoid Medicare fraud and abuse, see Chapter 8. For information on specific questions regarding Medicare billing, consult the *Medicare Carriers Manual,* which can be downloaded from the CMS Web site (http://www.cms.gov) or obtained from a local Medicare carrier, or call the

Medicare carrier in the geographic area of practice. Medicare carriers are companies that have contracts with CMS to administer Medicare payments to providers.

MEDICAID

The federal government has given most of the rule-making and administrative duties for Medicaid to the individual states, and, in most situations, state law controls Medicaid activities. However, the states must follow the Federal Code, 42 U.S.C.A. § 1396, in such matters as ensuring access to care and offering a choice of provider. Federal law provides that Medicaid will cover the services of pediatric NPs and family NPs, whether or not the NP is employed by or supervised by a physician [42 U.S.C.S. § 1396d(a)(xi)(21)].

The states also must follow CMS rules and regulations regarding administration of Medicaid. For example, states wishing to enroll all Medicaid recipients in managed care have had to apply to CMS for waivers that specify how the managed-care programs will be handled. It has been important for NPs in states that have applied for waivers to ensure that NPs are permitted to be "primary care providers." If NPs are not included as providers in the language of state waivers approved by CMS, they are in the position of being able to care for Medicaid patients covered by traditional Medicaid but not to care for patients in managed care. If all patients are in managed care, NPs who can care only for patients covered by traditional, fee-for-service Medicaid will find that there are no such patients.

NPs must apply to their state agency administering Medicaid for Medicaid provider numbers. For more information on billing Medicaid, see Chapter 9. For specific questions on Medicaid issues, contact the state Medicaid agency.

NURSING HOMES

Under federal law addressing patients covered by Medicare, the care of residents of a skilled nursing facility must be under the supervision of a physician [42 U.S.C.S. § 1395i-3(b)(6)(A)]. The law states, "Skilled nursing facilities must require that the medical care of every resident be provided under the supervision of a physician" [42 U.S.C.S. § 1395i-3(b)(6)(A)] and "provide for having a physician available to furnish necessary medical care in case of emergency" [42 U.S.C.S. § 1395i-3(b)(6)(B)]. Physicians may delegate tasks to other qualified health care providers (42 C.F.R. 483).

Under federal law addressing patients covered by Medicaid, the care of nursing home residents may be provided under the supervision of an NP. Medicaid law states:

> A nursing facility must require that the health care of every resident be provided under the supervision of a physician, or, at the option of a state, under the supervision of a nurse practitioner, clinical nurse

specialist, or physician assistant who is not an employee of the facility but who is working in collaboration with a physician.

Citation: 42 U.S.C.S. § 1396r(b)(6)(A).

Even if the care is supervised by an NP or a PA, a nursing facility must have a physician "available to furnish necessary medical care in case of emergency" [42 U.S.C.S. § 1396r(b)(6)(B)].

IN-OFFICE AND HOSPITAL LABORATORIES UNDER CLIA

Office laboratories, no matter how small or limited in scope, are subject to federal oversight under CLIA. State health departments often require office laboratories to meet certain requirements as well. Office laboratories are subject to state and federal inspection and approval. In offices where laboratory tests are limited to fecal occult blood (hemocult), urine pregnancy test, blood glucose, urinalysis (urine dip), and office microscopy, practices may obtain exemption from inspection. Nevertheless, offices must apply to CLIA for a letter of exemption.

SELF-REFERRAL BY HEALTH CARE PROVIDERS, UNDER THE STARK ACTS

CMS has released proposed rules regarding "Physicians' Referrals to Health Care Entities With Which They Have Financial Relationships" [63 Fed. Reg. 1659 (1998)]. These rules relate to the Ethics in Patient Referral Act of 1989 (42 U.S.C. § 1395nn), which was amended by the Omnibus Budget and Reconciliation Act of 1993 and incorporated into the Social Security Act [Social Security Act, 42 U.S.C.A. §§ 1877 & 1903(s)]. The acts are commonly referred to as the "Stark Acts."

Under the Stark Acts, a physician cannot refer a patient covered by Medicare to a clinical laboratory where the physician or an immediate family member of the physician has a financial relationship. Nor may a physician refer a patient to certain designated health services when the physician has a financial relationship with the facility offering the services. The designated health services include: (1) physical therapy services; (2) occupational therapy services; (3) radiation therapy services; (4) radiology services; (5) durable medical equipment and supplies; (6) parenteral and enteral nutrients; (7) prosthetics, orthotics, and prosthetic devices; (8) home health services; (9) outpatient prescription drugs; and (10) inpatient and outpatient hospital services. The Stark laws are aimed at physicians who own an interest in, for example, medical equipment companies or laboratories and are in a position to profit when the physician refers patients for additional services.

For the purposes of the Stark Acts, *referral* is defined broadly. A physician may make a referral simply by including a service in the plan of care.

The Stark Acts have wide-ranging application. It is still unclear, however, just how Stark applies to many situations.

CMS rules allow for certain exceptions from the self-referral prohibitions. For example, there is an exception for ownership and compensation for physicians' services "provided personally by or under the personal supervision of another physician in the same group practice . . . as the referring physician" [Social Security Act, 42 U.S.C.A. § 1877(b)(1)]. In other words, a physician may refer a patient to another physician in the same group practice without violating the self-referral law.

How Might Stark Affect NPs?

The Stark Acts are not aimed at nurse practitioners, but at physicians. However, if a physician requires a nurse practitioner employee to refer to an entity with which the physician employer has a financial relationship, then a nurse practitioner may become involved in an activity which violates the Stark Acts. If the referrals were found to be a violation of the Stark Act, the referrals would be imputed to the physician employing the nurse practitioner, rather than the nurse practitioner. On the other hand, if a nurse practitioner employee is free to refer to the entity of his or her choice, and the nurse practitioner independently chooses to refer to an entity in which his or her employer has a financial relationship, it is not clear that a Stark violation has taken place. The Office of the Inspector General has said that in such a case it would evaluate the specific facts of the situation.

Include attention to Stark and anti-kickback laws in a compliance program

Practices' compliance programs should focus on:

- Potential violations of Stark laws regarding self-referral
- Potential violations of anti-kickback laws
- Billing for services that are not medically necessary
- Billing twice for the same service
- Billing at a higher level code than justified by documentation or performance
- Noncompliance with the "incident to" rule

Availability of advisory opinions

Nurse practitioners and other health care providers wanting to start businesses that might lead to questions regarding the issues described above should consult an attorney.

Anti-kickback Statutes

Under Federal law, there are criminal penalties for individuals or entities that knowingly and willfully offer, pay, solicit, or receive remuneration (i.e., anything of value, in cash or in kind) in order to induce the referral of business reimbursable by a Federal health care program. Violations of the anti-kickback statute also may result in civil money penalties. The statute has been in existence since 1977. It applies to all kinds of health care providers and suppliers.

The law was enacted because Congress believed that payments tied to referrals increase the likelihood of overutilization of items and services, increase the cost of health care programs, lead to inappropriate referrals, and make competition unfair.

Examples of kickbacks include:

- Waiving deductibles and copayments for Medicare patients
- Paying a nurse practitioner or physician a fee for referring a patient
- Accepting a fee for referring a patient

Implications for NPs

The Federal prohibition on kickbacks applies to nurse practitioners. For example, what if a nurse practitioner started a practice, asked a physician to be the collaborator, and promised to refer at least 50 patients per year to the physician as compensation for the services involved in being the collaborator? The promise to refer, combined with the actual referral of patients covered by Medicaid or Medicare, may be evidence of kickbacks in violation of Federal law.

PRESCRIPTION OF CONTROLLED SUBSTANCES UNDER THE DEA

The Drug Enforcement Administration (DEA) licenses health care providers who prescribe controlled dangerous substances. The DEA licenses NPs as "mid-level practitioners" (21 C.F.R. §§ 1301, 1304, & 1306.3). The DEA will assign an NP a DEA number if the NP has no felony on record, if the NP has a practice site, and if state law permits NPs to prescribe controlled substances. Controlled substances may be issued only by a practitioner who is authorized to prescribe controlled substances by the jurisdiction in which the practitioner is licensed to practice and either registered or exempted from registration.

REPORTING TO THE NATIONAL PRACTITIONER DATA BANK

Under federal law (42 C.F.R. § 60) malpractice insurers must report damage awards paid on behalf of physicians, dentists, NPs, and some other health care providers to the NPDB, a national repository of information on health care providers. For more about the NPDB, see Chapter 7.

PATIENT CONFIDENTIALITY

Federal law requires NPs and other health care providers to protect patient privacy and confidentiality. Specific federal laws protect the privacy of patients with substance abuse problems (42 U.S.C. § 290dd-2), patients with mental health problems (42 U.S.C. § 9501), and patients who are residents of nursing homes [42 U.S.C. § 1395e-3(C)(x)(A)(iv)].

Patient Privacy

Congress mandated the Department of Health and Human Services to promulgate rules governing privacy in health care under the Health Insurance Portability and Accountability Act (HIPAA) of 1996. Incidents which inspired Congress to pass the privacy protection requirements include:

- A health system in Michigan accidentally posted the medical records of thousands of patients on the Internet (1999 report).
- A businessman purchased at auction the medical records of patients at a family practice in South Carolina, and attempted to sell them back to the former patients (1991 report).
- Johnson & Johnson marketed a list of 5 million elderly women who had been treated for incontinence (1998 report).

Under the Final Rule, any individual, organization, or facility which meets the definition of "covered entity" must:

- Appoint a privacy officer.
- Assess the office, hospital, or facility for potential for breaches of patient privacy.
- Issue policies regarding handling of and protection of patient information
- Conduct training for staff about the policies.
- Monitor office or facility procedures for compliance with policies.
- Get patients to authorize, in writing, any release of their individually identifiable information for marketing purposes.
- Notify patients, in writing, of their rights under the rules, and make a good faith effort to get patients to sign an acknowledgment that they have received notice of their rights.

"Covered entities" include the following:

- Health plans
- Health care clearinghouses
- Health care providers who transmit any health information in electronic form in connection with a transaction

"Health care providers" include:

- Hospitals
- Skilled nursing facilities
- Comprehensive outpatient rehabilitation facilities
- Home health agencies
- Hospice programs
- Nurse practitioners
- Certified nurse midwives
- Clinical nurse specialists
- Psychologists

- Clinical social workers
- Certified registered nurse anesthetists
- Physicians and physician assistants
- "And any other person or organization who furnishes, bills, or is paid for health care in the normal course of business."

An individual health care provider—a nurse practitioner, for example—need not personally transmit health information in electronic form for the rules to apply. If information is transmitted on the provider's behalf or by the provider's agency, the rules apply. The rules also apply to "business associates" of health care providers.

Basic requirements of the privacy rule are as follows:

- Providers and their staff are restricted to conveying the "minimum necessary information" about patients. "Minimum necessary" must be defined by organizational policy. Providers must establish policies that a) identify the persons or classes of persons in the workforce who need access to protected patient information to do their jobs, b) specify the information these workers may access, and c) specify how information is protected from inspection by unauthorized individuals.
- If a provider wants to release patient information for marketing purposes, the provider must first explain to the patient how the information will be used, to whom it will be disclosed, and the time frame. The patient needs to authorize use of the information, in writing. If the provider will be paid for releasing the patient's information, the provider must inform the patient of that fact.
- Providers may disclose health information to oversight agencies, such as the Center for Medicare and Medicaid Services (CMS) without patient authorization. No authorization is required for victims of abuse, neglect, or domestic violence when state law mandates that the provider report abuse. No separate authorization is required when information is used for public health purposes, or for organ and tissue donation. No authorization is required under certain circumstances involving law enforcement.
- There are special rules for psychotherapy notes. In general, patient authorization is required in order to disclose psychotherapy notes to carry out treatment, payment, or health care operations. Patients may authorize disclosure of their entire record. Such authorizations must include the name or class of the persons authorized to disclose and an expiration date or event.
- Providers must notify patients about how personal medical information may be used and disclosed, and how individuals may access their own information. Individuals have no right to three types of information about themselves: psychotherapy notes, information compiled in anticipation of civil or criminal litigation, and certain clinical laboratory information covered by the Clinical Laboratory Improvement Amendments.
- Providers must accommodate reasonable requests from patients who want to restrict use of their information.

For more information on the new rules, visit http:/www.aspe.dhhs.gov/admnsimp. A loose-leaf packet of policies, training, and forms appropriate for office practice is available for purchase from the Law Office of Carolyn Buppert, www.buppert.com.

DISCRIMINATION IN HIRING AND FIRING

Federal law prohibits discrimination based on race, color, sex, national origin, age, and disability. Title VII of the Civil Rights Act of 1964, which prohibits discrimination based on race, color, or national origin, applies to government employers and private employers with more than 15 employees. The Age Discrimination Act of 1967 prohibits discrimination based on age above 40 and applies to employers with more than 20 employees. The Equal Pay Act of 1963 prohibits wage discrimination between men and women and applies to most employers.

PEOPLE WITH DISABILITIES UNDER THE ADA

Title I of the Americans with Disabilities Act of 1990 prohibits private employers from discriminating against qualified individuals in hiring, firing, advancement, compensation, job training, and conditions of employment. A disabled person is one who has a physical or mental impairment that substantially limits one or more major life activities. The act applies to employers with more than 15 employees.

NOTE

1. *Medicare Carriers Manual,* Section 2050.3, 1997. Available from the Center for Medicare and Medicaid Services Web site: http://www.cms.gov. Accessed July 2003.

APPENDIX 4-A

Documentation Guidelines for Evaluation and Management Services

This is an update of the guidelines jointly produced by the American Medical Association (AMA) and the Health Care Financing Administration (HCFA) in May 1997. It appears on the CMS Web site at www.cms.gov. It incorporates revisions to the gastrointestinal section of the general multisystem exam and the skin section of the single-organ system exam of the skin. These revisions were approved by the AMA and CMS in November 1997. This is not the final version of the guidelines. This version of the guidelines will be reviewed and may be amended before Medicare carriers begin to use it in compliance activities. Nurse practitioners should check the CMS Web site periodically to determine whether revisions have been published.

FOREWORD

These guidelines were developed jointly by the American Medical Association (AMA) and the Health Care Financing Administration (HCFA) now known as the Center for Medicare and Medicaid Services (CMS). The stated goal was to provide physicians and claims reviewers with advice about preparing or reviewing documentation for Evaluation and Management services. In developing and testing the validity of these guidelines, special emphasis was placed on assuring that they:

- Are consistent with the clinical descriptors and definitions contained in CPT;
- Would be widely accepted by clinicians and minimize any changes in record-keeping practices; and
- Would be interpreted and applied uniformly by users across the country.

This edition contains a substantial amount of new material and a number of significant revisions in material that appeared in the first edition. Because of the extensive changes, the section on examination should be read in its entirety. In this edition:

Note: This is the most recent version of the guidelines, as of July 2003.

- The content of general multi-system examinations has been defined with greater clinical specificity.
- Documentation requirements for general multi-system examinations have been changed.
- For the first time, content and documentation requirements have been defined for examinations pertaining to ten organ systems. The content of these examinations was developed with the assistance of representatives from the specialties that frequently perform these examinations.
- Several editorial changes have been made in the definitions of the four types of examinations. This text also appears in CPT itself in the section headed "Evaluation and Management (E/M) Services Guidelines.
- The definition of an extended history of present illness has been expanded to include information about chronic or inactive conditions.

Documentation Guidelines for Evaluation and Management Services

I. INTRODUCTION

What Is Documentation and Why Is It Important?

Medical record documentation is required to record pertinent facts, findings, and observations about an individual's health history including past and present illnesses, examinations, tests, treatments, and outcomes. The medical record chronologically documents the care of the patient and is an important element contributing to high quality care. The medical record facilitates:

- The ability of the physician and other health care professionals to evaluate and plan the patient's immediate treatment, and to monitor his/her health care over time;
- Communication and continuity of care among physicians and other health care professionals involved in the patient's care;
- Accurate and timely claims review and payment;
- Appropriate utilization review and quality of care evaluations; and
- Collection of data that may be useful for research and education.

An appropriately documented medical record can reduce many of the "hassles" associated with claims processing and may serve as a legal document to verify the care provided, if necessary.

What Do Payers Want and Why?

Because payers have a contractual obligation to enrollees, they may require reasonable documentation that services are consistent with the insurance coverage provided. They may request information to validate:

- The site of service;
- The medical necessity and appropriateness of the diagnostic and/or therapeutic services provided; and/or
- That services provided have been accurately reported.

II. GENERAL PRINCIPLES OF MEDICAL RECORD DOCUMENTATION

The principles of documentation listed below are applicable to all types of medical and surgical services in all settings. For Evaluation and Management (E/M) services, the nature and amount of physician work and documentation varies by type of service, place of service, and the patient's status. The general principles listed below may be modified to account for these variable circumstances in providing E/M services.

1. The medical record should be complete and legible.
2. The documentation of each patient encounter should include:
   - Reason for the encounter and relevant history, physical examination findings and prior diagnostic test results;
   - Assessment, clinical impression, or diagnosis;
   - Plan for care; and
   - Date and legible identity of the observer.
3. If not documented, the rationale for ordering diagnostic and other ancillary services should be easily inferred.
4. Past and present diagnoses should be accessible to the treating and/or consulting physician.
5. Appropriate health risk factors should be identified.
6. The patient's progress, response to and changes in treatment, and revision of diagnosis should be documented.
7. The CPT and ICD-9-CM codes reported on the health insurance claim form or billing statement should be supported by the documentation in the medical record.

III. DOCUMENTATION OF E/M SERVICES

This publication provides definitions and documentation guidelines for the three key components of E/M services and for visits that consist predominately of counseling or coordination of care. The three *key* components—history, examination, and medical decision making—appear in the descriptors for office and other outpatient services, hospital observation services, hospital inpatient services, consultations, emergency department services, nursing facility services, domiciliary care services, and home services. While some of the text of CPT has been repeated in this publication, the reader should refer to CPT for the complete descriptors for E/M services and instructions for selecting a level of service. Documentation guidelines are identified by the symbol ***•DG.***

The descriptors for the levels of E/M services recognize seven components that are used in defining the levels of E/M services. These components are:

- History;
- Examination;

- Medical decision making;
- Counseling;
- Coordination of care;
- Nature of presenting problem; and
- Time.

The first three of these components (i.e., history, examination, and medical decision making) are the key components in selecting the level of E/M services. In the case of visits that consist *predominantly* of counseling or coordination of care, time is the key or controlling factor to qualify for a particular level of E/M service.

Because the level of E/M service is dependent on two or three key components, performance and documentation of one component (e.g., examination) at the highest level does not necessarily mean that the encounter in its entirety qualifies for the highest level of E/M service.

These Documentation Guidelines for E/M services reflect the needs of the typical adult population. For certain groups of patients, the recorded information may vary slightly from that described here. Specifically, the medical records of infants, children, adolescents, and pregnant women may have additional or modified information recorded in each history and examination area.

As an example, newborn records may include under history of the present illness (HPI) the details of mother's pregnancy and the infant's status at birth; social history will focus on family structure; family history will focus on congenital anomalies and hereditary disorders in the family. In addition, the content of a pediatric examination will vary with the age and development of the child. Although not specifically defined in these documentation guidelines, these patient group variations on history and examination are appropriate.

Documentation of History

The levels of E/M services are based on four types of history (Problem Focused, Expanded Problem Focused, Detailed, and Comprehensive). Each type of history includes some or all of the following elements:

- Chief complaint (CC);
- History of present illness (HPI);
- Review of systems (ROS); and
- Past, family, and/or social history (PFSH).

The extent of history of present illness, review of systems and past, family, and/or social history that is obtained and documented is dependent upon clinical judgment and the nature of the presenting problem(s). The chart below shows the progression of the elements required for each type of history. To qualify for a given type of history all three elements in the table must be met. (A chief complaint is indicated at all levels.)

History of Present Illness (HPI)	*Review of Systems (ROS)*	*Past, Family, and/or Social History (PFSH)*	*Type of History*
Brief	N/A	N/A	Problem Focused
Brief	Problem Pertinent	N/A	Expanded Problem Focused
Extended	Extended	Pertinent	Detailed
Extended	Complete	Complete	Comprehensive

- ***DG:*** *The CC, ROS, and PFSH may be listed as separate elements of history, or they may be included in the description of the history of the present illness.*
- ***DG:*** *An ROS and/or a PFSH obtained during an earlier encounter does not need to be rerecorded if there is evidence that the physician reviewed and updated the previous information. This may occur when a physician updates his or her own record or in an institutional setting or group practice where many physicians use a common record. The review and update may be documented by:*
  - *Describing any new ROS and/or PFSH information or noting there has been no change in the information; and*
  - *Noting the date and location of the earlier ROS and/or PFSH.*
- ***DG:*** *The ROS and/or PFSH may be recorded by ancillary staff or on a form completed by the patient. To document that the physician reviewed the information, there must be a notation supplementing or confirming the information recorded by others.*
- ***DG:*** *If the physician is unable to obtain a history from the patient or other source, the record should describe the patient's condition or other circumstance which precludes obtaining a history.*

Definitions and specific documentation guidelines for each of the elements of history are listed below.

Chief Complaint (CC)

The CC is a concise statement describing the symptom, problem, condition, diagnosis, physician recommended return, or other factor that is the reason for the encounter, usually stated in the patient's words.

- ***DG:*** *The medical record should clearly reflect the chief complaint.*

History of Present Illness (HPI)

The HPI is a chronological description of the development of the patient's present illness from the first sign and/or symptom or from the previous encounter to the present. It includes the following elements:

- Location,
- Quality,
- Severity,
- Duration,
- Timing,
- Context,
- Modifying factors, and
- Associated signs and symptoms.

Brief and *extended* HPIs are distinguished by the amount of detail needed to accurately characterize the clinical problem(s).

A *brief* HPI consists of one to three elements of the HPI.

•***DG:*** *The medical record should describe one to three elements of the present illness (HPI).*

An *extended* HPI consists of at least four elements of the HPI or the status of at least three chronic or inactive conditions.

•***DG:*** *The medical record should describe at least four elements of the present illness (HPI), or the status of at least three chronic or inactive conditions.*

Review of Systems (ROS)

An ROS is an inventory of body systems obtained through a series of questions seeking to identify signs and/or symptoms that the patient may be experiencing or has experienced.

For purposes of ROS, the following systems are recognized:

- Constitutional symptoms (e.g., fever, weight loss)
- Eyes
- Ears, nose, mouth, throat
- Cardiovascular
- Respiratory
- Gastrointestinal
- Genitourinary
- Musculoskeletal
- Integumentary (skin and/or breast)
- Neurological
- Psychiatric
- Endocrine
- Hematologic/lymphatic
- Allergic/immunologic

A *problem pertinent* ROS inquires about the system directly related to the problem(s) identified in the HPI.

• ***DG:*** *The patient's positive responses and pertinent negatives for the system related to the problem should be documented.*

An *extended* ROS inquires about the system directly related to the problem(s) identified in the HPI and a limited number of additional systems.

• ***DG:*** *The patient's positive responses and pertinent negatives for two to nine systems should be documented.*

A *complete* ROS inquires about the system(s) directly related to the problem(s) identified in the HPI *plus* all additional body systems.

• ***DG:*** *At least ten organ systems must be reviewed. Those systems with positive or pertinent negative responses must be individually documented. For the remaining systems, a notation indicating all other systems are negative is permissible. In the absence of such a notation, at least ten systems must be individually documented.*

Past, Family, and/or Social History (PFSH)

The PFSH consists of a review of three areas:

- Past history (the patient's past experiences with illnesses, operations, injuries, and treatments);
- Family history (a review of medical events in the patient's family, including diseases which may be hereditary or place the patient at risk); and
- Social history (an age appropriate review of past and current activities).

For certain categories of E/M services that include only an interval history, it is not necessary to record information about the PFSH. Those categories are subsequent hospital care, follow-up inpatient consultations and subsequent nursing facility care.

A *pertinent* PFSH is a review of the history area(s) directly related to the problem(s) identified in the HPI.

• ***DG:*** *At least one specific item from any of the three history areas must be documented for a pertinent PFSH.*

A *complete* PFSH is of a review of two or all three of the PFSH history areas, depending on the category of the E/M service. A review of all three history areas is required for services that by their nature include a comprehensive assessment or reassessment of the patient. A review of two of the three history areas is sufficient for other services.

• ***DG:*** *At least one specific item from two of the three history areas must be documented for a complete PFSH for the following categories of E/M services: office or other outpatient services, established patient; emergency department; domiciliary care, established patient; and home care, established patient.*

- ***DG:** At least one specific item from each of the three history areas must be documented for a complete PFSH for the following categories of E/M services: office or other outpatient services, new patient; hospital observation services; hospital inpatient services, initial care; consultations; comprehensive nursing facility assessments; domiciliary care, new patient; and home care, new patient.*

Documentation of Examination

The levels of E/M services are based on four types of examination:

- *Problem Focused*—a limited examination of the affected body area or organ system.
- *Expanded Problem Focused*—a limited examination of the affected body area or organ system and any other symptomatic or related body area(s) or organ system(s).
- *Detailed*—an extended examination of the affected body area(s) or organ system(s) and any other symptomatic or related body area(s) or organ system(s).
- *Comprehensive*—a general multi-system examination or complete examination of a single organ system and other symptomatic or related body area(s) or organ system(s).

These types of examinations have been defined for general multi-systems and the following single organ systems:

- Cardiovascular
- Ears, nose, mouth, and throat
- Eyes
- Genitourinary (female)
- Genitourinary (male)
- Hematologic/lymphatic/immunologic
- Musculoskeletal
- Neurological
- Psychiatric
- Respiratory
- Skin

A general multi-system examination or a single organ system examination may be performed by any physician regardless of specialty. The type (general multi-system or single organ system) and content of examination are selected by the examining physician and are based upon clinical judgment, the patient's history, and the nature of the presenting problem(s).

The content and documentation requirements for each type and level of examination are summarized below and described in detail in tables beginning below. In the tables, organ systems and body areas recognized by CPT for purposes of describing examinations are shown in the left column. The content, or individual elements, of the examination pertaining to that body area or organ system are identified by bullets (•) in the right column.

Parenthetical examples "(e.g., . . .)" have been used for clarification and to provide guidance regarding documentation. Documentation for each element must satisfy any numeric requirements (such as "Measurement of *any three of the following seven . . .*") included in the description of the element. Elements with multiple components but with no specific numeric requirement (such as "Examination of *liver* and *spleen*") require documentation of at least one component. It is possible for a given examination to be expanded beyond what is defined here. When that occurs, findings related to the additional systems and/or areas should be documented.

- ***DG:*** *Specific abnormal and relevant negative findings of the examination of the affected or symptomatic body area(s) or organ system(s) should be documented. A notation of "abnormal" without elaboration is insufficient.*
- ***DG:*** *Abnormal or unexpected findings of the examination of any asymptomatic body area(s) or organ system(s) should be described.*
- ***DG:*** *A brief statement or notation indicating "negative" or "normal" is sufficient to document normal findings related to unaffected area(s) or asymptomatic organ system(s).*

General Multi-System Examinations

General multi-system examinations are described in detail below. To qualify for a given level of multi-system examination, the following content and documentation requirements should be met:

- *Problem Focused Examination*—should include performance and documentation of one to five elements identified by a bullet (•) in one or more organ system(s) or body area(s).
- *Expanded Problem Focused Examination*—should include performance and documentation of at least six elements identified by a bullet (•) in one or more organ system(s) or body area(s).
- *Detailed Examination*—should include at least six organ systems or body areas. For each system/area selected, performance and documentation of at least two elements identified by a bullet (•) are expected. Alternatively, a detailed examination may include performance and documentation of at least twelve elements identified by a bullet (•) in two or more organ systems or body areas.
- *Comprehensive Examination*—should include at least nine organ systems or body areas. For each system/area selected, all elements of the examination

identified by a bullet (•) should be performed, unless specific directions limit the content of the examination. For each area/system, documentation of at least two elements identified by a bullet is expected.

Single Organ System Examinations

The single organ system examinations recognized by CPT are described in detail below. Variations among these examinations in the organ systems and body areas identified in the left columns and in the elements of the examinations described in the right columns reflect differing emphases among specialties. To qualify for a given level of single organ system examination, the following content and documentation requirements should be met:

- *Problem Focused Examination*—should include performance and documentation of one to five elements identified by a bullet (•), whether in a box with a shaded or unshaded border.
- *Expanded Problem Focused Examination*—should include performance and documentation of at least six elements identified by a bullet (•), whether in a box with a shaded or unshaded border.
- *Detailed Examination*—examinations other than the eye and psychiatric examinations should include performance and documentation of at least twelve elements identified by a bullet (•), whether in box with a shaded or unshaded border. Eye and psychiatric examinations should include the performance and documentation of at least nine elements identified by a bullet (•), whether in a box with a shaded or unshaded border.
- *Comprehensive Examination*—should include performance of all elements identified by a bullet (•), whether in a shaded or unshaded box. Documentation of every element in each box with a shaded border and at least one element in each box with an unshaded border is expected.

CONTENT AND DOCUMENTATION REQUIREMENTS

General Multi-System Examination

System/Body Area	*Elements of Examination*
Constitutional	• Measurement of **any three of the following seven** vital signs: 1) sitting or standing blood pressure, 2) supine blood pressure, 3) pulse rate and regularity, 4) respiration, 5) temperature, 6) height, 7) weight (May be measured and recorded by ancillary staff) • General appearance of patient (e.g., development, nutrition, body habitus, deformities, attention to grooming)

System/Body Area	*Elements of Examination*
Eyes	• Inspection of conjunctivae and lids • Examination of pupils and irises (e.g., reaction to light and accommodation, size and symmetry) • Ophthalmoscopic examination of optic discs (e.g., size, C/D ratio, appearance) and posterior segments (e.g., vessel changes, exudates, hemorrhages)
Ears, Nose, Mouth, and Throat	• External inspection of ears and nose (e.g., overall appearance, scars, lesions, masses) • Otoscopic examination of external auditory canals and tympanic membranes • Assessment of hearing (e.g., whispered voice, finger rub, tuning fork) • Inspection of nasal mucosa, septum, and turbinates • Inspection of lips, teeth, and gums • Examination of oropharynx: oral mucosa, salivary glands, hard and soft palates, tongue, tonsils, and posterior pharynx
Neck	• Examination of neck (e.g., masses, overall appearance, symmetry, tracheal position, crepitus) • Examination of thyroid (e.g., enlargement, tenderness, mass)
Respiratory	• Assessment of respiratory effort (e.g., intercostal retractions, use of accessory muscles, diaphragmatic movement) • Percussion of chest (e.g., dullness, flatness, hyperresonance) • Palpation of chest (e.g., tactile fremitus) • Auscultation of lungs (e.g., breath sounds, adventitious sounds, rubs)
Cardiovascular	• Palpation of heart (e.g., location, size, thrills) • Auscultation of heart with notation of abnormal sounds and murmurs Examination of: • Carotid arteries (e.g., pulse amplitude, bruits) • Abdominal aorta (e.g., size, bruits) • Femoral arteries (e.g., pulse amplitude, bruits) • Pedal pulses (e.g., pulse amplitude) • Extremities for edema and/or varicosities
Chest (Breasts)	• Inspection of breasts (e.g., symmetry, nipple discharge) • Palpation of breasts and axillae (e.g., masses or lumps, tenderness)
Gastrointestinal (Abdomen)	• Examination of abdomen with notation of presence of masses or tenderness • Examination of liver and spleen • Examination for presence or absence of hernia • Examination (when indicated) of anus, perineum and rectum, including sphincter tone, presence of hemorrhoids, rectal masses • Obtain stool sample for occult blood test when indicated

System/Body Area	*Elements of Examination*
Genitourinary	**MALE:** • Examination of the scrotal contents (e.g., hydrocele, spermatocele, tenderness of cord, testicular mass) • Examination of the penis • Digital rectal examination of prostate gland (e.g., size, symmetry, nodularity, tenderness) **FEMALE:** Pelvic examination (with or without specimen collection for smears and cultures), including: • Examination of external genitalia (e.g., general appearance, hair distribution, lesions) and vagina (e.g., general appearance, estrogen effect, discharge, lesions, pelvic support, cystocele, rectocele) • Examination of urethra (e.g., masses, tenderness, scarring) • Examination of bladder (e.g., fullness, masses, tenderness) • Cervix (e.g., general appearance, lesions, discharge) • Uterus (e.g., size, contour, position, mobility, tenderness, consistency, descent, or support) • Adnexa/parametria (e.g., masses, tenderness, organomegaly, nodularity)
Lymphatic	Palpation of lymph nodes in **two or more** areas: • Neck • Axillae • Groin • Other
Musculoskeletal	• Examination of gait and station • Inspection and/or palpation of digits and nails (e.g., clubbing, cyanosis, inflammatory conditions, petechiae, ischemia, infections, nodes) Examination of joints, bones, and muscles of **one or more of the following six** areas: 1) head and neck; 2) spine, ribs and pelvis; 3) right upper extremity; 4) left upper extremity; 5) right lower extremity; and 6) left lower extremity. The examination of a given area includes: • Inspection and/or palpation with notation of presence of any misalignment, asymmetry, crepitation, defects, tenderness, masses, effusions • Assessment of range of motion with notation of any pain, crepitation, or contracture • Assessment of stability with notation of any dislocation (luxation), subluxation, or laxity • Assessment of muscle strength and tone (e.g., flaccid, cog wheel, spastic) with notation of any atrophy or abnormal movements
Skin	• Inspection of skin and subcutaneous tissue (e.g., rashes, lesions, ulcers)

System/Body Area	Elements of Examination
	• Palpation of skin and subcutaneous tissue (e.g., induration, subcutaneous nodules, tightening)
Neurologic	• Test cranial nerves with notation of any deficits • Examination of deep tendon reflexes with notation of pathological reflexes (e.g., Babinski) • Examination of sensation (e.g., by touch, pin, vibration, proprioception)
Psychiatric	• Description of patient's judgment and insight Brief assessment of mental status including: • Orientation to time, place, and person • Recent and remote memory • Mood and affect (e.g., depression, anxiety, agitation)

Content and Documentation Requirements

Level of Exam	*Perform and Document:*
Problem Focused	**One to five** elements identified by a bullet.
Expanded Problem Focused	**At least six** elements identified by a bullet.
Detailed	**At least two** elements identified by a bullet **from each of six areas/systems** OR **at least twelve** elements identified by a bullet **in two or more areas/systems**.
Comprehensive	Perform **all elements** identified by a bullet in **at least nine** organ systems or body areas and document **at least two** elements identified by a bullet **from each of nine areas/systems**.

Cardiovascular Examination

System/Body Area	Elements of Examination
Constitutional	• Measurement of **any three of the following seven** vital signs: 1) sitting or standing blood pressure, 2) supine blood pressure, 3) pulse rate and regularity, 4) respiration, 5) temperature, 6) height, 7) weight (May be measured and recorded by ancillary staff) • General appearance of patient (e.g., development, nutrition, body habitus, deformities, attention to grooming)
Head and Face	
Eyes	• Inspection of conjunctivae and lids (e.g., xanthelasma)

System/Body Area	*Elements of Examination*
Ears, Nose, Mouth, and Throat	• Inspection of teeth, gums, and palate • Inspection of oral mucosa with notation of presence of pallor or cyanosis
Neck	• Examination of jugular veins (e.g., distension; a, v, or cannon a waves) • Examination of thyroid (e.g., enlargement, tenderness, mass)
Respiratory	• Assessment of respiratory effort (e.g., intercostal retractions, use of accessory muscles, diaphragmatic movement) • Auscultation of lungs (e.g., breath sounds, adventitious sounds, rubs)
Cardiovascular	• Palpation of heart (e.g., location, size, and forcefulness of the point of maximal impact; thrills; lifts; palpable S3 or S4) • Auscultation of heart including sounds, abnormal sounds, and murmurs • Measurement of blood pressure in two or more extremities when indicated (e.g., aortic dissection, coarctation) Examination of: • Carotid arteries (e.g., waveform, pulse amplitude, bruits, apical-carotid delay) • Abdominal aorta (e.g., size, bruits) • Femoral arteries (e.g., pulse amplitude, bruits) • Pedal pulses (e.g., pulse amplitude) • Extremities for peripheral edema and/or varicosities
Chest (Breasts)	
Gastrointestinal (Abdomen)	• Examination of abdomen with notation of presence of masses or tenderness • Examination of liver and spleen • Obtain stool sample for occult blood from patients who are being considered for thrombolytic or anticoagulant therapy
Genitourinary	
Lymphatic	
Musculoskeletal	• Examination of the back with notation of kyphosis or scoliosis • Examination of gait with notation of ability to undergo exercise testing and/or participation in exercise programs • Assessment of muscle strength and tone (e.g., flaccid, cog wheel, spastic) with notation of any atrophy and abnormal movements
Extremities	• Inspection and palpation of digits and nails (e.g., clubbing, cyanosis, inflammation, petechiae, ischemia, infections, Osler's nodes)

System/Body Area	Elements of Examination
Skin	• Inspection and/or palpation of skin and subcutaneous tissue (e.g., stasis dermatitis, ulcers, scars, xanthomas)
Neurological/ Psychiatric	Brief assessment of mental status including: • Orientation to time, place, and person • Mood and affect (e.g., depression, anxiety, agitation)

Content and Documentation Requirements

Level of Exam	*Perform and Document:*
Problem Focused	**One to five** elements identified by a bullet.
Expanded Problem Focused	**At least six** elements identified by a bullet.
Detailed	**At least twelve** elements identified by a bullet.
Comprehensive	Perform **all elements** identified by a bullet; document **every** element in each box with a shaded border and **at least one** element in each box with an unshaded border.

Ear, Nose, Mouth, and Throat Examination

System/Body Area	Elements of Examination
Constitutional	• Measurement of **any three of the following seven** vital signs: 1) sitting or standing blood pressure, 2) supine blood pressure, 3) pulse rate and regularity, 4) respiration, 5) temperature, 6) height, 7) weight (May be measured and recorded by ancillary staff) • General appearance of patient (e.g., development, nutrition, body habitus, deformities, attention to grooming) • Assessment of ability to communicate (e.g., use of sign language or other communication aids) and quality of voice
Head and Face	• Inspection of head and face (e.g., overall appearance, scars, lesions, and masses) • Palpation and/or percussion of face with notation of presence or absence of sinus tenderness • Examination of salivary glands • Assessment of facial strength
Eyes	• Test ocular motility including primary gaze alignment
Ears, Nose, Mouth, and Throat	• Otoscopic examination of external auditory canals and tympanic membranes including pneumo-otoscopy with notation of mobility of membranes

System/Body Area	*Elements of Examination*
	• Assessment of hearing with tuning forks and clinical speech reception thresholds (e.g., whispered voice, finger rub) • External inspection of ears and nose (e.g., overall appearance, scars, lesions, and masses) • Inspection of nasal mucosa, septum, and turbinates • Inspection of lips, teeth, and gums • Examination of oropharynx: oral mucosa, hard and soft palates, tongue, tonsils, and posterior pharynx (e.g., asymmetry, lesions, hydration of mucosal surfaces) • Inspection of pharyngeal walls and pyriform sinuses (e.g., pooling of saliva, asymmetry, lesions) • Examination by mirror of larynx including the condition of the epiglottis, false vocal cords, true vocal cords, and mobility of larynx (Use of mirror not required in children) • Examination by mirror of nasopharynx including appearance of the mucosa, adenoids, posterior choanae, and eustachian tubes (Use of mirror not required in children)
Neck	• Examination of neck (e.g., masses, overall appearance, symmetry, tracheal position, crepitus) • Examination of thyroid (e.g., enlargement, tenderness, mass)
Respiratory	• Inspection of chest including symmetry, expansion, and/or assessment of respiratory effort (e.g., intercostal retractions, use of accessory muscles, diaphragmatic movement) • Auscultation of lungs (e.g., breath sounds, adventitious sounds, rubs)
Cardiovascular	• Auscultation of heart with notation of abnormal sounds and murmurs • Examination of peripheral vascular system by observation (e.g., swelling, varicosities) and palpation (e.g., pulses, temperature, edema, tenderness)
Chest (Breasts)	
Gastrointestinal (Abdomen)	
Genitourinary	
Lymphatic	• Palpation of lymph nodes in neck, axillae, groin, and/or other location
Musculoskeletal	
Extremities	
Skin	
Neurological/ Psychiatric	• Test cranial nerves with notation of any deficits Brief assessment of mental status including: • Orientation to time, place, and person • Mood and affect (e.g., depression, anxiety, agitation)

Content and Documentation Requirements

Level of Exam	*Perform and Document:*
Problem Focused	**One to five** elements identified by a bullet.
Expanded Problem Focused	**At least six** elements identified by a bullet.
Detailed	**At least twelve** elements identified by a bullet.
Comprehensive	Perform **all elements** identified by a bullet; document **every** element in each box with a shaded border and **at least one** element in each box with an unshaded border.

Eye Examination

System/Body Area	*Elements of Examination*
Constitutional	
Head and Face	
Eyes	• Test visual acuity (Does not include determination of refractive error) • Gross visual field testing by confrontation • Test ocular motility including primary gaze alignment • Inspection of bulbar and palpebral conjunctivae • Examination of ocular adnexae including lids (e.g., ptosis or lagophthalmos), lacrimal glands, lacrimal drainage, orbits, and preauricular lymph nodes • Examination of pupils and irises including shape, direct and consensual reaction (afferent pupil), size (e.g., anisocoria), and morphology • Slit lamp examination of the corneas including epithelium, stroma, endothelium, and tear film • Slit lamp examination of the anterior chambers including depth, cells, and flare • Slit lamp examination of the lenses including clarity, anterior and posterior capsule, cortex, and nucleus • Measurement of intraocular pressures (except in children and patients with trauma or infectious disease) • Ophthalmoscopic examination through dilated pupils (unless contraindicated) of: – Optic discs including size, C/D ratio, appearance (e.g., atrophy, cupping, tumor elevation), and nerve fiber layer – Posterior segments including retina and vessels (e.g., exudates and hemorrhages)
Ears, Nose, Mouth, and Throat	

System/Body Area	*Elements of Examination*
Neck	
Respiratory	
Cardiovascular	
Chest (Breasts)	
Gastrointestinal (Abdomen)	
Genitourinary	
Lymphatic	
Musculoskeletal	
Extremities	
Skin	
Neurological/ Psychiatric	Brief assessment of mental status including: • Orientation to time, place, and person • Mood and affect (e.g., depression, anxiety, agitation)

Content and Documentation Requirements

Level of Exam	*Perform and Document:*
Problem Focused	**One to five** elements identified by a bullet.
Expanded Problem Focused	**At least six** elements identified by a bullet.
Detailed	**At least nine** elements identified by a bullet.
Comprehensive	Perform **all elements** identified by a bullet; document **every** element in each box with a shaded border and **at least one** element in each box with an unshaded border.

Genitourinary Examination

System/Body Area	*Elements of Examination*
Constitutional	• Measurement of **any three of the following seven** vital signs: 1) sitting or standing blood pressure, 2) supine blood pressure, 3) pulse rate and regularity, 4) respiration, 5) temperature, 6) height, 7) weight (May be measured and recorded by ancillary staff) • General appearance of patient (e.g., development, nutrition, body habitus, deformities, attention to grooming)

System/Body Area	*Elements of Examination*
Head and Face	
Eyes	
Ears, Nose, Mouth, and Throat	
Neck	• Examination of neck (e.g., masses, overall appearance, symmetry, tracheal position, crepitus) • Examination of thyroid (e.g., enlargement, tenderness, mass)
Respiratory	• Assessment of respiratory effort (e.g., intercostal retractions, use of accessory muscles, diaphragmatic movement) • Auscultation of lungs (e.g., breath sounds, adventitious sounds, rubs)
Cardiovascular	• Auscultation of heart with notation of abnormal sounds and murmurs • Examination of peripheral vascular system by observation (e.g., swelling, varicosities) and palpation (e.g., pulses, temperature, edema, tenderness)
Chest (Breasts)	[See genitourinary (female)]
Gastrointestinal (Abdomen)	• Examination of abdomen with notation of presence of masses or tenderness • Examination for presence or absence of hernia • Examination of liver and spleen • Obtain stool sample for occult blood test when indicated
Genitourinary	**MALE:** • Inspection of anus and perineum Examination (with or without specimen collection for smears and cultures) of genitalia including: • Scrotum (e.g., lesions, cysts, rashes) • Epididymides (e.g., size, symmetry, masses) • Testes (e.g., size, symmetry, masses) • Urethral meatus (e.g., size, location, lesions, discharge) • Penis (e.g., lesions, presence or absence of foreskin, foreskin retractability, plaque, masses, scarring, deformities) Digital rectal examination including: • Prostate gland (e.g., size, symmetry, nodularity, tenderness) • Seminal vesicles (e.g., symmetry, tenderness, masses, enlargement) • Sphincter tone, presence of hemorrhoids, rectal masses **FEMALE:** Includes **at least seven of the following eleven** elements identified by bullets: • Inspection and palpation of breasts (e.g., masses or lumps, tenderness, symmetry, nipple discharge) • Digital rectal examination including sphincter tone, presence of hemorrhoids, rectal masses Pelvic examination (with or without specimen collection for smears and cultures) including:

System/Body Area	*Elements of Examination*
	• External genitalia (e.g., general appearance, hair distribution, lesions) • Urethral meatus (e.g., size, location, lesions, prolapse) • Urethra (e.g., masses, tenderness, scarring) • Bladder (e.g., fullness, masses, tenderness) • Vagina (e.g., general appearance, estrogen effect, discharge, lesions, pelvic support, cystocele, rectocele) • Cervix (e.g., general appearance, lesions, discharge) • Uterus (e.g., size, contour, position, mobility, tenderness, consistency, descent, or support) • Adnexa/parametria (e.g., masses, tenderness, organomegaly, nodularity) • Anus and perineum
Lymphatic	• Palpation of lymph nodes in neck, axillae, groin, and/or other location
Musculoskeletal	
Extremities	
Skin	• Inspection and/or palpation of skin and subcutaneous tissue (e.g., rashes, lesions, ulcers)
Neurological/ Psychiatric	Brief assessment of mental status including: • Orientation (e.g., time, place, and person) • Mood and affect (e.g., depression, anxiety, agitation)

Content and Documentation Requirements

Level of Exam	*Perform and Document:*
Problem Focused	**One to five** elements identified by a bullet.
Expanded Problem Focused	**At least six** elements identified by a bullet.
Detailed	**At least twelve** elements identified by a bullet.
Comprehensive	Perform **all elements** identified by a bullet; document **every** element in each box with a shaded border and **at least one** element in each box with an unshaded border.

Hematologic/Lymphatic/Immunologic Examination

System/Body Area	*Elements of Examination*
Constitutional	• Measurement of **any three of the following seven** vital signs: 1) sitting or standing blood pressure, 2) supine blood pressure, 3) pulse rate and regularity, 4) respiration, 5) temperature, 6) height, 7) weight (May be measured and recorded by ancillary staff)

System/Body Area	*Elements of Examination*
	• General appearance of patient (e.g., development, nutrition, body habitus, deformities, attention to grooming)
Head and Face	• Palpation and/or percussion of face with notation of presence or absence of sinus tenderness
Eyes	• Inspection of conjunctivae and lids
Ears, Nose, Mouth, and Throat	• Otoscopic examination of external auditory canals and tympanic membranes • Inspection of nasal mucosa, septum, and turbinates • Inspection of teeth and gums • Examination of oropharynx (e.g., oral mucosa, hard and soft palates, tongue, tonsils, posterior pharynx)
Neck	• Examination of neck (e.g., masses, overall appearance, symmetry, tracheal position, crepitus) • Examination of thyroid (e.g., enlargement, tenderness, mass)
Respiratory	• Assessment of respiratory effort (e.g., intercostal retractions, use of accessory muscles, diaphragmatic movement) • Auscultation of lungs (e.g., breath sounds, adventitious sounds, rubs)
Cardiovascular	• Auscultation of heart with notation of abnormal sounds and murmurs • Examination of peripheral vascular system by observation (e.g., swelling, varicosities), and palpation (e.g., pulses, temperature, edema, tenderness)
Chest (Breasts)	
Gastrointestinal (Abdomen)	• Examination of abdomen with notation of presence of masses or tenderness • Examination of liver and spleen
Genitourinary	
Lymphatic	• Palpation of lymph nodes in neck, axillae, groin, and/or other location
Musculoskeletal	
Extremities	• Inspection and palpation of digits and nails (e.g., clubbing, cyanosis, inflammation, petechiae, ischemia, infections, nodes)
Skin	• Inspection and/or palpation of skin and subcutaneous tissue (e.g., rashes, lesions, ulcers, ecchymoses, bruises)
Neurological/ Psychiatric	Brief assessment of mental status including: • Orientation to time, place, and person • Mood and affect (e.g., depression, anxiety, agitation)

Content and Documentation Requirements

Level of Exam	*Perform and Document:*
Problem Focused	**One to five** elements identified by a bullet.
Expanded Problem Focused	**At least six elements** identified by a bullet.
Detailed	**At least twelve elements** identified by a bullet.
Comprehensive	Perform **all elements** identified by a bullet; document **every** element in each box with a shaded border and **at least one** element in each box with an unshaded border.

Musculoskeletal Examination

System/Body Area	*Elements of Examination*
Constitutional	• Measurement of **any three of the following seven** vital signs: 1) sitting or standing blood pressure, 2) supine blood pressure, 3) pulse rate and regularity, 4) respiration, 5) temperature, 6) height, 7) weight (May be measured and recorded by ancillary staff) • General appearance of patient (e.g., development, nutrition, body habitus, deformities, attention to grooming)
Head and Face	
Eyes	
Ears, Nose, Mouth, and Throat	
Neck	
Respiratory	
Cardiovascular	• Examination of peripheral vascular system by observation (e.g., swelling, varicosities) and palpation (e.g., pulses, temperature, edema, tenderness)
Chest (Breasts)	
Gastrointestinal (Abdomen)	
Genitourinary	
Lymphatic	• Palpation of lymph nodes in neck, axillae, groin, and/or other location
Musculoskeletal	• Examination of gait and station Examination of joint(s), bone(s), and muscle(s)/tendon(s) of **four of the following six** areas: 1) head and neck; 2) spine, ribs, and pelvis; 3) right upper extremity; 4) left upper extremity; 5) right lower extremity;

System/Body Area	*Elements of Examination*
	and 6) left lower extremity. The examination of a given area includes: • Inspection, percussion, and/or palpation with notation of any misalignment, asymmetry, crepitation, defects, tenderness, masses, or effusions • Assessment of range of motion with notation of any pain (e.g., straight leg raising), crepitation, or contracture • Assessment of stability with notation of any dislocation (luxation), subluxation, or laxity • Assessment of muscle strength and tone (e.g., flaccid, cog wheel, spastic) with notation of any atrophy or abnormal movements NOTE: For the comprehensive level of examination, all four of the elements identified by a bullet must be performed and documented for each of four anatomic areas. For the three lower levels of examination, each element is counted separately for each body area. For example, assessing range of motion in two extremities constitutes two elements.
Extremities	[See musculoskeletal and skin]
Skin	• Inspection and/or palpation of skin and subcutaneous tissue (e.g., scars, rashes, lesions, cafe-au-lait spots, ulcers) in **four of the following six** areas: 1) head and neck; 2) trunk; 3) right upper extremity; 4) left upper extremity; 5) right lower extremity; and 6) left lower extremity. NOTE: For the comprehensive level, the examination of four anatomic areas must be performed and documented. For the three lower levels of examination, each body area is counted separately. For example, inspection and/or palpation of the skin and subcutaneous tissue of two extremitites constitutes two elements.
Neurological/ Psychiatric	• Test coordination (e.g., finger/nose, heel/knee/shin, rapid alternating movements in the upper and lower extremities, evaluation of fine motor coordination in young children) • Examination of deep tendon reflexes and/or nerve stretch test with notation of pathological reflexes (e.g., Babinski) • Examination of sensation (e.g., by touch, pin, vibration, proprioception) Brief assessment of mental status including: • Orientation to time, place, and person • Mood and affect (e.g., depression, anxiety, agitation)

Content and Documentation Requirements

Level of Exam	*Perform and Document:*
Problem Focused	**One to five** elements identified by a bullet.
Expanded Problem Focused	**At least six** elements identified by a bullet.
Detailed	**At least twelve** elements identified by a bullet.

Comprehensive — Perform **all elements** identified by a bullet; document **every** element in each box with a shaded border and **at least one** element in each box with an unshaded border.

Neurological Examination

System/Body Area	*Elements of Examination*
Constitutional	• Measurement of **any three of the following seven** vital signs: 1) sitting or standing blood pressure, 2) supine blood pressure, 3) pulse rate and regularity, 4) respiration, 5) temperature, 6) height, 7) weight (May be measured and recorded by ancillary staff) • General appearance of patient (e.g., development, nutrition, body habitus, deformities, attention to grooming)
Head and Face	
Eyes	• Ophthalmoscopic examination of optic discs (e.g., size, C/D ratio, appearance) and posterior segments (e.g., vessel changes, exudates, hemorrhages)
Ears, Nose, Mouth, and Throat	
Neck	
Respiratory	
Cardiovascular	• Examination of carotid arteries (e.g., pulse amplitude, bruits) • Auscultation of heart with notation of abnormal sounds and murmurs • Examination of peripheral vascular system by observation (e.g., swelling, varicosities) and palpation (e.g., pulses, temperature, edema, tenderness)
Chest (Breasts)	
Gastrointestinal (Abdomen)	
Genitourinary	
Lymphatic	
Musculoskeletal	• Examination of gait and station Assessment of motor function including: • Muscle strength in upper and lower extremities • Muscle tone in upper and lower extremities (e.g., flaccid, cog wheel, spastic) with notation of any atrophy or abnormal movements (e.g., fasciculation, tardive dyskinesia)
Extremities	[See musculoskeletal]
Skin	

System/Body Area	*Elements of Examination*
Neurological / Psychiatric	Evaluation of higher integrative functions including: • Orientation to time, place, and person • Recent and remote memory • Attention span and concentration • Language (e.g., naming objects, repeating phrases, spontaneous speech) • Fund of knowledge (e.g., awareness of current events, past history, vocabulary) Test the following cranial nerves: • 2nd cranial nerve (e.g., visual acuity, visual fields, fundi) • 3rd, 4th, and 6th cranial nerves (e.g., pupils, eye movements) • 5th cranial nerve (e.g., facial sensation, corneal reflexes) • 7th cranial nerve (e.g., facial symmetry, strength) • 8th cranial nerve (e.g., hearing with tuning fork, whispered voice, and/or finger rub) • 9th cranial nerve (e.g., spontaneous or reflex palate movement) • 11th cranial nerve (e.g., shoulder shrug strength) • 12th cranial nerve (e.g., tongue protrusion) • Examination of sensation (e.g., by touch, pin, vibration, proprioception) • Examination of deep tendon reflexes in upper and lower extremities with notation of pathological reflexes (e.g., Babinski) • Test coordination (e.g., finger/nose, heel/knee/shin, rapid alternating movements in the upper and lower extremities, evaluation of fine motor coordination in young children)
Psychiatric	

Content and Documentation Requirements

Level of Exam	*Perform and Document:*
Problem Focused	**One to five** elements identified by a bullet.
Expanded Problem Focused	**At least six** elements identified by a bullet.
Detailed	**At least twelve** elements identified by a bullet.
Comprehensive	Perform **all elements** identified by a bullet; document **every** element in each box with a shaded border and **at least one** element in each box with an unshaded border.

Psychiatric Examination

System/Body Area	*Elements of Examination*
Constitutional	• Measurement of **any three of the following seven** vital signs: 1) sitting or standing blood pressure, 2) supine blood pressure, 3) pulse rate and regularity, 4) respiration, 5) temperature, 6) height, 7) weight (May be measured and recorded by ancillary staff) • General appearance of patient (e.g., development, nutrition, body habitus, deformities, attention to grooming)

System/Body Area	*Elements of Examination*
Head and Face	
Eyes	
Ears, Nose, Mouth, and Throat	
Neck	
Respiratory	
Cardiovascular	
Chest (Breasts)	
Gastrointestinal (Abdomen)	
Genitourinary	
Lymphatic	
Musculoskeletal	• Assessment of muscle strength and tone (e.g., flaccid, cog wheel, spastic) with notation of any atrophy and abnormal movements • Examination of gait and station
Extremities	
Skin	
Neurological	
Psychiatric	• Description of speech including: rate; volume; articulation; coherence; and spontaneity with notation of abnormalities (e.g., perseveration, paucity of language) • Description of thought processes including: rate of thoughts; content of thoughts (e.g., logical vs. illogical, tangential); abstract reasoning; and computation • Description of associations (e.g., loose, tangential, circumstantial, intact) • Description of abnormal or psychotic thoughts including: hallucinations; delusions; preoccupation with violence; homicidal or suicidal ideation; and obsessions • Description of the patient's judgment (e.g., concerning everyday activities and social situations) and insight (e.g., concerning psychiatric condition)

System/Body Area	*Elements of Examination*
	Complete mental status examination including: • Orientation to time, place, and person • Recent and remote memory • Attention span and concentration • Language (e.g., naming objects, repeating phrases) • Fund of knowledge (e.g., awareness of current events, past history, vocabulary) • Mood and affect (e.g., depression, anxiety, agitation, hypomania, lability)

Content and Documentation Requirements

Level of Exam	*Perform and Document:*
Problem Focused	**One to five** elements identified by a bullet.
Expanded Problem Focused	**At least six** elements identified by a bullet.
Detailed	**At least nine** elements identified by a bullet.
Comprehensive	Perform **all elements** identified by a bullet; document **every** element in each box with a shaded border and **at least one** element in each box with an unshaded border.

Respiratory Examination

System/Body Area	*Elements of Examination*
Constitutional	• Measurement of **any three of the following seven** vital signs: 1) sitting or standing blood pressure, 2) supine blood pressure, 3) pulse rate and regularity, 4) respiration, 5) temperature, 6) height, 7) weight (May be measured and recorded by ancillary staff) • General appearance of patient (e.g., development, nutrition, body habitus, deformities, attention to grooming)
Head and Face	
Eyes	
Ears, Nose, Mouth, and Throat	• Inspection of nasal mucosa, septum, and turbinates • Inspection of teeth and gums • Examination of oropharynx (e.g., oral mucosa, hard and soft palates, tongue, tonsils, and posterior pharynx)
Neck	• Examination of neck (e.g., masses, overall appearance, symmetry, tracheal position, crepitus) • Examination of thyroid (e.g., enlargement, tenderness, mass)

System/Body Area	*Elements of Examination*
	• Examination of jugular veins (e.g., distension; a, v, or cannon a waves)
Respiratory	• Inspection of chest with notation of symmetry and expansion • Assessment of respiratory effort (e.g., intercostal retractions, use of accessory muscles, diaphragmatic movement) • Percussion of chest (e.g., dullness, flatness, hyperresonance) • Palpation of chest (e.g., tactile fremitus) • Auscultation of lungs (e.g., breath sounds, adventitious sounds, rubs)
Cardiovascular	• Auscultation of heart including sounds, abnormal sounds, and murmurs • Examination of peripheral vascular system by observation (e.g., swelling, varicosities) and palpation (e.g., pulses, temperature, edema, tenderness)
Chest (Breasts)	
Gastrointestinal (Abdomen)	• Examination of abdomen with notation of presence of masses or tenderness • Examination of liver and spleen
Genitourinary	
Lymphatic	• Palpation of lymph nodes in neck, axillae, groin, and/or other location
Musculoskeletal	• Assessment of muscle strength and tone (e.g., flaccid, cog wheel, spastic) with notation of any atrophy and abnormal movements • Examination of gait and station
Extremities	• Inspection and palpation of digits and nails (e.g., clubbing, cyanosis, inflammation, petechiae, ischemia, infections, nodes)
Skin	• Inspection and/or palpation of skin and subcutaneous tissue (e.g., rashes, lesions, ulcers)
Neurological/ Psychiatric	Brief assessment of mental status including: • Orientation to time, place, and person • Mood and affect (e.g., depression, anxiety, agitation)

Content and Documentation Requirements

Level of Exam	*Perform and Document:*
Problem Focused	**One to five** elements identified by a bullet.
Expanded Problem Focused	**At least six** elements identified by a bullet.
Detailed	**At least twelve** elements identified by a bullet.
Comprehensive	Perform **all elements** identified by a bullet; document **every** element in each box with a shaded border and **at least one** element in each box with an unshaded border.

Skin Examination

System/Body Area	*Elements of Examination*
Constitutional	• Measurement of any **three of the following seven** vital signs: 1) sitting or standing blood pressure, 2) supine blood pressure, 3) pulse rate and regularity, 4) respiration, 5) temperature, 6) height, 7) weight (May be measured and recorded by ancillary staff) • General appearance of patient (e.g., development, nutrition, body habitus, deformities, attention to grooming)
Head and Face	
Eyes	• Inspection of conjunctivae and lids
Ears, Nose, Mouth, and Throat	• Inspection of lips, teeth, and gums • Examination of oropharynx (e.g., oral mucosa, hard and soft palates, tongue, tonsils, posterior pharynx)
Neck	• Examination of thyroid (e.g., enlargement, tenderness, mass)
Respiratory	
Cardiovascular	• Examination of peripheral vascular system by observation (e.g., swelling, varicosities) and palpation (e.g., pulses, temperature, edema, tenderness)
Chest (Breasts)	
Gastrointestinal (Abdomen)	• Examination of liver and spleen • Examination of anus for condyloma and other lesions
Genitourinary	
Lymphatic	• Palpation of lymph nodes in neck, axillae, groin, and/or other location
Musculoskeletal	
Extremities	• Inspection and palpation of digits and nails (e.g., clubbing, cyanosis, inflammation, petechiae, ischemia, infections, nodes)
Skin	• Palpation of scalp and inspection of hair of scalp, eyebrows, face, chest, pubic area (when indicated), and extremities Inspection and/or palpation of skin and subcutaneous tissue (e.g., rashes, lesions, ulcers, susceptibility to and presence of photo damage) in **eight of the following ten** areas: • Head, including the face • Neck • Chest, including breasts and axillae • Abdomen • Genitalia, groin, buttocks • Back

System/Body Area	*Elements of Examination*
	• Right upper extremity • Left upper extremity • Right lower extremity • Left lower extremity NOTE: For the comprehensive level, the examination of at least eight anatomic areas must be performed and documented. For the three lower levels of examination, each body area is counted separately. For example, inspection and/or palpation of the skin and subcutaneous tissue of the right upper extremity and the left upper extremity constitutes two elements. • Inspection of eccrine and apocrine glands of skin and subcutaneous tissue with identification and location of any hyperhidrosis, chromhidrosis, or bromhidrosis
Neurological/ Psychiatric	Brief assessment of mental status including: • Orientation to time, place, and person • Mood and affect (e.g., depression, anxiety, agitation)

Content and Documentation Requirements

Level of Exam	*Perform and Document:*
Problem Focused	**One to five** elements identified by a bullet.
Expanded Problem Focused	**At least six** elements identified by a bullet.
Detailed	**At least twelve** elements identified by a bullet.
Comprehensive	Perform **all elements** identified by a bullet; document **every** element in each box with a shaded border and **at least one** element in each box with an unshaded border.

Documentation of the Complexity of Medical Decision Making

The levels of E/M services recognize four types of medical decision making (straightforward, low complexity, moderate complexity, and high complexity). Medical decision making refers to the complexity of establishing a diagnosis and/or selecting a management option as measured by:

- The number of possible diagnoses and/or the number of management options that must be considered;
- The amount and/or complexity of medical records, diagnostic tests, and/or other information that must be obtained, reviewed, and analyzed; and
- The risk of significant complications, morbidity and/or mortality, as well as comorbidities, associated with the patient's presenting problem(s), the diagnostic procedure(s), and/or the possible management options.

The chart below shows the progression of the elements required for each level of medical decision making. To qualify for a given type of decision making, two of the three elements in the table must be either met or exceeded.

Number of Diagnoses or Management Options	*Amount and/or Complexity of Data To Be Reviewed*	*Risk of Complications and/or Morbidity or Mortality*	*Type of Decision Making*
Minimal	Minimal to None	Minimal	Straightforward
Limited	Limited	Low	Low Complexity
Multiple	Moderate	Moderate	Moderate Complexity
Extensive	Extensive	High	High Complexity

Each of the elements of medical decision making is described below.

Number of Diagnoses or Management Options

The number of possible diagnoses and/or the number of management options that must be considered is based on the number and types of problems addressed during the encounter, the complexity of establishing a diagnosis, an[illegible] the management decisions that are made by the physician.

Generally, decision making with respect to a diagnosed probl[illegible]asier than that for an identified but undiagnosed problem. The number [illegible]f diagnostic tests employed may be an indicator of the number of poss[illegible]noses. Problems which are improving or resolving are less complex than [illegible] which are worsening or failing to change as expected. The need to seek adv[illegible] from others is another indicator of complexity of diagnostic or manageme[illegible] problems.

- **•DG:** *For each encounter, an assessment, clinical impression, or diagnosis sho[illegible] documented. It may be explicitly stated or implied in documented de[illegible] regarding management plans and/or further evaluation.*
  - *For a presenting problem with an established diagnosis the record shoul[illegible]lect whether the problem is: a) improved, well controlled, resolving, or resc[illegible]; or, b) inadequately controlled, worsening, or failing to change as expecte[illegible]*
  - *For a presenting problem without an established diagnosis, the as[illegible]nent or clinical impression may be stated in the form of differential dia[illegible]es or as a "possible," "probable," or "rule out" (R/O) diagnosis.*
- **•DG:** *The initiation of, or changes in, treatment should be documented. [illegible]ment includes a wide range of management options including patient in[illegible]uctions, nursing instructions, therapies, and medications.*
- **•DG:** *If referrals are made, consultations requested, or advice sought, the record should indicate to whom or where the referral or consultation is made or from whom the advice is requested.*

Amount and/or Complexity of Data To Be Reviewed

The amount and complexity of data to be reviewed is based on the types of diagnostic testing ordered or reviewed. A decision to obtain and review old medical records and/or obtain history from sources other than the patient increases the amount and complexity of data to be reviewed.

Discussion of contradictory or unexpected test results with the physician who performed or interpreted the test is an indication of the complexity of data being reviewed. On occasion the physician who ordered a test may personally review the image, tracing, or specimen to supplement information from the physician who prepared the test report or interpretation; this is another indication of the complexity of data being reviewed.

- *DG: If a diagnostic service (test or procedure) is ordered, planned, scheduled, or performed at the time of the E/M encounter, the type of service, e.g., lab or X-ray, should be documented.*
- *DG: The review of lab, radiology, and/or other diagnostic tests should be documented. A simple notation such as "WBC elevated" or "chest X-ray unremarkable" is acceptable. Alternatively, the review may be documented by initialing and dating the report containing the test results.*
- *DG: A decision to obtain old records or a decision to obtain additional history from the family, caretaker, or other source to supplement that obtained from the patient should be documented.*
- *DG: Relevant findings from the review of old records, and/or the receipt of additional history from the family, caretaker, or other source to supplement that obtained from the patient should be documented. If there is no relevant information beyond that already obtained, that fact should be documented. A notation of "old records reviewed" or "additional history obtained from family" without elaboration is insufficient.*
- *DG: The results of discussion of laboratory, radiology, or other diagnostic tests with the physician who performed or interpreted the study should be documented.*
- *DG: The direct visualization and independent interpretation of an image, tracing, or specimen previously or subsequently interpreted by another physician should be documented.*

Risk of Significant Complications, Morbidity, and/or Mortality

The risk of significant complications, morbidity, and/or mortality is based on the risks associated with the presenting problem(s), the diagnostic procedure(s), and the possible management options.

- *DG: Comorbidities/underlying diseases or other factors that increase the complexity of medical decision making by increasing the risk of complications, morbidity, and/or mortality should be documented.*

- •*DG:* *If a surgical or invasive diagnostic procedure is ordered, planned, or scheduled at the time of the E/M encounter, the type of procedure, e.g., laparoscopy, should be documented.*
- •*DG:* *If a surgical or invasive diagnostic procedure is performed at the time of the E/M encounter, the specific procedure should be documented.*
- •*DG:* *The referral for or decision to perform a surgical or invasive diagnostic procedure on an urgent basis should be documented or implied.*

The following table may be used to help determine whether the risk of significant complications, morbidity, and/or mortality is *minimal, low, moderate,* or *high.* Because the determination of risk is complex and not readily quantifiable, the table includes common clinical examples rather than absolute measures of risk. The assessment of risk of the presenting problem(s) is based on the risk related to the disease process anticipated between the present encounter and the next one. The assessment of risk of selecting diagnostic procedures and management options is based on the risk during and immediately following any procedures or treatment. The highest level of risk in any one category (presenting problem(s), diagnostic procedure(s), or management options) determines the overall risk.

TABLE OF RISK

Level of Risk	*Presenting Problem(s)*	*Diagnostic Procedure(s) Ordered*	*Management Options Selected*
Minimal	• One self-limited or minor problem, e.g., cold, insect bite, tinea corporis	• Laboratory tests requiring venipuncture • Chest X-rays • EKG/EEG • Urinalysis • Ultrasound, e.g., echocardiography • KOH prep	• Rest • Gargles • Elastic bandages • Superficial dressings
Low	• Two or more self-limited or minor problems • One stable chronic illness, e.g., well controlled hypertension, noninsulin dependent diabetes, cataract, BPH • Acute uncomplicated illness or injury, e.g., cystitis, allergic rhinitis, simple sprain	• Physiologic tests not under stress, e.g., pulmonary function tests • Non-cardiovascular imaging studies with contrast, e.g., barium enema • Superficial needle biopsies • Clinical laboratory tests requiring arterial puncture • Skin biopsies	• Over-the-counter drugs • Minor surgery with no identified risk factors • Physical therapy • Occupational therapy • IV fluids without additives

Level of Risk	*Presenting Problem(s)*	*Diagnostic Procedure(s) Ordered*	*Management Options Selected*
Moderate	• One or more chronic illnesses with mild exacerbation, progression, or side effects of treatment • Two or more stable chronic illnesses • Undiagnosed new problem with uncertain prognosis, e.g., lump in breast • Acute illness with systemic symptoms, e.g., pyelonephritis, pneumonitis, colitis • Acute complicated injury, e.g., head injury with brief loss of consciousness	• Physiologic tests under stress, e.g., cardiac stress test, fetal contraction stress test • Diagnostic endoscopies with no identified risk factors • Deep needle or incisional biopsy • Cardiovascular imaging studies with contrast and no identified risk factors, e.g., arteriogram, cardiac catheterization • Obtain fluid from body cavity, e.g., lumbar puncture, thoracentesis, culdocentesis	• Minor surgery with identified risk factors • Elective major surgery (open, percutaneous, or endoscopic) with no identified risk factors • Prescription drug management • Therapeutic nuclear medicine • IV fluids with additives • Closed treatment of fracture or dislocation without manipulation
High	• One or more chronic illnesses with severe exacerbation, progression, or side effects of treatment • Acute or chronic illnesses or injuries that pose a threat to life or bodily function, e.g., multiple trauma, acute renal failure • MI, pulmonary embolus, severe respiratory distress, progressive severe rheumatoid arthritis, psychiatric illness with potential threat to self or others, peritonitis, acute renal failure • An abrupt change in neurologic status, e.g., seizure, TIA, weakness, sensory loss	• Cardiovascular imaging studies with contrast with identified risk factors • Cardiac electrophysiological tests • Diagnostic endoscopies with identified risk factors • Discography	• Elective major surgery (open, percutaneous, or endoscopic) with identified risk factors • Emergency major surgery (open, percutaneous, or endoscopic) • Parenteral controlled substances • Drug therapy requiring intensive monitoring for toxicity • Decision not to resuscitate or to de-escalate care because of poor prognosis

Documentation of an Encounter Dominated by Counseling or Coordination of Care

In the case where counseling and/or coordination of care dominates (more than 50 percent) of the physician/patient and/or family encounter (face-to-face time in the office or other outpatient setting, floor/unit time in the hospital or nursing facility), time is considered the key or controlling factor to qualify for a particular level of E/M services.

- ***DG:*** *If the physician elects to report the level of service based on counseling and/or coordination of care, the total length of time of the encounter (face-to-face or floor time, as appropriate) should be documented and the record should describe the counseling and/or activities to coordinate care.*

CHAPTER 5

Prescribing

Nurse practitioners (NPs) in 50 states and the District of Columbia have the ability to prescribe or otherwise arrange for a patient to get a prescription medication. The independence of NPs' prescriptive authority varies widely, and, in several states, words other than *prescribe* are used.

In eight states, NPs have explicit legal authority to "prescribe," with no requirement for physician involvement. In one state (Montana), NPs have explicit legal authority to prescribe, and physician involvement is required only insofar as an NP must have a quality assurance plan that provides for a system of referral to other health care providers and physician review of a percentage of an NP's charts. In 38 states, NPs have explicit legal authority to prescribe but must have a collaborative relationship with a specific physician. In one state (California), NPs may not prescribe but may "furnish" or "order" drugs. In two states (Michigan and Georgia), NPs do not have specific legal authority to prescribe, but the law permits physicians to delegate medical functions. In Michigan, if a physician chooses to delegate prescription writing to an NP, the physician may do so, and the NP may write prescriptions under delegated authority (Exhibit 5-1). In 32 states, prescribing is specifically included as an element in the NP scope of practice. In 21 states, protocols detailing how drugs are to be prescribed are required by law. See Exhibit 5-2 for the states that fall into each of these categories. Appendix 5-A presents laws on prescriptive authority for each state.

CONTROLLED SUBSTANCES

Controlled dangerous substances are narcotics, depressants, stimulants, and hallucinogenic drugs covered under the Controlled Substances Act, a federal law. In 49 states and the District of Columbia, NPs may prescribe controlled substances.

Exhibit 5-1 Forms of Prescriptive Authority

Explicit Legal Authority To Prescribe/No Physician Involvement Required
- Alaska
- District of Columbia
- Maine
- New Hampshire
- New Mexico
- Oregon
- Washington

Explicit Legal Authority To Prescribe/Physician Must Review a Percentage of NP's Charts as Part of Quality Assurance Plan
- Montana

Authority To "Furnish" Drugs/ Physician Delegation Required
- California

Physician May Delegate Authority To Prescribe under Protocols
- Georgia
- Michigan

Explicit Legal Authority To Prescribe/Physician Collaboration Required
- Alabama
- Arizona
- Arkansas
- Colorado
- Connecticut
- Delaware
- Florida
- Hawaii
- Idaho
- Illinois
- Indiana
- Iowa
- Kentucky
- Louisiana
- Maryland
- Massachusetts
- Minnesota
- Mississippi
- Missouri
- Nebraska
- Nevada
- New Jersey
- New York
- North Carolina
- North Dakota
- Ohio
- Oklahoma
- Pennsylvania
- Rhode Island
- South Carolina
- South Dakota
- Tennessee
- Texas
- Utah
- Vermont
- Virginia
- West Virginia
- Wisconsin
- Wyoming

Classification of Controlled Substances

There are five "schedules" of controlled substances:

- *Schedule I:* Schedule I substances have little or no accepted medical use in the United States and have high abuse potential. Examples are heroin, LSD, marijuana, mescaline, methaqualone, and peyote.
- *Schedule II:* Schedule II drugs have a high abuse potential with severe psychic or physical dependence liability and in general are substances that have therapeutic utility. Schedule II narcotics include morphine, codeine, fentanyl, hydromorphone (Dilaudid), levorphanol, meperidine (Demerol), methadone, oxycodone, and opium. Stimulants such as amphetamines are in Schedule II, as well as depressants such as pentobarbital.

Exhibit 5-2 State Regulations of NPs' Prescriptive Activity

NP May Prescribe Controlled Substances
- Alaska
- Arizona
- Arkansas (Not Schedule I-II)
- California (Not Schedule I-II)
- Colorado
- Connecticut
- Delaware
- District of Columbia
- Georgia
- Idaho
- Illinois (Not Schedule I-II)
- Indiana
- Iowa
- Kansas
- Louisiana
- Maine
- Maryland
- Massachusetts
- Michigan
- Minnesota
- Mississippi
- Montana
- Nebraska
- Nevada
- New Hampshire
- New Jersey
- New Mexico
- New York
- North Carolina
- North Dakota
- Ohio
- Oklahoma (Not Schedule I-II)
- Oregon
- Pennsylvania
- Rhode Island
- South Dakota
- Tennessee
- Texas (Schedules III-V)
- Utah
- Vermont
- Virginia
- Washington
- West Virginia (Not Schedule I-II)
- Wisconsin
- Wyoming

CDS Limited to Schedule V
- South Carolina

Physician's Name Required on Prescription
- Alabama
- Idaho
- Illinois
- Kansas
- Louisiana
- Massachusetts
- Missouri
- New Jersey
- Oklahoma
- Pennsylvania
- South Carolina
- Texas

- *Schedule III:* Schedule III drugs are stimulants and depressants with an abuse potential. Schedule III narcotics include mixtures of limited specified quantities of codeine with noncontrolled active ingredients, mixtures of amobarbital, pentobarbital, or secobarbital with other noncontrolled medicinal ingredients, and anabolic steroids.
- *Schedule IV:* Schedule IV drugs are: (a) depressants such as: alprazolam clonazepam, diazepam, and flurazepam; (b) stimulants such as phenteramine; and other substances such as pentazocine.
- *Schedule V:* The schedule V drugs include narcotic drugs not listed in another schedule, stimulants not listed in another schedule, and narcotic drugs containing non-narcotic medicinal ingredients.

A complete listing of the drugs controlled under the Controlled Substances Act may be found in Title 21, Code of Federal Regulations, Part 1300 to end, Sections 1308.11 through 1308.15. Prescribing references usually provide the class of each drug listed.

DEA Registration

The federal government—the Drug Enforcement Administration (DEA)—oversees NPs' prescribing of controlled substances. To prescribe controlled substances, an NP must register with the DEA and obtain a DEA number. The NP must use the DEA number on prescriptions for scheduled drugs.

DEA registration is one method of tracking health care providers' prescribing practices related to controlled substances. The DEA number is also a method of minimizing unauthorized prescribing: that is, a person who is not authorized to prescribe but who wants to write a prescription for a controlled substance, has a prescription pad, and signs the name of an authorized prescriber will be unable to get the prescription filled if it does not include a DEA number.

Federal registration is based on the applicant's complying with state and local laws. If a state requires a separate controlled substances license, an NP must obtain that license and submit a copy with the application for a DEA number. If state law does not authorize NPs to prescribe controlled substances, the DEA will not issue DEA numbers.

DEA registration costs $210 for a three-year term. States may charge for registration as well. For a DEA registration application, call 1-800-882-9539. Once a DEA number is issued, a renewal application is automatically issued 45 days prior to expiration. Registrants must report, in writing, any change in business location to the DEA. DEA registration is issued in the NP's name at the business address.

GUIDELINES FOR PRESCRIBING LEGALLY

The Physician Insurers Association of America reported that an analysis of malpractice claims identified the two most common medication errors made by physicians as (1) choosing the wrong drug and (2) failing to monitor side effects.[1]

NPs should follow these general guidelines when prescribing:

1. Prescribe the right medicine at the right time for the right indication for the right patient.
2. If there is a practice protocol or guidelines in the facility, follow it.
3. If there is no facility-wide protocol, adhere to the standard of care in prescribing. The standard of care for prescribing may be assumed to be the *Physician's Desk Reference.*
4. Before prescribing, ask a patient:
    - Are you pregnant?
    - Are you breastfeeding?

- Are you allergic to any medications?
- Have you taken [this medicine] before? Did it work? Did it give you any ill effects?
- Do you have any liver or kidney problems?
- What other medications are you on?
- What other medical problems do you have?

5. Address any cross-sensitivities. For example, if a patient is allergic to penicillin, an NP probably should not prescribe Keflex, which has cross-sensitivities with penicillin.
6. Address any contraindications. For example, a patient with chronic hepatitis should not be prescribed a medication that has potential for liver damage unless it is a life-and-death situation and there is no other choice.
7. Address any drug interactions. For example, theophylline is antagonized by phenytoin and potentiated by macrolide antibiotics.
8. Inform the patient of potential side effects, and ask whether the patient wants to accept the risk of experiencing those side effects.
9. Inform the patient to call or return if he or she notices any adverse change in his or her condition.

Other considerations when prescribing are:

- Can the patient afford the medication? If not, the NP should not count on the patient's getting the prescription filled.
- Is the drug to be prescribed in the formulary for the agency or health maintenance organization?
- Is there potential for abuse of the medication? For example, a depressed patient may overdose on a prescribed medication, and a patient with a history of substance abuse may be seeking to continue the habit through a request for pain medication.

NOTE

1. Common medication errors. *Clinician Reviews* 1997; 7(2):132.

APPENDIX 5-A

State-by-State Law Prescriptive Authority

ALABAMA

[The] joint committee shall recommend model practice protocols to be used by certified registered nurse practitioners and certified nurse midwives and a formulary of legend drugs that may be prescribed by these advanced practice nurses, subject to approval by both the State Board of Medical Examiners and the Board of Nursing. The joint committee shall also recommend rules and regulations to establish the ratio of physicians to certified registered nurse practitioners and certified nurse midwives; provided, however, that the rules and regulations shall not limit the ratio to less than two nurse practitioners or midwives to one physician or one certified registered nurse practitioner and one certified nurse midwife to one physician and shall provide for exceptions. The joint committee shall also recommend rules and regulations that establish the manner in which a collaborating physician may designate a covering physician when temporarily unavailable as the collaborating physician.

Citation: ALA. CODE, § 34-21-87.

(a) Certified registered nurse practitioners and certified nurse midwives, engaged in collaborative practice with physicians practicing under protocols approved in the manner prescribed by this article may prescribe legend drugs to their patients, subject to both of the following conditions:
  (1) The drug type, dosage, quantity prescribed, and number of refills shall be authorized in an approved protocol signed by the collaborating physician; and
  (2) The drug shall be on the formulary recommended by the joint committee and adopted by the State Board of Medical Examiners and the Board of Nursing.

Source: © Carolyn Buppert 2003.

(b) A certified registered nurse practitioner or a certified nurse midwife may not initiate a call-in prescription in the name of a collaborating physician for any drug, whether legend or controlled substance, which the nurse practitioner or certified nurse midwife is not authorized to prescribe under the protocol signed by the collaborating physician and certified registered nurse practitioner or certified nurse midwife and approved under this section unless the drug is specifically ordered for the patient by the physician, either in writing or by a verbal order which has been reduced to writing, and which has been signed by the physician within a time specified in the rules and regulations approved by the State Board of Medical Examiners and the Board of Nursing.

(c) Registered nurses and licensed practical nurses are authorized to administer any legend drug that has been lawfully ordered or prescribed by an authorized practitioner including certified registered nurse practitioners, certified nurse midwives, and/or assistants to physicians.

Citation: ALA. CODE § 34-21-86.

Certified registered nurse practitioners may be granted prescriptive authority upon submission of evidence of completion of an academic course in pharmacology or evidence of integration of pharmacology theory and clinical application in the certified nurse practitioner curriculum.

The drug type, dosage, quantity prescribed, and number of refills shall be authorized in an approved protocol. . . .

The drug shall be included in the formulary recommended by the Joint Practice Committee and adopted by the Board of Nursing and the State Board of Medical Examiners.

When prescribing legend drugs, a certified registered nurse practitioner shall use a prescription form which includes . . . the name, medical practice site address and telephone number of the collaborating physician or covering physician . . . the words "Product Selection Permitted" printed on one side of the prescription form directly beneath the signature line; the words "Dispense as written" printed on one side of the prescription form directly beneath the signature line.

Citation: ALA. ADMIN. CODE r. 610-X-9-17.

ALASKA

The board will, in its discretion, authorize an advanced nurse practitioner or "ANP" to prescribe and dispense legend drugs in accordance with applicable state and federal laws.

A registered nurse who applies for authorization to prescribe and dispense drugs . . . shall provide evidence of completion of 15 contact hours of education in pharmacology and clinical management of drug therapy within the 2-year period immediately before the date of application.

Citation: ALAS. ADMIN. CODE tit. 12, § 44.440.

There is no requirement for physician collaboration.

ARIZONA

A. The Board shall authorize an RNP to prescribe and dispense medication within the RNP's scope of practice only if the RNP:
   1. Is a professional nurse currently licensed in Arizona in good standing and authorized by the Board to practice within a specialty area identified in R4-19-501;
   2. Submits a completed, notarized application on a form provided by the Board containing the following information:
      a. Name, address, and home phone number;
      b. Professional nurse license number;
      c. Nurse practitioner specialty;
      d. Certification number;
      e. Business address and phone number;
      f. Length of time that applicant has practiced as an RNP and whether full or part time;
      g. If a faculty member, the number of hours of direct patient contact during the year preceding the date of application;
      h. Chronological listing of continuing education obtained by the applicant in pharmacology or clinical management of drug therapy or both in the last two years;
      i. Whether the applicant intends to apply for a DEA number to prescribe controlled substances;
      j. Authority for which the applicant is applying; and
      k. Applicant's sworn statement verifying the truthfulness of the information provided.
   3. Submits evidence of completion of a minimum of 45 contact hours of education in pharmacology or clinical management of drug therapy or both:
      a. An applicant shall complete:
         i. At least six of the 45 hours in the 12-month period immediately prior to the application date; and
         ii. All 45 hours within the two-year period before the application date.
      b. One-half (22 hours) of the required contact hours may be from mediated instruction and self-study.

   c. If documented, contact hours may consist of hours of the initial presentations of an RNP who leads, instructs, or lectures to groups of health professionals on pharmacy-related topics in continuing education activities.
   d. An RNP whose primary responsibility is the education of health professionals does not earn contact hours for time expended on normal teaching duties within a learning institution.

B. An applicant who is denied medication P & D authority may request a hearing by filing a written request with the Board within 10 days of service of the Board's order denying the application for P & D authority. Board hearings shall comply with 41 A.R.S. 6, Article 10, and 4 A.A.C. 19, Article 6.

C. An RNP with P & D authority may:
   1. Prescribe medications, medical devices, and appliances;
   2. Provide for refill of prescription-only medications for one year from the date of the prescription.

D. An RNP with P & D authority who wishes to prescribe a controlled substance shall apply to the DEA to obtain a DEA registration number before prescribing a controlled substance. The RNP shall file the DEA registration number with the Board.

E. An RNP with a DEA registration number may prescribe a Class II controlled substance as defined in the Federal Controlled Substance Act, 21 U.S.C. § 801 et seq., or Arizona's Uniform Controlled Substance Act, 36 A.R.S. 27, but shall not prescribe refills of the prescription.

F. An RNP with a DEA registration number may prescribe a Class III or IV controlled substance, as defined in the Federal Controlled Substance Act or Arizona's Uniform Controlled Substances Act, and may prescribe a maximum of five refills in six months.

G. An RNP with a DEA registration number may prescribe a Class V controlled substance, as defined in the Federal Controlled Substance Act or Arizona's Uniform Controlled Substance Act, and may prescribe refills for a maximum of one year.

H. An RNP with P & D authority shall ensure that all prescription orders contain the following:
   1. The RNP's name, address, phone number, and specialty area;
   2. The prescription date;
   3. The name and address of the patient;
   4. The full name, strength, dosage form, and directions for use;
   5. Two signature lines for the prescriber with "dispense as written" under the left signature line and "substitution permissible" under the right; and
   6. The DEA registration number, if applicable.

I. The Board of Nursing shall annually send a list of registered nurse practitioners with P & D authority to the Board of Pharmacy, the Board of Medical Examiners, and the Board of Osteopathic Examiners in Medicine and Surgery.

J. An RNP shall not prescribe or dispense medications without prior Board authority. The Board may impose a civil penalty for each violation, suspend the RNP's P & D authority, and impose other sanctions under A.R.S. § 32-1606(C). In determining the appropriate sanction, the Board shall consider factors such as the number of violations, the severity of the violation and the potential or existence of patient harm.

Citation: ARIZ. ADMIN. CODE R4-19-507.

ARKANSAS

An advanced practice nurse may receive and prescribe drugs, medications, or therapeutic devices appropriate to an advanced practice nurse's area of practice.

Citation: ARK. CODE ANN. § 17-87-310(b)(1).

An advanced practice nurse may prescribe schedule III-V drugs.

Citation: ARK. CODE ANN. § 17-87-310(b)(2).

Prescriptive authority requires:

- Proof of completion of a board-approved advanced pharmacology course that includes preceptorial experience in the prescription of drugs, medicine, and therapeutic devices;
- A collaborative practice with a physician, who has a practice comparable in scope, specialty or expertise to that of the advanced practice nurse on file with the board.

Citation: ARK. CODE § 17-87-310.

CALIFORNIA

Neither this chapter nor any other provision of law shall be construed to prohibit a nurse practitioner from furnishing or ordering drugs or devices when all of the following apply:

(a) The drugs or devices are furnished or ordered by a nurse practitioner in accordance with standardized procedures or protocols developed by the nurse practitioner and his or her supervising physician and surgeon under any of the following circumstances:

1. When furnished or ordered incidental to the provision of family planning services.

2. When furnished or ordered incidental to the provision of routine health care or prenatal care.
3. When rendered to essentially healthy persons.

(b) The nurse practitioner is functioning pursuant to standardized procedure, as defined by Section 2725, or protocol. The standardized procedure or protocol shall be developed and approved by the supervising physician and surgeon, the nurse practitioner, and the facility administrator or his or her designee.

(c) The standardized procedure or protocol covering the furnishing of drugs or devices shall specify which nurse practitioner may furnish or order drugs or devices, which drugs or devices may be furnished or ordered, under what circumstances, the extent of physician and surgeon supervision, the method of periodic review of the nurse practitioner's competence, including peer review, and review of the provision of the standardized procedure.

(d) The furnishing or ordering of drugs or devices by a nurse practitioner occurs under physician and surgeon supervision. Physician and surgeon supervision shall not be construed to require the physical presence of the physician, but does include: (1) collaboration on the development of the standardized procedure, (2) approval of the standardized procedure, and (3) availability by telephonic contact at the time of patient examination by the nurse practitioner.

(e) For purposes of this section, no physician and surgeon shall supervise more than four nurse practitioners at one time.

(f) Drugs or devices furnished or ordered by a nurse practitioner may include Schedule III through Schedule V controlled substances under the California Uniform Controlled Substances Act . . . and shall be further limited to those drugs agreed upon by the nurse practitioner and physician and surgeon and specified in the standardized procedure. When Schedule III controlled substances . . . are furnished or ordered by a nurse practitioner, the controlled substances shall be furnished or ordered in accordance with a patient specific protocol approved by the treating or supervising physician. A copy of the section of the nurse practitioner's standardized procedure relating to controlled substances shall be provided upon request, to any licensed pharmacist who dispenses drugs or devices, when there is uncertainty about the nurse practitioner furnishing the order.

(g) The board has certified that in accordance with Section 2836.3 that the nurse practitioner has satisfactorily completed (1) at least six month's physician and surgeon-supervised experience in the furnishing or ordering of drugs or devices and (2) a course in pharmacology covering the drugs or devices to be furnished or ordered under this section. The board shall establish the requirements for satisfactory completion of this subsection.

(h) Use of the term "furnishing" in this section, in health facilities defined in subdivisions (b), (c), (d), (e), and (i) of Section 1250 of the Health and Safety Code, shall include (1) the ordering of a drug or device in accordance with the standardized procedure and (2) transmitting an order of a supervising physician and surgeon.

(i) "Drug order" or "order" for purposes of this section means an order for medication which is dispensed to or for an ultimate user, issued by a nurse practitioner as an individual practitioner, within the meaning of Section 1306.02 of Title 21 of the Code of Federal Regulations. Notwithstanding any other provision of law, (1) a drug order issued pursuant to this section shall be treated in the same manner as a prescription of the supervising physician; (2) all references to "prescription" in this code and the Health and Safety Code shall include drug orders issued by nurse practitioners; and (3) the signature of a nurse practitioner on the drug order issued in accordance with this section shall be deemed to be the signature of a prescriber for purposes of this code and the Health and Safety Code.

Citation: CAL. BUS. & PROF. CODE § 2836.1.

COLORADO

An advanced practice nurse (APN) may be granted authority to prescribe prescription drugs and controlled substances to provide treatment for persons requiring routine health maintenance or routine preventive care. An APN may be granted authority to prescribe drugs and controlled substances to provide treatment for persons requiring care for an acute self-limiting condition, care for a chronic condition that has stabilized, or terminal comfort care.

Citation: COLO. REV. STAT. ANN. § 12-38-111.6.

An advanced practice nurse applying for prescriptive authority shall provide evidence to the board of the following:

- A graduate degree in a nursing specialty
- Satisfactory completion of specific educational requirements in the use of controlled substances and prescription drugs, as established by the board, either as part of a degree program or in addition to a degree program
- Post-graduate experience as an advanced practice nurse in a relevant clinical setting, as defined by the board, consisting of not less than 1800 hours to be completed within the immediately preceding 5-year period. The board shall define the requirements for such experience to include:

(I) Satisfactory completion of a structured plan;
(II) Adequate interaction between the advanced practice nurse, the physician, and any other health care professional;
(III) Experience with specific drugs relevant to the scope of practice of the advanced practice nurse; and
(IV) Any other requirement the board deems relevant and necessary.

Citation: COLO. REV. STAT. ANN. § 12-38-111.6 and COLO. CODE REGS. § 716-1.

Applicants for prescriptive authority shall:
- Be listed in the Advanced Practice registry;
- Have completed a graduate degree in a nursing specialty;
- Have completed an advanced health/physical and psychological assessment which consists of a minimum of 45 clock hours;
- Have completed advanced pathophysiology/psychopathology which consists of a minimum of 45 clock hours;
- Have completed advanced pharmacology with a minimum of 45 clock hours;
- Have completed precepted experience with weekly interaction between nurse and preceptor; and
- Have experience with specific drugs.

Citation: BOARD RULES, CH. XV.

CONNECTICUT

Policies shall be in place to insure that prescribing activities are reviewed by the physician directing the prescribing in a manner that is consistent with the type of setting in which care is rendered. Such policies shall provide for a periodic review consistent with the type of setting and the nature of patients' health care needs.

Citation: CONN. GEN. STAT. ANN. § 20-87a-5.

All prescription forms used by an Advanced Practice Registered Nurse shall satisfy the requirements of section 20-101c of the general statutes and contain the name, address, and telephone number of the Advanced Practice Registered Nurse who is prescribing medical therapeutics and corrective measures.

An Advanced Practice Registered Nurse who has received a license pursuant to section 20-94a of the general statutes shall use the abbreviation "A.P.R.N." when engaging in any activity authorized under any state or federal statute or regulation that governs practice under such license.

Citation: CONN. GEN. STAT. ANN. § 20-87a-6.

DELAWARE

Advanced practice nursing is the application of nursing principles . . . and includes: . . . [f]or those advanced practice nurses performing independent acts of diagnosis and/or prescription with the collaboration of a licensed physician, dentist, podiatrist, or licensed Delaware health care delivery system, without written guidelines or protocols and within the scope of practice as defined in the rules and regulations promulgated by the Joint Practice Committee and approved by the Board of Medical Practice.

Citation: DEL. CODE ANN. tit. 24, § 1902(d)(1).

The Joint Practice Committee with the approval of the Board of Medical Practice shall have the authority to grant, restrict, suspend or revoke practice or independent practice authorization and the Joint Practice Committee with the approval of the Board of Medical Practice shall be responsible for promulgating rules and regulations to implement the provisions of this chapter regarding "advanced practice nurses" who have been granted authority for independent practice and/or independent prescriptive authority.

Citation: DEL. CODE ANN. tit. 24, § 1906(20).

Those individuals who wish to engage in independent practice without written guidelines or protocols and/or wish to have independent prescriptive authority shall apply for such privilege or privileges to the Joint Practice Committee and do so only in collaboration with a licensed physician, dentist, podiatrist, or licensed health care delivery system. This does not include those individuals who have protocols and/or waiver approved by the Board of Medical Practice.

Citation: DEL. CODE ANN. tit. 24, § 1902(d)(2).

DISTRICT OF COLUMBIA

An advanced practice registered nurse (APRN) may initiate, monitor, and alter drug therapies.

Citation: D.C. CODE ANN. § 3-1206.4.

The APRN may perform actions of medical diagnosis, treatment, prescription, and other functions authorized by this subchapter.

Citation: D.C. CODE ANN. § 3-1206.1.

A nurse practitioner shall have the authority to prescribe legend drugs and controlled substances, Schedules II through V, [subject to certain conditions].

Citation: MUNICIPAL REGS § 5909-5910.

FLORIDA

The scope of practice for all categories of advanced registered nurse practitioner (ARNP) shall include those functions which the ARNP has been educated to perform including the monitoring and altering of drug therapies, and initiation of appropriate therapies, according to the established protocol and consistent with the practice setting.

Citation: FLA. ADMIN. CODE CH. 64B9-4.009.

GEORGIA

A physician may delegate to a physician assistant in accordance with job description or nurse recognized by the Georgia Board of Nursing as certified nurse midwife, certified registered nurse practitioner or clinical nurse specialist, psychiatric/mental health, in accordance with nurse protocol, the authority to order controlled substances selected from a formulary of such drugs established by the Composite State Board of Medical Examiners and the authority to order dangerous drugs. . . .

A physician may delegate to a nurse or physician assistant the authority to order dangerous drugs, medical treatments, or diagnostic studies and a nurse or physician's assistant is authorized to dispense dangerous drugs, in accordance with dispensing procedures and under the authority of an order issued in conformity with a nurse protocol or job description, if that nurse or physician's assistant orders or dispenses those dangerous drugs, medical treatments, or diagnostic studies. [Statute lists further conditions pertinent to specific practice settings; i.e. employee of public health department, any 501(c)(3) organization, the public health service, outpatient department of a hospital].

Citation: GA. CODE ANN. § 43-34-26.1.

HAWAII

NPs have prescriptive authority.

Citation: HAW. Rev. STAT. ANN. § 457-8.6.

To be eligible for prescriptive authority, an APRN shall submit a completed application prescribed by the department and shall submit evidence of satisfying the following requirements:

1. Current and unencumbered recognition as an APRN by the board of nursing in accordance with Chapter 457, HRS, and Chapter 16-89;
2. An official transcript of a master's degree in clinical nursing or nursing science sent directly from the school to the department;

3. Current certification in the nursing practice specialty sent directly to the department from a recognized national certifying body, or if currently licensed by the state department of health, in accordance with Chapter 321, HRS, and Chapter 11-141, evidence of a valid unencumbered license;
4. Successful completion of one of the following within the three-year time period immediately preceding the date of application for prescriptive authority;
   A. At least thirty contact hours, as part of a master's degree program from an accredited college or university, of advanced pharmacology education, including advanced pharmacotherapeutics that is integrated into the curriculum; or
   B. At least thirty contact hours of advanced pharmacology, including advanced pharmacotherapeutics, from an accredited college or university; or
   C. At least thirty contact hours of continuing education approved by board-recognized national certifying bodies in advanced pharmacology, including advanced pharmacotherapeutics related to the applicant's scope of nursing practice specialty.
5. Verification of one thousand hours of clinical experience in an institution as a recognized APRN practitioner in the applicant's nursing practice specialty, within a three-year time period immediately preceding the date of application;
6. A collegial working relationship agreement in compliance with section 16-89C-10, between a physician, who is currently licensed in the State where such license is unencumbered and where such license excludes a limited or temporary license, and a recognized APRN to be granted prescriptive authority; and
7. Payment of a non-refundable application fee.

Citation: HAW. ADMIN. R. § 16-89C-5.

(a) The board of medical examiners shall determine the drugs or categories of drugs listed in the exclusionary formulary for recognized APRNs granted prescriptive authority and shall review or revise the formulary at least every two years. The formulary, entitled "Exclusionary Formulary," dated January 9, 1998, attached to this chapter as Exhibit A and made a part of this chapter, lists the drugs or categories of drugs that shall not be prescribed by the APRN recognized to prescribe by the department.
(b) The Exclusionary Formulary, and any revised formularies, shall be made available to licensed pharmacies at no cost.
(c) Recognized APRNs with prescriptive authority shall not prescribe any substance included in Schedules I, II, III, IV, or V of Chapter 329, HRS.

(d) The recognized APRN with prescriptive authority shall comply with all applicable state and federal laws and rules relating to prescribing, administering, dispensing, and distributing of drugs.
(e) Prescriptions ordered by a recognized APRN with prescriptive authority shall be filled according to the terms of the prescription. In addition to the requirements of section 328-16(b)(1), HRS, a prescription shall also provide the APRN-Rx designation and number of the recognized APRN with prescriptive authority as assigned by the department, and the name and phone number of the collegial working relationship physician. Drugs shall be dispensed in accordance with all applicable laws.

Citation: HAW. ADMIN. R. § 16-89C-15.

Prescriptive authority renewal for recognized advanced practice registered nurses.

(a) Prescriptive authority for recognized APRNs shall expire on December 31 of every odd-numbered year and shall be renewed biennially. In each odd-numbered year, the department shall make available an application for renewal of license before the deadline set forth by the department to every person to whom prescriptive authority was issued or renewed during the biennium. In addition to satisfying the renewal requirements of a APRN in section 16-89-87, the APRN seeking renewal of prescriptive authority shall also submit the following:
    (1) Evidence of current certification in the nursing practice specialty by a recognized national certifying body, or if licensed by the state department of health in accordance with Chapter 321, HRS, and Chapter 11-141, evidence of current licensure;
    (2) Documentation of successful completion, during the prior biennium, of thirty contact hours of continuing education in the practice specialty area, and eight contact hours in pharmacology, including pharmacotherapeutics, related to the applicant's practice specialty area, approved by board recognized national certifying bodies, the American Nurses Association, the American Medical Association, or accredited colleges or universities. Verification of successful completion of continuing education required for recertification by a recognized national certifying body, within the current renewal biennium, may be accepted in lieu of the thirty hours of continuing education required for renewal;
    (3) Notarized statement signed by the renewing recognized APRN with prescriptive authority, the physician, and interim physician attesting that the collegial working relationship agreement on file with the department is still in effect and that the parties are in compliance with section 16-89C-10; and

(4) The renewal fee established for prescriptive authority renewal.

(b) Failure, neglect, or refusal to renew the prescriptive authority by a recognized APRN on or before December 31 of each odd-numbered year shall result in automatic forfeiture of prescriptive authority. Prescriptive authority may be restored within six months, in compliance with subsection (a) and additional payment of a restoration fee. Failure to restore within the time frame provided shall constitute an automatic termination of the prescriptive authority. Thereafter, to be eligible for prescriptive authority, the applicant shall meet the requirements of section 16-89C-5, and submit documentation of successful completion during the prior two years of thirty contact hours of continuing education in the practice specialty area and eight contact hours in pharmacology, including pharmacotherapeutics, approved by board recognized national certifying bodies, the American Nurses Association, the American Medical Association, or accredited colleges or universities.

(c) Any recognized APRN subject to this chapter who fails to renew his or her prescriptive authority and continues to practice as a recognized APRN with prescriptive authority shall be considered an illegal practitioner and shall be subject to penalties provided for by law.

Citation: HAW. ADMIN. R. § 16-89C-20.

IDAHO

Nurse practitioners . . . may perform comprehensive health assessments, diagnosis, health promotion, and the direct management of acute and chronic illness and disease which may include the prescribing of pharmacologic and nonpharmacologic treatments as defined by rules of the board.

Citation: IDAHO CODE § 54-1402(1)(c).

An advanced practice professional nurse who applies for authorization to prescribe pharmacologic and non-pharmacologic agents within the scope of practice for the advanced practice category shall:

i. Be currently licensed as an advanced practice professional nurse in Idaho; and
ii. Provide evidence of completion of thirty (30) contact hours of post-basic education in pharmacotherapeutics . . .

Citation: IDAHO ADMIN. CODE 23.01.01.315.01.

The advanced practice professional nurse when exercising prescriptive and dispensing authority is accountable for:

a. Patient selection;
b. Problem identification through appropriate assessment;
c. Medication and device selection;
d. Patient education for use of therapeutics;
e. Evaluation of outcome; and
f. Recognition and management of complications and untoward reactions.

Citation: IDAHO ADMIN. CODE 23.01.01.315.06.

ILLINOIS

(Section scheduled to be repealed on January 1, 2008)

(a) A collaborating physician may, but is not required to, delegate limited prescriptive authority to an advanced practice nurse as part of a written collaborative agreement. This authority may, but is not required to, include prescription and dispensing of legend drugs and legend controlled substances categorized as Schedule III, IV, or V controlled substances, as defined in Article II of the Illinois Controlled Substances Act.

(b) To prescribe Schedule III, IV, or V controlled substances under this Section, an advanced practice nurse must obtain a mid-level practitioner controlled substance license. Medication orders shall be reviewed periodically by the collaborating physician.

(c) The collaborating physician shall file with the Department notice of delegation of prescriptive authority and termination of such delegation, in accordance with rules of the Department. Upon receipt of this notice delegating authority to prescribe Schedule III, IV, or V controlled substances, the licensed advanced practice nurse shall be eligible to register for a mid-level practitioner controlled substance license under Section 303.05 of the Illinois Controlled Substances Act.

(d) Nothing in this Act shall be construed to limit the delegation of tasks or duties by a physician to a licensed practical nurse, a registered professional nurse, or other personnel.

Citation: 225 ILL. COMP. STAT. 65/15-20.

a) A collaborating physician who delegates limited prescriptive authority to an advanced practice nurse shall include that delegation in the written collaborative agreement. The prescriptive authority may include prescription and dispensing of legend drugs and legend controlled substances categorized as Schedule III, IV, or V controlled substances, as defined in the Illinois Controlled Substances Act [720 ILCS 570]. The authority to prescribe Schedule II controlled substances may not be delegated by the collaborating physician.

b) An APN who has been given controlled substances prescriptive authority shall be required to obtain an Illinois mid-level practitioner controlled substance license in accordance with 77 Ill. Adm. Code 3100. The physician shall file a notice of delegation of prescriptive authority with the Department. The delegation of authority form shall be submitted to the Department prior to the issuance of a controlled substance license.
c) The APN may only prescribe and dispense within the scope of practice of the collaborating physician.
d) All prescriptions written and signed by an advanced practice nurse shall indicate the name of the collaborating physician. The collaborating physician's signature is not required. The advanced practice nurse shall sign his/her own name.
e) An APN may receive and dispense samples per the collaborative agreement.
f) Medication orders shall be reviewed periodically by the collaborating physician.

Citation: ILL. ADMIN. CODE. tit. 68 § 1305.40.

INDIANA

An advanced practice nurse may be authorized to prescribe legend drugs including controlled substances if the advanced practice nurse does the following:

- Submits an application;
- Submits proof of an active, unrestricted Indiana registered nurse license;
- Submits proof of having met the requirements of all applicable laws for practice as advanced practice nurse in the state of Indiana;
- Submits proof of a baccalaureate or higher degree in nursing;
- Submits proof of having successfully completed a graduate level pharmacology course, consisting of at least two (2) semester hours of academic credit from a college or university accredited by the commission on Recognition of Postsecondary Accreditation within five (5) years of the date of application; or as part of a degree program, with clear and convincing proof of subsequent collaborative experience as an advanced practice nurse within the last five (5) years, if the course was completed more than five (5) years, but not more than eight (8) years, prior to the date of application;
- Submits proof of collaboration with a licensed practitioner, in form of a written practice agreement that sets forth the manner in which the advanced practice nurse and licensed practitioner will cooperate, coordinate, and consult with each other in the provision of health care to patients.

Written practice agreements for advanced practice nurses applying for prescriptive authority shall not be valid until prescriptive authority is granted by the board.

Citation: IND. ADMIN. CODE tit. 848, r. 5-1-1.

IOWA

Notwithstanding subsection 1, but subject to the limitations contained in subsections 2 and 3 [see subsections 2 and 3 below], a registered nurse who is licensed and registered as an advanced registered nurse practitioner and who qualifies for and is registered in a recognized nursing specialty may prescribe substances or devices, including controlled substances or devices, if the nurse is engaged in the practice of a nursing specialty under rules adopted by the board of nursing in consultation with the board of pharmacy examiners.

Subsection 2. A pharmacist, physician, dentist, or podiatrist who dispenses prescription drugs, including but not limited to controlled substances, for human use, may delegate nonjudgmental dispensing functions to staff assistants only when verification of the accuracy and completeness of the prescription is determined by the pharmacist or practitioner in the pharmacist's or practitioner's physical presence. . . .

Subsection 3. A physician's assistant or registered nurse may supply when pharmacist services are not reasonably available or when it is in the best interests of the patient, on the direct order of the supervising physician, a quantity of properly packaged and labeled prescription drugs, controlled substances, or contraceptive devices necessary to complete a course of therapy. However, a remote clinic, staffed by a physician's assistant or registered nurse, where pharmacy services are not reasonably available, shall secure the regular advice and consultation of a pharmacist regarding the distribution, storage, and appropriate use of such drugs, substances, and devices.

Citation: IOWA CODE § 147.107.

"Prescriptive authority" is the authority granted to an ARNP registered in Iowa in a recognized nursing specialty to prescribe, deliver, distribute, or dispense prescription drugs, devices, and medical gases when the nurse is engaged in the practice of that nursing specialty. Registration as a practitioner with the Federal Drug Enforcement Administration and the Iowa board of pharmacy examiners extends this authority to controlled substances. ARNPs shall obtain a copy of the Iowa Pharmacy Law and Informational Manual. ARNPs are encouraged to subscribe to the Iowa Board of Pharmacy Newsletter.

Citation: IOWA ADMIN. CODE r. 655-7.1(152).

KANSAS

An advanced registered nurse practitioner may prescribe drugs pursuant to a written protocol as authorized by a responsible physician.

Citation: KAN. STAT. ANN. § 65-1130(d).

Each written protocol pursuant to which an advanced registered nurse practitioner may transmit prescription orders shall:
(1) Specify for each classification of disease or injury the corresponding class of drugs for which the advanced registered nurse practitioner is permitted to transmit a prescription order;
(2) Be maintained in either a looseleaf notebook or a book of published protocols;
(3) Be kept at the advanced registered nurse practitioner's principal place of practice.

Each advanced registered nurse practitioner shall ensure that each protocol is reviewed by the advanced registered nurse practitioner and physician at least annually. Each prescription order in written form shall meet the following requirements:
(1) Include the name, address, and telephone number of the practice location of the advanced registered nurse practitioner;
(2) Include the name, address, and telephone number of the responsible physician;
(3) Be signed by the advanced registered nurse practitioner with the letters A.R.N.P.;
(4) Be from a class of drugs prescribed pursuant to protocol; and
(5) Contain any D.E.A. registration number issued to the advanced registered nurse practitioner when a controlled substance, as defined in K.S.A. 65-4101(e) and amendments thereto, is prescribed.

Nothing in this regulation shall be construed to prohibit any registered nurse or licensed practical nurse or advanced registered nurse practitioner from conveying a prescription order orally or administering a drug if acting under the lawful direction of a person licensed to practice either medicine and surgery or dentistry, or certified as an advanced registered nurse practitioner.

Citation: KAN. ADMIN. REGS. 60-11-104a.

An advanced registered nurse practitioner may prescribe drugs pursuant to a written protocol as authorized by a responsible physician. Each written protocol shall contain a precise and detailed medical plan of care for each classification of disease or injury for which the advanced registered nurse practitioner is authorized to prescribe and shall specify all drugs which may be prescribed by the advanced registered nurse practitioner. Any written prescription order shall include the name,

address, and telephone number of the responsible physician. The advanced registered nurse practitioner may not dispense drugs, but may request, receive, and sign for professional samples and may distribute professional samples to patients pursuant to a written protocol as authorized by a responsible physician. In order to prescribe controlled substances, the advanced registered nurse practitioner shall
(1) register with the federal drug enforcement administration; and
(2) notify the board of the name and address of the responsible physician or physicians. In no case shall the scope of authority of the advanced registered nurse practitioner exceed the normal and customary practice of the responsible physician. An advanced registered nurse practitioner certified in the category of registered nurse anesthetist while functioning as a registered nurse anesthetist under K.S.A. 1988 Supp. 65-1151 to 65-1164, including, and amendments thereto, shall be subject to the provisions of K.S.A. 1988 Supp. 65-1151 and 65-1164, inclusive and amendments thereto, with respect to drugs and anesthetic agents and shall not be subject to the provisions of this subsection. For the purposes of this subsection, "responsible physician" means a person licensed to practice medicine and surgery in Kansas who has accepted responsibility for the protocol and the actions of the advanced registered nurse practitioner when prescribing drugs. As used in this section, "drug" means those articles and substances defined as drugs in K.S.A. 1998 Supp.

Citation: KAN. ADMIN. REGS. 60-11-104 (d).

KENTUCKY

Practice of an Advanced Registered Nurse Practitioner shall include prescribing treatments, drugs and devices, and ordering diagnostic tests which are within the scope and standard of practice of the ARNP.

Citation: 201 KY. ADMIN. REGS. 20:057.

LOUISIANA

An advanced practice registered nurse with limited prescriptive authority approved by the committee may prescribe drugs and therapeutic devices as indicated by clinical practice guidelines and the parameters of the collaborative practice agreement.

An APRN may not prescribe controlled substances, unless explicitly authorized by the Joint Committee.

The collaborating physician's name and office address must appear on the prescription.

Requirements for prescriptive privileges:

- RN licensure
- APRN licensure

- 500 hours of clinical practice as a licensed APRN within the 6 months preceding application
- 36 hours of education in pharmacotherapeutics
- 12 hours of pathophysiology
- Collaborative practice agreement
- Each year . . . 6 hours of continuing education in pharmacology or pharmacologic management.

Citation: LA. ADMIN. CODE tit. 46 § XLVII.4513.

MAINE

Certified nurse practitioners and certified nurse midwives are authorized to prescribe the following:

1. Over the counter drugs
2. Appliances and devices
3. Drugs related to the specialty area of certification
4. Drugs prescribed off label according to common and established standards of practice.

Regardless of the schedules indicated on the certificate issued by the Drug Enforcement Administration, the certified nurse practitioner and certified nurse midwives shall prescribe only those controlled drugs from Schedules II, III, IV, and V. A Drug Enforcement Agency (D.E.A.) number is required to prescribe these drugs.

Citation: CODE ME. R. § 02 380 008.

MARYLAND

A nurse practitioner may prescribe drugs, independently, under the terms and conditions set forth in a written agreement with a physician.

Citation: MD. REGS. CODE tit. 10 § 27.07.02(4).

MASSACHUSETTS

A nurse practitioner may issue written prescriptions and order tests and therapeutics pursuant to guidelines mutually developed and agreed upon by the nurse and the supervising physician in accordance with regulations promulgated jointly by the board and the board of registration in pharmacy. A prescription made by a nurse practitioner shall include the name of the physician with whom guidelines approved by said board and said board of registration in medicine pursuant to section 80B.

Citation: MASS. ANN. LAWS, CH. 112, § 80E.

A nurse engaged in prescriptive practice means one who is authorized to practice in an expanded role, one who has a minimum of 24 contact hours in pharmacotherapeutics which are beyond those acquired in a generic nursing program and one with a valid registration with the Massachusetts Department of Public Health and where required by the Drug Enforcement Administration.

Citation: MASS. REGS. CODE tit. 244, § 4.05.

Guidelines for prescriptive practice shall:

- Include a defined mechanism to monitor prescribing practices, including documentation of review with a supervising physician at least every 3 months;
- Include protocols for initiation of intravenous therapies and Schedule II drugs;
- Specify the frequency of review of initial prescription of controlled substances; the initial prescription of Schedule II drugs must be reviewed within 96 hours;
- Conform to M.G.L. c94C, the regulations of the Department of Public Health at 105 CMR 700.000 et seq., and M.G.L. c. 112 §§ 80E or 80G, as applicable.

Citation: MASS. REGS. CODE tit. 244, § 4.22.

MICHIGAN

A licensee who holds a license other than a health profession subfield license may delegate to a licensed or unlicensed individual who is otherwise qualified by education, training, or experience the performance of selected acts, tasks, or functions where the acts, tasks, or functions fall within the scope of practice of the licensee's profession and will be performed under the licensee's supervision. An act, task, or function shall not be delegated under this section which, under standards of acceptable and prevailing practice, requires the level of education, skill, and judgment required of a licensee under this article.

Citation: MICH. COMP. LAWS § 333.16215(1).

A supervising physician may delegate in writing to a registered professional nurse the ordering, receipt, and dispensing of complimentary starter dose drugs other than controlled substances.

Citation: MICH. COMP. LAWS § 333.17212(1).

MINNESOTA

A nurse practitioner who has a written agreement with a physician based on standards established by the Minnesota Nurses Association and the Minnesota Medical Association that defines the delegated responsibilities related to the prescription of drugs and therapeutic devices, may prescribe and administer drugs and therapeutic devices within the scope of the written agreement and within practice as a nurse practitioner. The written agreement required under this subdivision shall be based on standards established by the Minnesota Nurses Association and the Minnesota Medical Association as of January 1, 1996, unless both associations agree to revisions.

Citation: MINN. STAT. ANN. § 148.235.

MISSISSIPPI

Nurse practitioners practicing in other specialty areas [other than as nurse anesthetists] must practice according to a Board-approved protocol which has been mutually agreed upon by the nurse practitioner and a Mississippi licensed physician whose practice or prescriptive authority is not limited as a result of a voluntary order or legal/regulatory order. The protocol must outline diagnostic and therapeutic procedures and categories of pharmacologic agents which may be ordered, administered, dispensed, and/or prescribed for patients with diagnoses identified by the nurse practitioner.

Citation: MISS. NURSING REGS. CH. IV, § 2.3c.(2).

Authorized nurse practitioners may prescribe Schedules II-V. [Detailed requirements omitted.]

Citation: MISS. NURSING REGS. CH. IV, § 2.4.

Pursuant to a physician's order, a nurse practitioner may call in a prescription for any schedule of controlled substances or administer any schedule of controlled substances, but only after the physician has made an independent determination as to the need for the controlled substance and this is documented in the patient records.

Citation: MISS. NURSING REGS. CH. IV, § 2.3c(4).

MISSOURI

The methods of treatment and the authority to administer, dispense, or prescribe drugs delegated in a collaborative practice arrangement between a collaborating physician and collaborating registered professional nurse or advanced practice nurse shall be within the scope of practice of each professional and shall be consistent with each professional's skill, training, education, and competence.

Citation: MO. CODE REGS. ANN. tit. 4, § 200-4.200(3)(A).

The collaborating physician shall consider the level of skill, education, training, and competence of the collaborating registered professional nurse or advanced practice nurse and ensure that the delegated responsibilities contained in the collaborative practice arrangement are consistent with that level of skill, education, training, and competence.

Citation: MO. CODE REGS. ANN. tit. 4, § 200-4.200(3)(B).

The methods of treatment and authority to administer, dispense, or prescribe drugs delegated to the collaborating registered professional nurse or advanced practice nurse in a collaborative practice arrangement shall also be consistent with the scope of practice of the collaborating physician.

Citation: MO. CODE REGS. ANN. tit. 4, § 200-4.200(3)(C).

The methods of treatment, including any authority to administer and dispense drugs, delegated in a collaborative practice arrangement between a collaborating physician and a collaborating registered professional nurse shall be delivered only pursuant to a written agreement, jointly agreed upon protocols, or standing orders that shall describe a specific sequence of orders, steps, or procedures to be followed in providing patient care in specified clinical situation.

Citation: MO. CODE REGS. ANN. tit. 4 § 200-4.200(3)(F).

Methods of treatment delegated and authority to administer, dispense, or prescribe drugs shall be subject to the following:

1. The physician retains the responsibility for ensuring the appropriate administering, dispensing, prescribing, and control of drugs utilized pursuant to a collaborative practice arrangement in accordance with all state and federal statutes, rules, or regulations;
2. All labeling requirements outlined in section 338.059, RSMo shall be followed;
3. Consumer product safety laws and Class B container standards shall be followed when packaging drugs for distribution;
4. All drugs shall be stored according to the United States Pharmacopeia (USP) recommended conditions;
5. Outdated drugs shall be separated from the active inventory;
6. Retrievable dispensing logs shall be maintained for all prescription drugs dispensed and shall include all information required by state and federal statutes, rules, or regulations;
7. All prescriptions shall conform to all applicable state and federal statutes, rules or regulations and shall include the name, address, and telephone number of the collaborating physician and collaborating advanced practice nurse.

Citation: MO. CODE REGS. ANN. tit. § 200-4.200(I).

An advanced practice nurse shall not, under any circumstances, prescribe controlled substances. The administering or dispensing of a controlled substance by a registered professional nurse or advanced practice nurse in a collaborative practice arrangement shall be accomplished only under the direction and supervision of the collaborating physician, or other physician designated in the collaborative practice agreement, and shall occur on a case-by-case determination of the patient's needs following verbal consultation between collaborating physician and collaborating registered professional nurse or advanced practice nurse. The required consultation and the physician's directions for administering or dispensing of controlled substances shall be recorded in the patient's chart and in the appropriate dispensing log. These recordings shall be made by the collaborating registered professional nurse or advanced practice nurse and shall be consigned by the collaborating physician following a review of the records.

Citation: MO. CODE REGS. ANN. tit. § 200-4.200(I)9.

An advanced practice nurse or registered professional nurse in a collaborative practice arrangement may only dispense starter doses of medication to cover a period of time for seventy-two (72) hours or less with the exception of Title X family planning providers or publicly funded clinics in community health settings that dispense medications free of charge.

Citation: MO. CODE REGS. ANN. tit. § 200-4.200(I)10.

MONTANA

Initial application requirements for prescriptive authority:

- Evidence of completion of 15 continuing education hours in pharmacology . . . within a 3-year period immediately prior to the date the application is received at the board office. This requirement is in addition to the education necessary for an advanced practice registered nurse to obtain original certification. Six of the 15 continuing education hours must have been obtained within one year immediately prior to the date the application is received at the board office. One-third of all continuing education hours must be face-to-face meetings or interaction;
- A copy of the original certification document from the advanced practice registered nurse's certifying body;
- A brief description of the proposed practice;
- A method of referral and documentation in client records;
- A method of quality assurance used to evaluate advanced practice registered nurse.

Citation: MONT. ADMIN. R. 8.32.1504.

The advanced practice registered nurse with prescriptive authority who wishes to prescribe Schedule II-V drugs will comply with federal drug enforcement administration requirements. . . . An advanced practice registered nurse with prescriptive authority who also possesses inpatient care privileges will practice pursuant to a written agreement between the agency and the advanced practice registered nurse which is consistent with the rules, regulations, and guidelines set forth in 37-8-202(5) and 37-2-104, MCA, and ARM 8.32.301 through 8.32.303, and this subchapter.

Citation: MONT. ADMIN. R. 8.32.1505.

An advanced practice registered nurse with prescriptive privilege will have a referral process to licensed physicians and a method for documentation of referral in client records.

Citation: MONT. ADMIN. R. 8.32.1507.

An advanced practice registered nurse with prescriptive authority will submit a method of quality assurance for evaluation of the advanced practice registered nurse's practice. The method of quality assurance will include:

- 30 charts or 5% of all charts handled by the advanced practice registered nurse, whichever is less, must be reviewed quarterly. Review shall be accomplished through the use of a mixture of peer review and review by a physician of the same specialty, as appropriate;
- Use of standards which apply to the APN's area of practice;
- Concurrent or retrospective review of the practice;
- Use of preestablished criteria;
- Written evaluation of a review with steps for corrective activities if indicated and follow-up.

Citation: MONT. ADMIN. R. 8.32.1508.

NEBRASKA

Advanced practice registered nurse practice means health promotion, health supervision, illness prevention and diagnosis, treatment and management of common health problems and chronic conditions including:

(1) Assessing patients, ordering diagnostic tests and therapeutic treatments, synthesizing and analyzing data, and applying advanced nursing principles;

(2) Dispensing, incident to practice only, sample medications. . . .

(3) Prescribing therapeutic measures and medications, except controlled substances listed in Schedule II, related to health conditions within the scope of practice. An advanced practice registered nurse

may prescribe controlled substances listed in Schedule II used for pain control for a maximum 72 hour supply if any subsequent renewal of such prescription is by a licensed physician.

Citation: NEB. REV. STAT. ANN. § 71-1721.

NEVADA

An applicant for a certificate of recognition as an advanced practitioner of nursing will be authorized to issue written prescriptions for poisons, dangerous drugs, and devices only if he:

a. Is authorized to do so by the board; and
b. Submits an application for authority to issue written prescriptions for poisons, dangerous drugs, or devices to the board.
c. Has successfully completed a program [meeting specified requirements].

In addition to the information contained in the application for a certificate of recognition as an advanced practitioner of nursing, the applicant for authority to write a prescription for poisons, dangerous drugs, and devices must include:

d. Documentation of 1,000 hours of active practice in the immediately preceding 2 years as an advanced practitioner of nursing under a collaborating physician. The documentation must consist of a signed statement from the collaborating physician indicating to the board that the applicant is competent to prescribe those drugs listed in his protocols.

Citation: NEV. ADMIN. CODE CH. 632, § 632.257.

An advanced practitioner of nursing may only prescribe poisons, dangerous drugs, or devices which are currently within the standard of medical practice in his identified medical speciality; and listed in his protocols.

Citation: NEV. ADMIN. CODE CH. 632, § 632.259.

The state board of nursing will issue a certificate to dispense controlled substances, poisons, dangerous drugs, and devices to an advanced practitioner of nursing if the practitioner (a) successfully completes an examination administered by the state board of nursing in Nevada law relating to pharmacy; and (b) submits to the board of nursing his affidavit verifying that he has made application with the state board of pharmacy for a certificate of registration.

Citation: NEV. ADMIN. CODE CH. 632, § 632.2595.

NEW HAMPSHIRE

An advanced registered nurse practitioner shall have plenary authority to possess, compound, prescribe, administer, dispense and distribute controlled and noncontrolled drugs to patients from the official formulary established by the joint health council and within the scope of the ARNP's practice as defined by the Board of Nursing.

Citation: N.H. REV. STAT. ANN. § 326-B:10.

NEW JERSEY

A nurse practitioner may order medications and devices in the inpatient setting, subject to the following conditions:

- Controlled substances may be ordered (a) to continue or reissue an order or prescription for a controlled dangerous substance originally ordered or prescribed by the collaborating physician or to otherwise adjust the dosage of that medication, provided there is prior consultation with the collaborating physician . . . (b) for a patient in an end of life situation. . . .
- The order is written in accordance with standing orders or joint protocols developed in agreement between a collaborating physician and the advanced practice nurse, or pursuant to the specific direction of a physician;
- The advanced practice nurse authorizes the order by signing his own name, printing the name and certification number, and printing the physician's name;
- The physician is present or readily available through electronic communications;
- The charts and records of the patients treated by the nurse practitioner are periodically reviewed by the collaborating physician and the nurse practitioner; and
- The joint protocols developed by the collaborating physician and the NP are reviewed, updated, and signed at least annually by both parties.

Citation: N.J. STAT. ANN. § 45:11-49.

An advanced practice nurse may prescribe medications and devices in all other medically appropriate settings, subject to the following conditions:

- Controlled substances may be prescribed (a) to continue or reissue an order or prescription for a controlled dangerous substance originally ordered or prescribed by the collaborating physician or to otherwise adjust the dosage of that medication, provided there is prior consultation with the collaborating physician . . . (b) for a patient in an end of life situation. . . .

- The prescription is written in accordance with standing orders or joint protocols developed in agreement between a collaborating physician and the advanced practice nurse, or pursuant to the specific direction of a physician;
- The advanced practice nurse authorizes the prescription by signing his own name, printing the name and certification number, and printing the physician's name;
- The physician is present or readily available through electronic communications;
- The charts and records of the patients treated by the nurse practitioner are periodically reviewed by the collaborating physician and the nurse practitioner; and
- The joint protocols developed by the collaborating physician and the NP are reviewed, updated, and signed at least annually by both parties.

Citation: N.J. STAT. ANN. § 45:11-49.

Every nurse practitioner issuing prescriptions and orders or dispensing medications in any setting other than a licensed acute care or long-term care facility shall provide the following on all said prescriptions and orders:

1. The prescriber's full name, address, telephone number, license number, certificate number, and academic degree. This information shall be printed on all prescriptions/orders;
2. The full name, age, and address of the patient;
3. The date of issuance of prescription/order;
4. The signature of prescriber, handwritten as "R.N., N.P.C.," or "R.N., C.N.S., C."; and
5. The full name and academic degree of the collaborating physician. For prescriptions only, the address and telephone number of the collaborating physician shall be printed. . . .

Citation: N.J. ADMIN. CODE tit.13, § 37-7.7.

NEW MEXICO

Certified nurse practitioners may . . . practice independently and make decisions regarding health care needs of the individual, family or community and carry out health regimens, including the prescription and distribution of dangerous drugs and controlled substances included in Schedules II through V of the Controlled Substances Act. . . .

Citation: N.M. STAT. ANN. § 61-3-23.2.B(2), C and D.

NEW YORK

Prescriptions for drugs, devices, and immunizing agents may be issued by a nurse practitioner . . . in accordance with the practice agreement and practice protocols. The nurse practitioner shall obtain a certificate from the department upon successfully completing a program including an appropriate pharmacology component, or its equivalent, as established by the commissioner's regulations, prior to prescribing under this subdivision. The certificate issued under section 6910 shall state whether the nurse practitioner has successfully completed such a program or equivalent and is authorized to prescribe under this subdivision.

Citation: N.Y. EDUC. LAW § 6902.3(b).

NORTH CAROLINA

Drugs and devices that may be prescribed by the nurse practitioner in each practice site shall be included in the written standing protocols as outlined in Paragraph (i), Subparagraph (2) of this rule.

Controlled Dangerous Substances (Schedules 2, 2N, 3, 3N, 4, 5) defined by the State and Federal Controlled Substances Act may be prescribed or ordered as established in written protocols, providing all of the following restrictions are met:

1. The nurse practitioner has an assigned DEA number which is entered on each prescription for a controlled substance;
2. Dosage units for Schedule 2, 2N, 3, and 3N are limited to a 30-day supply; and
3. The prescription or order for Schedule 2, 2N, 3, and 3N may not be refilled. [Additional conditions omitted.]

Citation: N.C. ADMIN. CODE tit. 21, r. 36.0227(h).

NORTH DAKOTA

The advanced practice registered nurse with prescriptive authority may prescribe drugs as defined by Chapter 43-15-01 pursuant to applicable state and federal laws.

Citation: N.D. ADMIN. CODE § 54-05-03.1-10.

OHIO

Under a certificate to prescribe issued under Section 4723.48 of the Revised Code, a . . . certified nurse practitioner is subject to all of the following:

(A) The nurse shall not prescribe any drug or therapeutic device that is not included in the types of drugs and devices listed on the formulary established in rules adopted under Section 4723.50 of the Revised Code;

(B) The nurse's prescriptive authority shall not exceed the prescriptive authority of the collaborating physician or podiatrist;

(C) The nurse may prescribe a Schedule II controlled substance as specified in division (A)(2) of section 3719.06 of the Revised Code, but shall not prescribe a Schedule II controlled substance in collaboration with a podiatrist;

(D) The nurse may personally furnish to a patient a sample of any drug or therapeutic device included in the types of drugs and devices listed in the formulary. . . .

Citation: OHIO REV. CODE ANN. § 4723.481.

OKLAHOMA

An advanced registered nurse practitioner shall be eligible to obtain recognition as authorized by the Board to prescribe, as defined by rules promulgated by the Board . . . subject to the medical direction of a supervising physician.

Citation: OKLA. STAT. ANN. tit. 59, § 567.3a.(6).

OREGON

The Oregon State Board of Nursing may grant to a nurse practitioner the privilege of writing prescriptions described in the formulary.

Citation: OR. REV. STAT. § 678.290.

The nurse practitioner is independently responsible and accountable for the continuous and comprehensive management of a broad range of health care, which may include:

. . . Prescription and/or administration of therapeutic devices and measures, including legend drugs and controlled substances as provided in OAR 851-050-0131 and dispensing drugs as provided in OAR 851-050-0133, 0134, and 0145, consistent with the definition of the practitioner's specialty category and scope of practice.

Citation: OR. ADMIN R. 851-050-0005.

The formulary for nurse practitioners with prescriptive authority . . . is based on the following premises:

Nurse practitioner may provide care for specialized client populations within each nurse practitioner's category/scope of practice.

Nurse practitioner prescribing is limited by the nurse practitioner's scope of practice and knowledge base within that scope of practice.

Nurse practitioners may prescribe drugs appropriate for patients within their scope of practice as defined by OAR 851-050-0005.

Nurse practitioners may prescribe drugs for conditions the nurse practitioner does not routinely treat within the scope of their practice provided there is ongoing consultation/collaboration with another health care provider who has the authority and experience to prescribe the drug(s).

Nurse practitioners will be held strictly accountable for their prescribing decisions.

All drugs in the formulary shall have Food and Drug Administration approval.

Nurse practitioners with prescriptive authority are authorized to prescribe:

- All over the counter drugs;
- Appliances and devices;
- The following drugs as listed in Drug Facts and Comparisons dated January 2003. [list omitted]

Citation: OR. ADMIN. R. 851-050-0131.

PENNSYLVANIA

A certified registered nurse practitioner (C.R.N.P.)—a registered nurse . . . who, while functioning in the expanded role as a professional nurse, performs acts of medical diagnosis or prescription of medical therapeutics or corrective measures in collaboration with and under the direction of a physician licensed to practice medicine in this Commonwealth.

Citation: 49 PA CODE § 21.251.

A certified registered nurse practitioner may prescribe medical therapeutic or corrective measures if the nurse is acting in accordance with the provision of Section 8.3 of this Act.

Citation: ACT 206 of 2002 § 8.2.

RHODE ISLAND

Citation for prescriptive authority is General Laws of Rhode Island, 5-34-39.

Prescriptive privileges for certified registered nurse practitioners shall be granted under the governance and supervision of the division of professional regulations, board of nurse regulation and nursing education and include prescription of legend medications and prescription of controlled dangerous substances from Schedules II, III, IV, and V that are established in regulation by the director with advice of the formulary committee. . . .

. . . A certified registered nurse practitioner is permitted to prescribe from a formulary established by the formulary committee in accordance with annually updated guidelines, written in collaboration with the medical director or physician consultant of their individual establishments.

To qualify for prescriptive privileges, an applicant must submit . . . evidence of completion of 30 hours of education in pharmacology within the 3-year period immediately prior to the date of application.

To maintain prescribing privileges, the certified registered nurse practitioner must submit evidence of 30 hours of continuing education in pharmacology every 6 years.

Citation: R.I. GEN. LAWS § 5-34-39.

SOUTH CAROLINA

A nurse practitioner or clinical nurse specialist practicing in an extended role shall perform delegated medical acts pursuant to an approved written protocol between the nurse and the physician.

Citation: 26 S.C. CODE ANN. REGS. 91-6h.1.

Standards for authorized prescriptions by the nurse practitioner with prescriptive authority.

1. Prescriptions for authorized drugs and devices shall comply with all applicable state and federal laws.
2. Prescriptions shall be limited to drugs and devices utilized to treat common well-defined medical problems within the specialty field of the nurse practitioner as authorized by the physician and listed in the approved written protocols. A listing of classifications of drugs as authorized by physicians and listed in approved written protocols will be established jointly by the Board of Nursing, Board of Medical Examiners, and Board of Pharmacy.
3. Controlled substances in Schedules II through IV cannot be prescribed. Controlled substances in Schedule V may be prescribed if listed in the approved written protocols, and as authorized by 44-53-300 of the South Carolina Code of Laws, 1976, as amended.
4. Prescriptions shall be signed by the nurse practitioner with the prescriber identification number assigned by the Board. The prescription form shall include the nurse practitioner's and physician's name, address, and phone number preprinted on the form and shall comply with the provisions of 39-24-40, South Carolina Code of Laws, 1976, as amended. Prescriptions shall designate a specific number of refills. There shall be no nonspecific refill indications.
5. Any drugs or devices prescribed by the nurse practitioner shall be documented in the patient record of the practice and a copy shall be available for review and audit purposes.

6. The nurse practitioner or clinical nurse specialist who holds prescriptive authority may request, receive, and sign for professional samples, except for controlled substances in Schedules II through IV, and may distribute professional samples to patients as listed in the approved written protocols subject to federal and state regulations.

Citation: 26 S.C. Code Ann. Regs. 91-6k.

SOUTH DAKOTA

An NP may accept the delegation of prescription of medications, including controlled drugs or substances listed on Schedule II for one period of not more than forty-eight hours, for treatment of causative factors and symptoms.

Citation: S.D. Codified Laws § 36-9A-12(2).

TENNESSEE

The nurse practitioner who holds a certificate of fitness shall be authorized to prescribe and/or issue controlled substances listed in Schedules II, III, IV, and V of title 39, chapter 17, part 4, upon join adoption of physician supervisory rules concerning controlled substances pursuant to subsection (d).

Citation: Tenn. Code Ann. § 63-7-123(2).

Any prescription written and signed or drug issued by a nurse practitioner under the supervision and control of a supervising physician shall be deemed to be that of the nurse practitioner. Every prescription issued by a nurse practitioner pursuant to this section shall be entered in the medical records of the patient and shall be written on a preprinted prescription pad bearing the name, address, and telephone number of the supervising physician and of the nurse practitioner, and the nurse practitioner shall sign each prescription so written. Where the preprinted prescripton pad contains the names of more than one (1) physician, the nurse practitioner shall indicate on the prescription which of those physicians is the nurse practitioner's primary supervising physician by placing a checkmark beside or a circle around the name of that physician.

Citation: Tenn. Code Ann. § 63-7-123(b)(3).

The Nurse Practice Act T.C.A. § 63-7-101 et seq. requires a certification process for a nurse practitioner to prescribe and/or issue noncontrolled legend drugs.

Process includes:

Certification by the Tennessee Board of Nursing to prescribe and/or issue noncontrolled legend drugs shall authorize a nurse practitioner to prescribe and/or issue such drugs.

A nurse who has been issued a certificate of fitness as a nurse practitioner shall file a notice with the Primary Care Advisory Board pursuant to T.C.A. § 68-1-701 containing;

a. Name of nurse practitioner;
b. A copy of the formulary describing the categories of legend drugs to be prescribed and/or issued; and
c. Name of the licensed physician having the supervision, control, and responsibility for prescriptive services rendered.

Citation: TENN. COMP. R. & REGS. CH 1000-4-.01.

TEXAS

(a) The advanced practice nurse with a valid prescription authorization number:
  (1) Shall carry out or sign prescription drug orders for only those drugs that are:
    (A) Authorized by Protocols or other written authorization for medical aspects of patient care; and
    (B) Prescribed for patient populations within the accepted scope of professional practice for the advanced practice nurse's specialty area; and
  (2) Shall comply with the requirements for adequate physician supervision published in the rules of the Board of Medical Examiners relating to Delegation of the Carrying Out of Signing of Prescription Drug Orders to Physician Assistants and Advanced Practice Nurses as well as other applicable laws.

(b) Protocols or other written authorization shall be defined in a manner that promotes the exercise of professional judgment by the advanced practice nurse commensurate with the education and experience of that person.
  (1) A protocol or other written authorization:
    (A) Is not required to describe the exact steps that the advanced practice nurse must take with respect to each specific condition, disease, or symptom; and
    (B) May state types or categories of medications that may be prescribed or contain the types or categories of medications that may not be prescribed.
  (2) Protocols or other written authorization:

(A) Shall be written, agreed upon and signed by the advanced practice nurse and the physician;
(B) Reviewed and signed at least annually; and
(C) Maintained in the practice setting of the advanced practice nurse. . . .

Citation: 22 TEX. ADMINISTRATIVE CODE § 222.4.

UTAH

"Practice of an advanced practice registered nursing" means the practice of nursing within the generally recognized scope of advanced practice registered nursing as defined in division rule and consistent with professionally recognized preparation and education standards of an advanced practice registered nurse by a person licensed under this chapter as an advanced practice registered nurse. Advanced practice registered nursing includes:
(a) Maintenance and promotion of health and prevention of disease;
(b) Diagnosis, treatment, correction, consultation, or referral for common health problems; and
(c) Prescription or administration of prescription drugs or devices, including local anesthesia, Schedule IV-V controlled substances; and Schedule II-V controlled substances in accordance with a consultation and referral plan.

Citation: UTAH CODE ANN. § 58-31b-102(16).

VERMONT

Prescriptions may be written and signed by the APRN for those medications covered in practice guidelines and in compliance with all other state laws and regulations. A list of endorsed APRNS will be made available to the Vermont Board of Pharmacy.

Advanced practice registered nurses may initiate written or oral orders in accordance with practice guidelines which may be carried out by other health care providers.

The APRNs shall retain professional accountability for APN care when delegating interventions.

Citation: VT. CODE Rules, CH. 4.VIII.C.4.h. and i.

VIRGINIA

In accordance with the provisions of this section and pursuant to the requirements of Chapter 33 (§ 54.1-3300 et seq.) of this title, a licensed nurse practitioner, other than a certified registered nurse anesthetist, shall have the authority to prescribe controlled substances and devices as set forth in Chapter 34 (§ 54.1-3400 et seq.) of this title as follows: (i) Schedule V and VI controlled substances on and after July 1, 2000; (ii) Schedules IV through VI on and after January 1, 2002; and (iii) Schedules II through VI controlled substances on and after July 1, 2003. Nurse practitioners shall have such prescriptive authority upon the provision to the Board of Medicine and the Board of Nursing of such evidence as they may jointly require that the nurse practitioner has entered into and is, at the time of writing a prescription, a party to a written agreement with a licensed physician, which provides for the direction and supervision by such physician of the prescriptive practices of the nurse practitioner. Such written agreements shall include the controlled substances the nurse practitioner is or is not authorized to prescribe and may restrict such prescriptive authority as deemed appropriate by the physician providing direction and supervision. . . .

Citation: VA. CODE ANN. § 54.1-2957.01.A.

The following restriction shall apply to any nurse practitioner authorized to prescribe drugs and devices pursuant to this section:

1. The nurse practitioner shall disclose to his patients the name, address, and telephone number of the supervising physician, and that he is a licensed nurse practitioner.
2. Physicians, other than physicians employed by, or under contract with, local health departments, federally funded comprehensive primary care clinics, or nonprofit health care clinics or programs to provide supervisory services, shall not supervise and direct at any one time more than four nurse practitioners. In the case of nurse practitioners other than nurse midwives, the supervising physician shall regularly practice in any location in which the nurse practitioner exercises prescriptive authority pursuant to this section. A separate office for the nurse practitioner shall not be established. . . .
3. Physicians employed by, or under contract with, local health departments, federally funded comprehensive primary care clinics, or nonprofit health care clinics or programs to provide supervisory services, shall not supervise and direct at any one time more than four nurse practitioners who provide services on behalf of such entities. Such physicians either shall regularly practice in such settings or shall make periodic site visits to such settings as required by regulations promulgated pursuant to this section. . . .

Citation: VA. CODE ANN. § 54.1-2957.01.E.

A nurse practitioner with prescriptive authority may prescribe only within the scope of a written practice agreement with a supervising physician.

A new practice agreement shall be submitted:

1. With the initial application for prescriptive authority; or
2. With the application for each biennial renewal, if there have been any changes in supervision, authorization, or scope of practice; or
3. At any time a change in the primary supervising physician shall occur.

The practice agreement shall contain the following:

1. A description of the prescriptive authority of the nurse practitioner within the scope allowed by law and the practice of the nurse practitioner.
2. An authorization for categories of drugs and devices within the requirements of § 54.1-2957.01 of the Code of Virginia.
3. The signatures of the primary supervising physician and any secondary physician who may be regularly called upon in the event of the absence of the primary physician.

Citation: 17 VA. ADMIN. CODE 90-40-90.

Physicians who enter into a practice agreement with a nurse practitioner for prescriptive authority shall:

1. Supervise and direct, at any one time, no more than four nurse practitioners with prescriptive authority.
2. Regularly practice in any location in which the licensed nurse practitioner exercises prescriptive authority. A separate practice setting may not be established for the nurse practitioner. Exceptions to this requirement are as follows:
   a. A separate office practice may be established for a certified nurse midwife or for a nurse practitioner employed by or under contract with local health department, federally funded comprehensive primary care clinics, or nonprofit health care clinics or programs.
   b. Physicians who do not regularly practice at the same location with the nurse practitioner and who provide supervisory services to such separate practices shall make regular site visits for consultation and direction for appropriate patient management. The site visits shall occur in accordance with the practice agreement, but no less frequently than once a quarter.
3. Conduct a monthly, random review of patient charts on which the nurse practitioner has entered a prescription for an approved drug or device.

Citation: VA. ADMIN. CODE 90-40-100.

WASHINGTON

An advanced registered nurse practitioner under his or her license may perform for compensation nursing care, as that term is usually understood, of the ill, injured, or infirm and in the course thereof, she or he may do the following things that shall not be done by a person not so licensed, except as provided in RCS 18.79.260 and 18.79.270:

(1) Perform specialized and advanced levels of nursing as recognized jointly by the medical and nursing professions, as defined by the commission;
(2) Prescribe legend drugs and Schedule V controlled substances, as defined in the Uniform Controlled Substances Act, chapter 69.50 RCS, and Schedule II through IV subject to RCW 18.79.240(1)(r) or (s) within the scope of practice defined by the commission;
(3) Perform all acts provided in RCS 18.79.260;
(4) Hold herself or himself out to the public or designate herself or himself as an advanced registered nurse practitioner or as a nurse practitioner.

Citation: WASH. REV. CODE 18.79.250.

The dispensing of Schedules II through IV controlled substances subject to RCW 18.79.240(1)(s) is limited to a maximum of a seventy-two-hour supply of the prescribed controlled substance.

Citation: WASH. Rev. CODE 18.79.255.

An advanced registered nurse practitioner licensed under chapter 18.79. RCW when authorized by the nursing commission may prescribe drugs pursuant to applicable state and federal laws. The ARNP when exercising prescriptive authority is accountable for competency in:

1. Patient selection;
2. Problem identification through appropriate assessment;
3. Medication and/or device selection;
4. Patient education for use of therapeutics:
5. Knowledge of interactions of therapeutics, if any;
6. Evaluation of outcome; and
7. Recognition and management of complications and untoward reactions.

Citation: WASH. ADMIN. CODE 246-840-400.

WEST VIRGINIA

The board may, in its discretion, authorize an advanced nurse practitioner to prescribe prescription drugs in a collaborative relationship with a physician licensed to practice in West Virginia and in accordance with applicable state and federal laws. An authorized advanced nurse practitioner may write or sign prescriptions or transmit prescriptions verbally or by other means of communication.

For purposes of this section an agreement to a collaborative relationship for prescriptive practice between a physician and an advanced nurse practitioner shall be set forth in writing. . . .

Collaborative agreements shall include, but not be limited to, the following:

1. Mutually agreed upon written guidelines or protocols for prescriptive authority as it applies to the advanced nurse practitioner's clinical practice;
2. Statements describing the individual and shared responsibilities of the advanced nurse practitioner and the physician pursuant to the collaborative agreement between them;
3. Periodic and joint evaluation of prescriptive practice; and
4. Periodic and joint review and updating of the written guidelines or protocols.

The board shall promulgate legislative rules . . . governing the eligibility and extent to which an advanced nurse practitioner may prescribe drugs. Such rules shall provide, at minimum, a state formulary classifying those categories of drugs which shall not be prescribed by advanced nurse practitioners, including, but not limited to, Schedules I and II of the Uniform Controlled Substances Act, anticoagulants, antineoplastics, radio-pharmaceuticals, and general anesthetics. Drugs listed under Schedule III shall be limited to a seventy-two hour supply without refill. . . .

Citation: W.V. CODE ANN. § 30-7-15.

WISCONSIN

The board shall grant a certificate to issue prescription orders to an advanced practice nurse who meets the education, training, and examination requirements established by the board for a certificate to issue prescription orders. . . .

Citation: WIS. STAT. § 441.16.

Advanced practice nurse prescribers shall communicate with patients through the use of modern communication techniques.

Advanced practice nurse prescribers shall facilitate collaboration with other health care professionals, at least 1 of whom shall be a physician, through the use of modern communication techniques.

Advanced practice nurse prescribers shall facilitate referral of patient health care records to other health care professionals and shall notify patients of their right to have their health care records referred to other health care professionals.

Advanced practice nurse prescribers shall provide a summary of a patient's health care records, including diagnosis, surgeries, allergies, and current medications to other health care providers as a means of facilitation case management and improved collaboration.

Citation: WIS. ADMIN. CODE § N8.10(2), (3), and (4).

WYOMING

"Advanced practitioner of nursing" means a registered professional nurse who performs advanced nursing acts and who may perform medical acts including prescribing or providing prepackaged medications, except Schedule I drugs as defined in W.S. 35-7-1013 and 35-7-1014, in collaboration with a licensed or otherwise legally authorized physician or dentist, in such manner to assure quality and appropriateness of services rendered.

Citation: WYO. STAT. ANN. § 33-21-120.

The board may authorize an advanced practitioner of nursing or "APN" to prescribe drugs, within the recognized scope of advanced specialty practice. . . .

Citation: WYO. BOARD OF NURSING RULES, CH. 4, § 8(a).

CHAPTER 6

Hospital Privileges

It is a tradition of medicine that a patient who needs to be admitted to a hospital is admitted through the patient's primary physician, who visits the patient in the hospital and coordinates the care. That tradition is now being challenged by the realization that the tradition is highly inefficient. More and more, "hospitalists," that is, physicians and nurse practitioners who specialize in the care of hospitalized patients, are taking over this aspect of primary care practice.

Hospital privileges were so termed because hospitals "awarded" the status of admitting physician to community physicians who had gone through a hospital's screening process. The screening process, administered by the physicians who already had privileges, was partly focused on credentialing and partly focused on keeping competing specialists out.

With the number of hospital days declining, that is, the duration a patient remains in the hospital, hospitals are more interested in broadening their market. While hospitals will want to be sure that the providers ordering hospital care are competent and adequately credentialed, a hospital wanting to maximize its business also will want to maximize the number of providers who can bring patients to a hospital. Therefore, hospitals are becoming more open to giving nurse practitioners (NPs) admitting privileges.

ARE HOSPITAL PRIVILEGES AN ISSUE FOR NPs?

NPs can perform primary care without hospital privileges as long as they arrange for patients who need hospitalization to be covered by a provider with hospital privileges or a hospitalist. Nevertheless, if a health plan requires that its primary care providers (PCPs) have hospital privileges, then NPs will need hospital privileges to be PCPs.

Physicians, when arguing to health plans that only physicians should be PCPs, have used hospital privileges as a way to distinguish themselves from NPs. NPs, they argue, do not have admitting privileges and therefore should not be PCPs. Two things are left unsaid. First, some NPs have admitting privileges.

Second, many primary care physicians are declining to pursue hospital practice and hospital privileges because of the inefficiencies of having to be in two places—office and hospital—at once.

DO PCPS NEED HOSPITAL PRIVILEGES?

A patient in need of hospitalization who is being cared for by an NP or a physician PCP can be accommodated in several ways. One approach is for the PCP who has hospital privileges to admit patients and continue to manage care during hospitalization. The PCP coordinates specialty consultation, writes admission and discharge orders, takes calls from hospital nurses about the patient's progress, and evaluates the patient on site once or twice a day, or more as needed.

A second possible approach is for a PCP to turn the care of patients in need of hospitalization over to a physician who has admitting privileges and who does hospital-based care, and to have patients admitted under that physician's care. The care of the patient returns to the PCP's direction after discharge. In this case, the PCP might visit the hospitalized patient, but the visit would be a social or courtesy visit rather than a medical visit. Physicians who advocate this arrangement are seeking reimbursement for social visits.

A third approach is for a PCP to admit to a hospital's staff hospitalists.[1] The third approach makes sense. The arguments in its favor are: (1) patients get round-the-clock access to a physically present provider of medical care; (2) the hospitalists devote all of their attention, every day, to hospitalized patients; (3) the community-based PCP need not feel torn between visiting hospitalized patients and conducting office visits; (4) the expertise of PCPs is not spread thin by the necessity of being an expert on hospital care; (5) admission and discharge are more efficient because hospitalists are on site to do the initial and discharge evaluation and order writing; and (6) nursing care is more efficient because nurses need not deal with off-site attending PCPs. At a time when hospital days are being monitored by health plans, it is the hospitalists who have the most potential for keeping utilization at a safe minimum.

There is only one strong argument against hospitalists. A patient may have established a close relationship with his or her PCP and presumably trusts his or her PCP. When hospitalized, the patient may feel more comfortable with the PCP directing the patient's care. The counterarguments are: (1) there is nothing to prevent the PCP from visiting or calling the patient who is hospitalized, (2) the PCP presumably has chosen a competent hospital with a competent hospitalist, (3) patients are accustomed to being referred to specialists and may likewise feel comfortable with being referred to hospitalists, and (4) many consumers of health care no longer have the close one-on-one relationship with one PCP, since they are signed on with a managed care plan that may have teams of PCPs.

WHAT IF HEALTH PLANS REQUIRE PCPs TO HAVE ADMITTING PRIVILEGES?

Health plans have medical directors. Medical directors usually are physicians. Physician medical directors may believe that the traditional way of handling hospitalized patients—attendance by the internist—is best, or they may believe that requiring PCPs to have hospital privileges is a way to ensure that only physicians will be PCPs.

On the other hand, health plan executives who are not physicians may respond positively to an argument that a PCP will do better to devote efforts to keeping patients out of the hospital by being available in the office for telephone and in-person communication with ambulatory patients and other providers. As long as a health plan's patients will be attended to by qualified providers, the health plan may not insist that the PCP be the in-hospital provider. As more and more data emerge about the effectiveness of hospitalists, managed care organizations are backing down from any requirement that PCPs must have admitting privileges.

DO NPs NEED HOSPITAL PRIVILEGES FOR ADVANCEMENT OF THE PROFESSION?

There are two arguments supporting the assertion that NPs who wish to be PCPs should seek hospital privileges.

First, it is a credential that carries weight among professionals. It is something professional groups boast about and battle about, and something that individual professionals strive for. Physicians sometimes use NPs' lack of hospital privileges as an argument that NPs should not be designated PCPs by managed care organizations. If the majority of NPs had hospital privileges, physicians would not be able to use the hospital privilege argument against NPs.

Second, some health plans and managed care organizations want their PCPs to have admitting privileges. If that is the case, and an NP wants to be a PCP, the NP will need to get hospital privileges.

DO INDIVIDUAL NPs NEED HOSPITAL PRIVILEGES?

The NP who does not need hospital privileges to be a PCP may not want them. For an individual NP weighing the pros and cons of hospital privileges, the issues are:

- Whether an NP needs hospital privileges to be an effective PCP;
- Whether local health plans require PCPs to have admitting privileges;
- Whether patients are better served by hospitalists or by attendance by their PCP;
- Whether hospitalists are available in a local hospital;
- Whether NP applications for hospital privileges are being accepted or denied by a local hospital.

An NP debating whether to apply for admitting privileges should consider what privileges will allow an NP to do, what not having privileges will keep an NP from doing, how difficult it will be to get admitting privileges, and what alternatives there are to the NP's personally admitting patients to hospitals. For example, answer the questions:

- Does a managed care organization with whom the provider wants to associate require admitting privileges?
- Is there a physician with admitting privileges who will take on an NP's patients when they need hospitalization?
- Does the local hospital have hospitalists who manage inpatient care?

Some NPs have found that the physicians they work with want them to have admitting privileges and support those NPs' applications. In other cases, physicians themselves have decided not to concentrate on admitted patients, but rather to work with other inpatient-oriented physicians to care for admitted patients. Further, while some NPs are educated in acute care-oriented graduate programs, others consider themselves experts on primary care only. Hospital care is, by definition, secondary, not primary care. An NP may wish to concentrate on primary care and may not wish to spread professional interests too thin.

Finally, an NP should look at the economics of taking on hospital visits. Managing hospitalized patients can take a large portion of an NP's day, and if there are few patients in the hospital, reimbursement may not be rewarding. For example, if a hospital visit can be billed at $50 but it takes 15 minutes to see the patient, 5 minutes to discuss the care with nursing staff and/or write orders and note, and 20 minutes each way between office and hospital, an NP will net only $50 per hour. In the office, an NP can bring in approximately $40 per 20-minute visit, or $120 per hour. A hospitalist can bill the $50 for the 20-minute visit but can also bill $50 for visits to other hospitalized patients and can bring in $150 per hour.

WHO HAS HOSPITAL PRIVILEGES?

Traditionally, only physicians had hospital privileges. Privileges were granted or denied on the basis of criteria to which only the hospital and physicians involved were privy. Physicians who were denied hospital privileges—often not because of any lack of expertise, but because a hospital already had one endocrinologist, or one radiation oncologist—sought admission by suing the hospital or by lobbying for legislation requiring impartial third-party review of hospital privilege denials. For example, the following New York law protects physicians, podiatrists, optometrists, and dentists from discrimination from hospitals in the matter of staff privileges:

> A hospital may not refuse to act upon an application for staff membership or professional privileges, or deny privileges for a physician, podiatrist, optometrist or dentist, without stating the reasons therefor,

> or if the reasons stated are unrelated to standards of patient care, patient welfare, the objectives of the institution or the character or competency of the applicant.
>
> *Citation:* N.Y. PUB. HEALTH LAW § 2801-b.1.

The law also states that "if a hospital does not follow proper procedure, above, the physician, podiatrist, etc. may file a complaint with the public health council, which will make a prompt investigation and may recommend that the hospital review its actions" (N.Y. PUB. HEALTH LAW § 2801-b.2. & 3).

Historically, dentists, podiatrists, optometrists, and clinical psychologists did not have admitting privileges. Recently, those professions have made progress in obtaining hospital privileges. Their organizations and individuals applied pressure through the courts and the legislature and eventually, in some states at least, got admitting privileges.

Nurse midwives have admitting privileges in some states. For example, in Oregon, nurse midwives (and NPs) have had statutorily permitted hospital privileges since the mid-1970s. The permissive legislation was passed at a time when midwives were needed in rural areas because obstetricians found that malpractice insurance was too expensive and gave up delivering babies. The Oregon legislature was convinced that nurse midwives needed admitting privileges to give rural Oregonians the ability to have attended deliveries. When the issue came before the Oregon legislature, the Oregon Nurses Association suggested that the legislature take the opportunity to permit all NPs, not just nurse midwives, to have admitting privileges. The bill passed. The law states:

> The rules of any hospital in this state may grant admitting privileges to NPs licensed and certified under ORS 678.375 for purposes of patient care, subject to hospital and medical staff bylaws, rules, and regulations governing admissions and staff privileges.
>
> Rules shall be in writing and may include, but need not be limited to:
>
> - Limitations on the scope of privileges;
> - Monitoring and supervision of nurse practitioners in the hospital by physicians who are members of the medical staff;
> - A requirement that an NP co-admit patients with a physician who is a member of the medical staff; and
> - Qualifications of NPs to be eligible for privileges including but not limited to requirements of prior clinical and hospital experience.[2]
>
> *Citation:* OR. REV. STAT. § 441.064.

The rules also may regulate the admissions and the conduct of NPs while using the facilities of the hospital and may prescribe procedures whereby an NP's privileges may be suspended or terminated. The hospital may refuse such privileges to NPs only upon the same basis that privileges are refused to other medical providers.

DOES FEDERAL LAW SUPPORT FULL HOSPITAL PRIVILEGES FOR NPs?

Federal law states that every hospitalized patient covered by Medicare must be under the care of a physician [42 U.S.C.S. § 1395x(e)(4)]. The Federal government has defined *physician* as a licensed doctor of medicine, osteopathy, dental surgery or dental medicine, podiatric medicine, chiropractic, or optometry (42 C.F.R. § 410.20). In 1994, clinical psychologists got an amendment to the Social Security Act to add language to federal Medicare law that allows hospitalized patients to be under the care of a clinical psychologist [42 U.S.C.S. § 1395x(e)(4)].

Federal regulation requires that every Medicare patient be "under the care of a doctor of medicine or osteopathy who may delegate tasks to other qualified health care personnel to the extent recognized under State law or a State's regulatory mechanism" (62 Fed. Reg. 224: 66756; proposed change to 42 C.F.R. § 482.20).

NPs who deliver care to hospitalized patients presumably fall under the delegation rule.

WHAT DOES IT MEAN TO HAVE HOSPITAL PRIVILEGES?

When a patient is admitted to a hospital, the admitting provider is the contact person for the hospital regarding the patient's care while hospitalized. Reports are given to the admitting provider, and it is agreed that decisions, such as readiness for discharge, are made by the admitting provider.

Unless a provider has privileges, some hospitals will not allow that provider to review a patient's chart, much less order treatments. Part of the rationale for this is patient confidentiality. It is the hospital's responsibility to protect the confidentiality of admitted patients. There have to be limits set upon who can have access to confidential documents. It would be inefficient for an administrator or nurse to have to decide on a visit-by-visit basis whether any particular provider should have access to patient records. Therefore, hospitals have developed systems for granting of admitting privileges to providers who have been screened and credentialed. By hospital policy, providers with privileges have full access to information about the patients they admit, have decision-making authority and ordering authority, and may have a variety of other privileges, such as designated parking spaces, eating areas, and educational programs, as a matter of policy.

LEVELS OF PRIVILEGE

Hospitals may have levels of privileges, which they may designate as *associate, affiliate, independent,* or some other term.

Associate privileges may mean that privileges are less than full. For example, providers who have associate privileges may be able to review the records but not write orders. Or, they may be able to review charts and write orders but not admit. Each hospital has its own policies on this matter. Some NPs who have admitting privileges have full privileges, and some NPs have limited privileges.

THE APPLICATION PROCESS

Often the medical staff governing body—traditionally physicians—decides which other providers may have hospital privileges. The medical staff governing body is a separate entity from hospital administration. It may be subject to the requirements of accreditation organizations, state laws, and federal laws.

Competency and experience are the general criteria that a medical staff group will look at in granting or denying privileges. Many hospitals require an applicant to be recommended by a present member of the medical staff, and, after research into credentials is done, a vote is taken on the applicant. Because of this club-type aspect of the privileging process, some qualified applicants have been denied privileges in the past because of non-competency–related personality issues, such as competition, personal bias, or prejudice.

Physician-oriented professional associations often have taken on the task of urging that privileging decisions be based on competency rather than friendship or lack thereof. Accrediting organizations also evaluate the emphasis on competency and experience in a hospital's privileging process as part of the accreditation review.

EXPENSE

There may be an application fee or annual fee for hospital privileges.

DENIAL OF PRIVILEGES

The lack of discussion in professional publications and at NP conferences would suggest that NPs are not applying for privileges in great numbers. Some NPs have had admitting privileges for years. Some NPs are applying for and receiving admitting privileges. Some NPs have lost admitting privileges when they left physician practices.

While there is a multitude of reported court decisions regarding other classes of health care providers who were denied privileges—family physicians, optometrists, and chiropractors, for example—there are no reported opinions regarding denial of admitting privileges to NPs.

Federal law regarding conditions of participation in Medicare state that a medical staff governing body must ensure that the accordance of staff membership or professional privileges in the hospital is not dependent solely upon certification, fellowship, or membership in a specialty body or society [42 C.F.R. 482.12(a)7]. It is not certain how this law relates to nonphysicians or whether NPs have challenged the law in court to find out whether it relates to NPs.

EXPECT CHANGE

Hospital admissions are declining around the nation. Hospitals are finding new product lines. Hospitals are consolidating, merging, and closing. It is in the interest of hospitals to draw patients from as many sources as possible. Therefore, hospitals may be opening their staff privileges to more classes of health care providers. If NPs decide they need hospital privileges, they should call the intended hospital, ask about the process, and apply.

NOTES

1. Henry, L. A. Working with Hospitalists. Fam Pract Manag 1997; 4:32–34, 37–42.

2. American Medical Association. Council on Ethical and Judicial Affairs, Opinion 4.07.

CHAPTER 7

Negligence and Malpractice

Nurse practitioners (NPs) carrying out their daily routine have one thing that appears on their "to do" list every single day: "Do no harm." Nevertheless, when an NP, or any other health care provider, makes hundreds of decisions a day, it is inevitable that mistakes will be made.

For example, researchers studying medical errors at a major teaching hospital followed nurses and doctors for nine months on three surgical units. They found that some medical error was made with almost half of the patients and that at least 18 percent of the patients had a serious consequence. Only 1 percent of these patients sued for malpractice, however.[1]

Though malpractice lawsuits against NPs are rare, the financial and emotional sequelae of being sued are so dire that it is worth dealing with this subject in depth. The incidence of lawsuits against NPs is difficult to state accurately, for a variety of reasons.

First, a filed lawsuit has no meaning other than to state that a person believes him- or herself to have been harmed. The belief may be unfounded. The blame may be placed on the wrong person. The complaint may not even meet the definition of malpractice. So, tracking the incidence of filed suits is of very limited value.

Second, some suits that are filed and that name NPs, do so not because the plaintiff believes an NP caused harm, but because an NP is a member of a team of caregivers who are being sued and because at the early stages of a lawsuit it is not clear who is responsible. On the other hand, some NPs who actually have been negligent may not be sued, for a variety of reasons.

Third, unless an insurance company reports a damage award—a successful lawsuit or a settlement for damages—against an NP to the National Practitioner Data Bank (NPDB), a lawsuit may come to light only if one searches county or insurance company records. Insurance companies are required to report damage awards to the NPDB. If a suit is filed but the plaintiff is unsuccessful in proving the necessary elements for malpractice, there will be no report filed with the NPDB. Keeping a national tally of unsuccessful lawsuits filed against NPs is almost impossible.

This said, one snapshot of the incidence of successful lawsuits against NPs placed the rate at 0.6 per 1,000 NPs, as compared with 38 per 1,000 for physicians.[2]

WHAT CAN HAPPEN TO AN NP WHO IS SUED?

An NP who is sued may feel like leaving the profession, may doubt his or her ability to make decisions, may resort to over-referring and seeking unnecessary consultation, may find that his or her insurance rates are increased, may miss days of work while testifying, may have to pay some legal expenses, and may have to mount a defense before the state licensing board.

Boards of nursing do not automatically investigate NPs who have lost malpractice lawsuits. However, if someone involved with the case reports the NP to the board of nursing, and the negligence approaches the level of gross negligence, the board of nursing will investigate. Gross negligence, for a professional, is the intentional failure to perform a professional duty in reckless disregard of the consequences.

LIFE CYCLE OF A LAWSUIT

A lawsuit starts with filing of pleadings with the state court, usually in the county where the incident occurred. Some states direct malpractice actions to an arbitration panel. The case is presented to the arbitration panel, and the panel makes a decision in favor of one party. Either party may appeal, in which case there will be a trial. A judge or jury decides in favor of one party. Either party may then appeal to a higher state court. Rarely, a party will seek an appeal to a federal court. Federal courts may accept or refuse appeals from the state courts. It is possible that a malpractice case could go to the US Supreme Court, but highly unlikely. Usually, the highest state court of appeals is the highest level of consideration of a malpractice case, and often the parties will let the matter drop after the state trial court case. Because the holdings of state trial courts are not published, the public cannot easily access information on malpractice trials unless there is an appeal. The opinions of appeals courts are published, and that is the information attorneys and professionals can use to gain insight into malpractice cases.

WHAT IS MALPRACTICE?

Malpractice is the failure of a professional to exercise that degree of skill and learning commonly applied by the average prudent, reputable member of the profession. Negligence is the predominant legal theory of malpractice liability. Negligence includes failure to follow up, failure to refer when necessary, failure to disclose necessary information to a patient, and failure to give necessary care.

ELEMENTS OF MALPRACTICE

For success, plaintiff must prove the following elements:

1. NP owed plaintiff a duty.
2. NP's conduct fell below the standard of care.
3. NP's conduct caused plaintiff's injury.
4. Plaintiff was injured.

Duty

A duty is established when there is a provider-patient relationship. A visit to the NP's office by a patient establishes an NP's duty to a patient. But there need not be an office visit to establish duty. Duty can be established by a telephone conversation or casual discussion with a patient or with someone who is not officially a patient. If an NP gives professional advice or treatment in any setting, a duty may be established. If an injured party has reason to believe that there was a provider-patient relationship, there may in fact be such a relationship, even if the provider did not think of the interaction in that way.

What Is the Standard of Care for NPs?

NPs are duty bound to use such reasonable, ordinary care, skill, and diligence as NPs in good standing in the same general type of practice in similar cases.

An NP is held to the standard of care of a reasonably prudent NP, and not necessarily to the standard of care expected of a physician. In many situations, however, the standards of care for MDs and NPs will be identical. For example, an NP doing primary care can be expected to be held to the same standard as a physician doing primary care.

If an NP is sued for malpractice, the standard of care will be argued in court. If an NP believes that she or he met the standard of care, the NP's attorney will enlist expert witnesses, usually other NPs, who will give testimony describing the steps that a reasonably prudent NP would take in a similar situation. The plaintiff's attorney also will enlist expert witnesses, who can be expected to testify that the standard of care called for other measures than those performed by the defendant NP. A judge or jury will accept either the plaintiff or the defendant's explanation of the standard of care and will then decide whether the defendant NP met that standard.

Causation of Injury

For malpractice to have occurred, a breach of the standard of care must have caused an injury to the plaintiff. For example, a patient visits an NP and is diagnosed with otitis media. The NP prescribes penicillin, to which the patient is allergic, as is marked on the patient's chart. The patient leaves the clinic with penicillin, but before she takes the penicillin, she is stung by a bee on the front steps of the clinic. She has an allergic reaction to the bee sting, falls, and hits her head, causing a permanent scar on her face. The patient sues the clinic and the NP, claiming that the NP had a duty to the patient, the NP breached the standard of care (by prescribing penicillin for a penicillin-allergic patient), and the patient suffered an injury. All of the above claims are true, but there is no malpractice because the breach of the standard of care (prescribing penicillin to an allergic patient) did not cause the injury (the wound to the head).

Injury

A provider may be terribly negligent, but if there is no injury, there is no malpractice. For example, if an NP prescribes penicillin to a patient who is allergic, and the patient takes the penicillin but has no reaction that injures the patient, then there is no malpractice, even though the standard of care has been breached and even though, if an injury occurred, there would have been a causal relationship between breach of the standard of care and injury.

EXAMPLES OF LAWSUITS AGAINST NPS

Missed Diagnosis

Example 1: The patient, a middle-aged man, began experiencing chest pain at work. He called the clinic and got an appointment for 4 PM. He worked until 4 PM and went to the clinic. An NP evaluated the patient, took a history and examined him, and conferred with a physician. The NP diagnosed muscle spasm and initiated treatment with Valium.

The patient went home, went to sleep, and awakened at 1 AM with severe chest pain. He went to the emergency department, where he was examined by a physician. A chest X-ray was taken. The physician diagnosed muscle spasm. He ordered Demerol, intramuscularly, and prescribed oral codeine.

At noon the next day, the patient's chest pain returned and was more severe. He went to the emergency department. An electrocardiogram was done, which showed a myocardial infarction. Finally, a correct diagnosis was made. The patient recovered but did not return to full-time work for 18 months. The patient sued for lost wages and won against the NP, the physicians, and Kaiser [*Fein v. Permanente Med. Group*, 38 Cal. 3d 137, 695 P.2d 665, 211 Cal. Rptr. 369 (1985)].

What NPs Can Learn from This Case: Rule out the worse diagnosis early on, especially if it can be done easily and inexpensively, as with an electrocardiogram.

Example 2: An NP saw a young married female patient for symptoms of cramps, headache, dysmenorrhea, and lesions on the perineum during menses. The NP examined the patient and, on the basis of the physical exam, diagnosed genital herpes. The NP counseled the patient about causes, prevention, and treatment. A physician working with the NP prescribed an antiviral medication appropriate for treating genital herpes.

The symptoms continued. The patient saw another physician, who correctly diagnosed the lesions as severe candidiasis.

The patient sued the NP and the employing MD, claiming pain and suffering and expenses of treatment. The patient's husband claimed loss of society, companionship, and conjugal relationship with his wife.

The court dismissed the case against the NP but found that the MD associated with the NP had breached the standard of care. The plaintiff won against the MD.

The physician appealed the case, asking whether the NP's mistake was correctly imputed to the physician. The appeals court said it was [*Adams v. Kreuger*, 124 Idaho 74, 856 P.2d 864 (1993)].

What NPs Can Learn from This Case:

1. The diagnosis of a sexually transmitted disease carries with it an emotional component. A patient surely will discuss the matter with the partner, and relationships may break up as a result. Confirm physical exam findings with laboratory testing, especially when diagnosing sexually transmitted diseases.
2. Some courts do not consider NPs to be professionally responsible for their judgments.

Example 3: A patient came to a medical office for a history and physical. An NP took the history and noted that there was a remote history of ulcer, with no recent complaints. The patient came back later complaining of back pain. A physician read the NP's history and began the patient on aspirin. The patient developed a gastrointestinal bleed. The patient sued the NP for failing to diagnose an ulcer and sued the physician for failing to order an endoscopy before starting the patient on aspirin. The court found for the NP and the physician. The court found that the patient had failed to prove a connection between the patient's gastrointestinal bleed and the failure to diagnose the ulcer or order an endoscopy earlier [*Topp v. Logan*, 197 Ill. App. 3d 285, 554 N.E.2d 454, 143 Ill. Dec. 519 (App. Ct. 1 Dist. 1990)].

What NPs Can Learn from This Case: Not every bad outcome is someone's fault. There must be causation between a breach in the standard of care and a poor outcome. See malpractice element 3, above.

Example 4: A patient saw a family NP for a complaint of discharge and constant scabbing of one of her nipples, of several months' duration. The NP ordered topical and oral antibiotics and a mammogram, which was negative. The patient returned seven months later with continuing pain and discharge from the same nipple. The NP referred the patient to a dermatologist. The patient did not see the dermatologist.

Four months later, the patient saw her gynecologist, who again treated her breast symptoms with antibiotics, and assured her that she did not have cancer.

The patient saw the NP several more times during the year following the first visit. Reasons for the patient's visits were varied. Eighteen months after the first visit, the patient came to the NP with unmistakable masses in her breast. The NP referred the patient to a surgical oncologist, who diagnosed Paget's disease. The cancer had metastasized, and the patient died shortly after the diagnosis. The patient's family sued the NP, the patient's family practitioner, and the gynecologist, and won damages against all three providers. The court said all three providers had breached the standard of care [*Jenkins v. Payne*, 465 S.E.2d 795 (Va. 1996)].

What NPs Can Learn from This Case: An NP must follow up symptoms from past visits, even when a patient does not continue to complain about the symptom. In this case, the NP should have continued to ask, on subsequent visits, whether the breast discharge had resolved and whether the patient had followed up with the dermatologist. Unless the patient stated that the breast discharge and scabbing had resolved (in which case the NP should have documented resolution of the symptom), the NP should have followed up with biopsy when the symptoms did not respond to the initial antibiotics.

Failure To Refer

Example 1: A 36-year-old pregnant patient received prenatal care at a women's health center from an NP and an MD. On the first prenatal visit, the woman told the NP she would like an amniocentesis. The NP explained that it was a very dangerous procedure and did not refer the woman to anyone to talk about amniocentesis.

Later in her pregnancy, the woman was examined by an MD at the center. The patient again introduced the subject of amniocentesis. The MD asked why she was worried, as 37 years of age was the age when one becomes concerned about Down syndrome. The physician dropped the matter, and so did the patient.

After the baby was born and it was discovered that the baby had Down syndrome, a geneticist took the mother aside and asked whether she had heard of amniocentesis. She said she had discussed it with the physician, and he had said it was unnecessary. The geneticist said that by the time she had talked to the doctor, it would have been too late for amniocentesis.

The patient sued the NP and MD at the women's center, claiming that they had failed to properly advise her with respect to amniocentesis and genetic counseling. The patient claimed that if she had been properly advised she would have had an amniocentesis, it would have revealed that the fetus had Down syndrome, and she would have had an abortion.

The trial court found in favor of both the NP and the MD. The appeals court reversed the trial court, saying that the MD had breached the standard of care—that at 36 to 37 years of age, an amniocentesis was indicated if the patient had a high level of concern.

The NP was not held liable because the patient had testified at trial that after her conversation with the NP, she still was determined to get the amniocentesis, and that the conversation with the NP did not affect her decision to go for amniocentesis [*Azzolino v. Dingfelder*, 71 N.C. App. 289, 322 S.E. 2d 567 (Ct. App. 1984)].

What NPs Can Learn from This Case:

1. Providers must practice within the standard of care.
2. When a patient asks for a specific test, strongly consider getting the test, especially when some providers' interpretations of the standard of care would call for getting the test.
3. This NP escaped liability because the patient did not place great weight on the NP's opinion. That is a hollow victory for the NP.

Negligent Practice Involving IUDs

Example 1: Insertion of IUD into a Pregnant Woman. The patient, who had a history of irregular menstrual cycles and menses during pregnancy, visited Planned Parenthood on August 22. The patient listed her last menstrual period as August 8. An NP and patient discussed birth control methods. The patient chose IUD. The NP told the patient to return during her next menses for IUD insertion. The NP and patient discussed the need for birth control in the interim. The patient chose abstinence. The patient's next menstruation was on October 22. The patient visited Planned Parenthood on October 24. The NP cursorily examined the patient and inserted an IUD. The patient had vaginal bleeding for the next two weeks. The patient reported bleeding to the clinic and was told that this was not unusual. Shortly thereafter, the patient had a miscarriage. The patient sued the NP for negligent insertion of an IUD into a pregnant patient. The patient won the case against the NP and Planned Parenthood [*Planned Parenthood v. Vines*, 543 N.E. 2d 654 (Ind. App. 1989)].

What NPs Can Learn from This Case:

A pregnancy test and careful evaluation of regularity of menses for the past three months is always indicated prior to IUD insertion.

Example 2: Negligent Attention to Patient Complaint. The patient had an IUD placed in 1972. In 1974, the patient read an article in the *New York Times* about the Dalkon Shield. The patient consulted her physician and told him she was having uterine bleeding. The physician reassured her about the Dalkon Shield and told her not to worry about the bleeding. In 1975, the patient noted a foul vaginal odor "like dead fish." The patient called the clinic and talked with an NP. The NP advised the patient to douche with yogurt. One week later, the patient called the clinic to complain of severe abdominal pain. The NP told the patient the pain was probably caused by the gastrointestinal flu, and to call again if the patient became febrile. The patient came to the clinic one week later. On examination, pelvic abscesses were found. The patient had a hysterectomy. The patient sued the NP and the clinic. The patient won the case [*Gagino v. Harvard Community Health Plan*, 403 N.E.2d 1166 (1980)].

The defendants appealed. The appeals court noted: (1) Yogurt douche is a lay remedy, inappropriate for treating this patient's complaint. (2) A delay of 48 hours in scheduling an examination was substandard care. (3) There was no documentation of a telephone conversation between the NP and the patient. (4) The medical records were difficult to read.

What NPs Can Learn from This Case:

1. Always document telephone conversations with patients.
2. Consult a patient's chart when giving telephone advice. If the NP had documented in the chart and consulted the chart, the NP would have put the sequence of complaints together and most likely would have considered pelvic infection rather than gastrointestinal flu.
3. A patient with an IUD and abdominal pain requires an examination within 24 hours.
4. Sloppy record keeping hurts NPs if a matter goes to court.

Example 3: Lack of Adequate Counseling. The patient requested and had an IUD inserted by an NP. The NP highly recommended the Dalkon Shield, saying it was almost as effective as birth control pills. The patient got pregnant. The NP told the patient she should have an abortion to avoid the "risk of blood poisoning." The patient saw a physician for an abortion. The physician told the patient she could leave the IUD in and go on with the pregnancy. The patient decided against continuing the pregnancy and had an abortion. Seven years later, the patient watched a "60 Minutes" television segment on the Dalkon Shield. The patient was especially interested in the statement that the manufacturer had concealed the side effects of IUDs and that the pregnancy rate actually was higher than originally stated. The patient then sued the NP for understating risks of pregnancy with IUD. The judge dismissed the case because the statute of limitations had run: that is, the patient waited too long before initiating legal action [*Snow v. A.H. Robins Co., Inc.*, 211 Cal. 165 CA 3d 120 (3rd App.) Rptr. 271 (1985)].

What NPs Can Learn from This Case:

Sometimes a lawsuit will arise from circumstances beyond the NP's control. That is, problems with the Dalkon Shield were not recognized until patients began to sue and the media began to cover the problem. An NP recommending an IUD may be practicing prudently at the time, but new information may provide basis for malpractice litigation at a later date.

THE NATIONAL PRACTITIONER DATA BANK

The NPDB is a repository for damage award data; that is, payments from professional liability insurance companies on behalf of their clients to injured parties for successful malpractice claims. NPDB also records adverse actions against providers by licensing boards, hospitals, and professional quality assurance committees.

The NPDB is under the responsibility of the US Department of Health and Human Services. It was established under a law that intended to encourage hospitals, state licensing boards, and other health care entities to discipline those who engage in unprofessional behavior and to restrict the ability of incompetent physicians, dentists, and other health care practitioners to move from state to state without disclosure of the practitioner's previous dangerous performance.

Under the law, any malpractice insurer who pays any amount to a plaintiff on behalf of an NP in a malpractice case must report that payment to the NPDB. If an NP pays an injured patient directly to settle a matter, that payment need not be reported. The insurer must also report damage awards to state licensing boards. A malpractice insurer must report to the NPDB any amount of dollars paid on behalf of a client to a plaintiff. If a health care provider pays an injured party directly, that need not be reported. In addition, state licensing boards are required to report adverse licensure actions, hospitals are required to report adverse clinical privilege actions, and professional societies are required to report adverse professional society membership actions.

Hospitals must check the NPDB data every two years before granting clinical privileges. Certain agencies may check the NPDB data. The general public does not have access to the NPDB data. Individual NPs may see their NPDB file and add a brief comment to give the NP's version of an incident.

WORKING WITH PRACTICE GUIDELINES

An NP may be following practice guidelines as a matter of law, policy, or good practice. Some states require an NP to establish practice protocols or guidelines, with or without a physician's input.

NPs should consult state law to determine whether written guidelines are required. General guidelines for writing guidelines include:

1. Do not write guidelines so detailed that the guidelines cannot reasonably be followed in everyday practice.
2. Base guidelines on widely used resources, and reference those resources in the guidelines.
3 Practices may adopt an already published set of guidelines.
4. Follow the guidelines.
5. If the guidelines are inappropriate for a particular patient, document why an alternative tack is being taken.
6. If guidelines are not followed because a patient will not comply, document efforts to follow guidelines and patient noncompliance.

The Agency for Healthcare Research and Quality (AHRQ), a federal agency that establishes guidelines for practice and conducts research into what works and what does not work in health care prevention and treatment, has established guidelines for the care of certain conditions. An NP who is caring for patients with conditions addressed by AHRQ would be wise to follow the AHRQ guidelines or to document why the guidelines are inappropriate to a particular patient. AHRQ changes its guidelines fairly frequently to keep up with new evidence. Visit the AHRQ web site at www.ahrq.gov to check for new and retired guidelines.

HOW TO PREVENT LAWSUITS

1. Be careful about establishing patient-provider relationships. If an NP gives medical advice, the NP has a patient and should exercise all of the cautions and standards that the NP would exercise with a patient in the office or hospital.
2. Know the standard of care and practice within it.
3. If practice guidelines or protocols have been adopted by the office or agency, follow them.
4. If in doubt, take the conservative approach.
5. Rule out the worst diagnoses early on.
6. Know the limits of training and expertise.
7. Follow up.

WHAT TO DO IF SUED

1. Call the NP's professional liability insurance company to report the lawsuit.
2. Do not talk about the suit with anyone but the NP's attorney. Specifically, do not talk with the plaintiff-patient or the plaintiff's attorney.
3. Consider retaining the NP's own attorney if the suit is against a group.
4. Never change a record after learning of a lawsuit (or for any other reason).
5. A deposition—a pretrial information-gathering session—can be as important as a trial in terms of need for preparation. What an NP says in deposition can lock the NP into what he or she may say at trial.
6. Think carefully before agreeing to settle. Settlement awards will appear on an NP's NPDB record.

COMMUNICATION

Researchers who compared the time physicians spent with patients with malpractice history found that primary care doctors with two or more malpractice claims against them spent 15 minutes on average with each patient, whereas doctors with no malpractice claims against them spent an average of 18.3 minutes with each patient. Quality-of-care ratings for the sued physicians were as good as ratings for physicians who had not been sued.[3]

It is no news to experienced NPs that good provider-patient communication means better outcomes and higher patient satisfaction. Good communication also means fewer lawsuits. Satisfied patients generally do not sue.

LIABILITY OF COLLABORATING PHYSICIANS

While in the past some courts have found physicians liable for the negligent acts of NPs, in each of these cases there was some element of physician involvement in the misdiagnosis. Nevertheless, physicians cannot expect to be fully free from threat of lawsuit for the acts of the NPs they collaborate with or supervise until the legal requirements for collaboration are lifted.

Medical practices and agencies that set policies calling for supervision of NPs and other advanced practice nurses can expect to be held liable when NPs are not, in fact, supervised.

Consider the following example: A Texas hospital had a contract with a group of anesthesiologists to provide anesthesia services. The anesthesia group employed certified registered nurse anesthetists (CRNAs). The contract between hospital and anesthesia group stated that all CRNAs would be supervised by the anesthesia group. The hospital's written policies and procedures required "direct and personal" supervision of CRNAs by physicians. Hospital policy also required that (1) patients be fully informed about the anesthesia providers who would be providing care, (2) an anesthesiologist prepare and evaluate patients about to have surgery, (3) CRNAs document and discuss the evaluation of their patients with a supervising anesthesiologist or surgeon, and (4) the supervising physician countersign all orders for medications.

One night, a CRNA, working without an anesthesiologist on site, attempted to intubate a patient having respiratory distress during a Caesarean section. The CRNA called the anesthesiologist on call to come in right away. The anesthesiologist immediately headed for the hospital. The CRNA eventually was able to intubate, but the patient suffered irreversible brain injury.

The patient and her husband made a settlement with the CRNA and physician. The plaintiff's suit against the hospital went to trial. The plaintiffs argued that the hospital was negligent for failing to adopt, implement, and enforce appropriate policies relating to providing an anesthesiologist, having an anesthesiologist evaluate the patient, supervising the CRNA, disclosing that a nurse was providing anesthesia; failing to exercise care in credentialing; and failing to ensure proper quality assurance and peer review in the anesthesia department.

The jury found that the hospital had not followed its own policies. The jury also found that the CRNA and physician were not negligent but found that the hospital was negligent, that the hospital's negligence was the cause of the patient's injuries, and that the hospital was liable for the injury to the patient.

The hospital appealed the case. The appeals court upheld the jury's decision [*Denton Reg. Med. Ctr. v. LaCroix*, No. 2-95-003-CV (Tex. Ct. App. June 26, 1997)].

A physician is not automatically liable for negligence of an NP with whom the physician has a written agreement to collaborate when called upon. Some neglect by the physician has to be proven.

On the other hand, if a physician is required, by policy or law, to supervise, then a physician has the responsibilities of supervisors in general. In general, employers and supervisors must determine that their employees or supervisees are adequately trained and competent in the areas in which they practice. If employees or supervisees are not adequately trained or competent, then the employer or supervisor is obligated to provide further training and guidance or to replace the employee or supervisee. If policies are called for, by law or higher policy, supervisors are responsible for ensuring that policies are in place. If supervisors know that policies are not being followed by employees or supervisees, it is the supervisors' responsibility to monitor supervised personnel until policies are followed, or to replace the personnel.

Guidelines for physicians who are required by law or policy to collaborate or supervise NPs and who want to avoid malpractice based on the negligence of an employed NP include:

1. Ascertain that the NP is licensed, and verify the NP's education, training, and malpractice history.
2. Co-manage patients with the NP until the physician can confirm that the NP is professionally competent.
3. Consult state law to determine whether co-signature of NPs' notes is required and whether there are time limits on co-signatures. Conform with state requirements.
4. Consult state law regarding scope of NP practice. Do not encourage the NP to go further than scope of practice allows unless the physician develops written protocols or is physically present.
5. Telephone diagnosis is risky for both the physician and the NP. If an after-hours call is a necessity of practice, establish a second level of call whereby NPs taking call can get backup.
6. Consult state law to determine whether an NP is independent, or dependent upon physician collaboration or supervision. If supervision is required by law, determine whether direct or indirect supervision is required. "Direct supervision" of an NP requires a physician to be immediately and physically available should the need arise. "Indirect supervision" or "general supervision" requires that the physician be on the premises or available by telephone in a timely and consistent manner.
7. If practice guidelines or protocols exist, follow them.
8. Consider supporting NP organizations in their efforts to eradicate legal requirements of supervision or collaboration. Support legal language that places responsibility for an NP's actions squarely on the NP. A physician who employs an NP who is independently responsible for the NP's actions is less likely to be vicariously liable for an NP's malpractice, and a physician can spend less time in supervisory activities.

MALPRACTICE INSURANCE

An NP cannot control everything. Everyone makes mistakes. Insurance provides a comfort factor that is well worth the money.

Four frequently asked questions about malpractice insurance are: (1) Do I need to have my employer cover me under the hospital/university/practice policy? (2) Will I be more likely to be sued if I have malpractice insurance? (3) Should I get "claims made" or "occurrence" insurance? and (4) Which company's policy is best?

Do I Need Insurance If My Employer Covers Me under the Hospital, University, or Practice Policy?

NPs who treat patients outside of their work settings or who moonlight definitely need individual insurance policies. For example, many NPs are approached by neighbors, friends, and relatives for a prescription. The wise NP will not only treat each of these encounters as thoroughly as if the friend was a patient at the office (or decline to become involved at all), but have malpractice insurance to cover the possibility of a mistake.

An NP who neither moonlights nor treats neighbors and friends may still want an individual policy, even if an employer covers an NP under an umbrella policy. Why? Because a lawsuit fractures collegial alliances. The human tendency is to deny one's own liability and blame others. In such an environment, each health care provider needs an advocate to protect his or her interests. Insurance will pay for that defense.

Will I Be More Likely To Be Sued If I Have Malpractice Insurance?

Possibly. But that is not a good reason to forego insurance. Patients do not usually know whether an NP has malpractice insurance. An injured patient who consults an attorney usually files suit before the patient or his or her attorney knows the insured status of the health care provider being sued. Information about the insurance usually comes out in the discovery process in preparation for trial.

However, an NP who tells patients about his or her malpractice coverage may provide an incentive for a litigious patient or may relieve a reluctant patient from any feeling of guilt over suing a respected health care provider.

Should I Get "Claims Made" or "Occurrence" Insurance?

Get "occurrence," which covers any incident that occurred while the NP was insured. Under a "claims made" policy, an NP is covered only when the insurance policy is active, no matter when the incident occurred. If an NP retires, leaves the profession, or no longer has need for active insurance, the NP must nevertheless keep a claims made insurance policy active to receive coverage for incidents that happened in years past. A claims made policy is extended through purchasing of a "tail" policy.

Which Company's Policy Is Best?

NPs should choose a company that is located in the United States (in case the NP has to sue the insurance company), has been in business at least 10 years, and has a stable financial rating.

An NP will be able to judge the quality of his or her insurer only after a lawsuit is over. There are no surveys of sued NPs that provide guidance as to which company provides the best service.

NOTES

1. Andrews, LB. An alternative strategy for studying adverse events in medical care. Lancet 1997; 349: 309–313.
2. Data for a period studied between March 1992 and July 1993; Birkholz, G. Malpractice data from the National Practitioner Data Bank. Nurse Pract 1995; 20:32–35.
3. Levinson, W., Roter, D., Mullooly, J., Dull, V., Frankel, R. The relationship with malpractice claims among primary care physicians and surgeons." JAMA 1997; 227:553–559.

RESOURCES

The Gold Sheet, newsletter from the Law Office of Carolyn Buppert. www.buppert.com.

Medical Malpractice Verdicts, Settlements, and Experts, newsletter, Lewis Fasha, 901 Church St., Nashville, TN 37203, 800-298-6288.

CHAPTER 8

Risk Management

Risk management is what one does to avoid problems later. Compare risk management to preventive medicine; risk management is preventive law.

Nurse practitioners (NPs) are at risk for two categories of professional mishap: clinical mishap and business mishap. There can be great overlap between clinical and business problems; that is, a clinical problem can turn into a business problem and then into a legal problem. For example, when an NP makes a clinical error and a patient discovers the error, the patient is quite likely to tell friends, relatives, and coworkers. Then the problem has evolved into a business problem for the NP. The friends, relatives, and coworkers of that patient are unlikely to visit the NP. If the patient is harmed by the NP's error and files a lawsuit based on malpractice, the NP also has a legal problem.

Any NP faces certain risks associated with practice:

- Risk of making a clinical error.
- Risk of being sued for malpractice when there was no clinical error.
- Risk of public perception that the NP is a poor-quality provider.
- Risk of breaching patient confidentiality and/or privacy.
- Risk of failing to inform patients fully about treatment and to get informed consent to treatment.
- Risk of failing to disclose information that patients need to get follow-up.
- Risk of poor quality ratings.
- Risk of disciplinary action.
- Risk of Medicare fraud for upcoding a patient visit.
- Risk of business failure for downcoding patient visits.

Whether any of these risks becomes an actual problem is largely up to the NP.

RISK OF MAKING A CLINICAL ERROR

Medical professionals who have been sued report that the experience soured their attitude toward their professions. NPs are rarely sued. Nevertheless, a lawsuit, even a lawsuit where the NP is found to be not liable, is a devastating personal experience. Therefore, every nurse practitioner should incorporate into his or her practice an awareness of how to avoid malpractice.

NPs will maintain their positive attitudes toward their profession by practicing litigation avoidance techniques just as they would advocate preventive medicine and health care maintenance to their patients. Avoidance measures include exercising caution about establishing patient-provider relationships and, when a patient-provider relationship has been established, practicing consistently in conjunction with the accepted standard of care for NPs.

What Is Malpractice?

Malpractice is a failure of professional skill that results in injury, loss, or damage. To prove malpractice, a patient/plaintiff must prove:

1. The existence of a client/professional relationship.
2. Behavior below the appropriate standard of care for professionals dealing in like circumstances.
3. A causal link between the practitioner's failure to conform to treatment standards and harm to the patient.
4. Actual injury to the patient.

For more information on medical malpractice, see Chapter 7.

Existence of a Professional Relationship

A patient-provider relationship is established when a patient arrives at an NP's office for a visit, when an NP undertakes the care of a hospitalized patient, or when an NP makes a home visit to a patient. However, patient-provider relationships also can arise in other, not-so-obvious ways, including:

- Over the telephone
- At a social gathering
- By supervising another's treatment
- By providing sample medication
- By giving advice or opinions to family or friends

When Is a Person a "Patient"?

Consider the following example: NP Jones receives a message to call Nurse Smith at home. Nurse Smith is a former colleague of NP Jones, and Jones remembers Smith as a very talented and competent nurse. Smith is calling about a personal health matter. Smith's son, James, age 6, has an earache. James has had several earaches in the past, all caused by infections, all cleared by amoxicillin. James is otherwise completely healthy, reports Smith.

Smith is working the evening shift, and James is in first grade all day. Smith does not have time to see James's pediatrician until the end of the month, two weeks away. Nor does Smith want to pay the $20 copay to see the pediatrician. NP Jones remembers that he met James once at a picnic but has never seen James in the office. Smith recalls that she has always respected NP Jones's judgment. Smith asks NP Jones, a family NP, to prescribe amoxicillin for James. Smith is asking a favor, as she and NP Jones both know that Smith's insurance with an HMO will not reimburse NP Jones for an office visit.

Is six-year-old James NP Jones's patient? Yes, if NP Jones calls in a prescription for James.

Risk Management by Limiting Patient Relationships

If NP Jones gives any advice to Smith or prescribes any medication, NP Jones has taken on a professional relationship with James, and James is NP Jones's patient. NP Jones will then be liable for any breach in the standard of care that leads to an injury to James. It does not matter that James is the patient of another provider. It does not matter that NP Jones will receive no compensation for treating James. It does not matter that the interaction is solely telephone advice.

NP Jones, to protect himself (manage his risk), should either: (1) politely refuse to give advice, other than that Smith should call James's pediatrician, or (2) require Smith to bring James to NP Jones's office to go through the usual new-patient evaluation before Jones prescribes an antibiotic or otherwise treats James. NP Jones should then follow up with James as NP Jones would with any of his patients.

For 95 out of 100 times that NP Jones is presented with a situation like this, NP Jones could proceed to treat the child over the telephone with no ill effects to the child or to NP Jones's malpractice history. However, NP Jones will be liable in court for the 5 percent of cases where: (1) the mother makes an erroneous diagnosis; (2) the mother does not know that the organism in the child's ear is resistant to the antibiotic used in the past; or (3) there is some other problem that NP Jones would have elicited with a careful history and physical examination.

In short, NPs should say "no" to all requests they receive for care that skirts the normal, safe evaluation process. The lesson of this case may seem elementary to experienced NPs. However, it is included because the pressure is great to deliver care to people who "just want a little advice" but are not "patients." It is easy for an NP to forget that the NP bears professional responsibility for any health care advice given to anyone.

What Is the Standard of Care for NPs?

The standard of care in any clinical situation is discovered by answering the question: What reasonable and ordinary care, skill, and diligence would be given by practitioners in good standing, in the same geographic area, in the same general type of practice in similar cases?

NPs are held to the standard of care of the reasonable and diligent NP. Is this the same standard that pertains to physicians? It may be. If the NP is performing primary care services, for example, the standard of care for an NP and for a physician performing those services will be the same standard.

Consider the example of *Fein v. Kaiser Permanente* given in Chapter 7. The *Fein* case is a good illustration of a missed diagnosis. In that case, Mr. Fein, a middle-aged attorney, called a Kaiser clinic at midday complaining of chest pains. He got a 4 PM appointment, at which time he was evaluated by an NP, who incorrectly diagnosed musculoskeletal pain. Mr. Fein was having a myocardial infarction. Later in the evening, Mr. Fein was evaluated by a physician, who also incorrectly diagnosed Mr. Fein's chest pain. It was not until Mr. Fein's third visit that an electrocardiogram was done.

The NP easily could have ruled out myocardial infarction through an electrocardiogram at the first visit. That would be risk management. A prudent NP faced with a middle-aged male patient with chest pain would rule out myocardial infarction before diagnosing musculoskeletal pain. In this case, the NP and physician shared the same standard of care.

How Does an NP Keep Up with the Standard of Care?

Sources of information about standards of care for any specific disease or health care maintenance effort include:

- Textbooks and reference books
- Professional journals
- Respected colleagues
- Continuing-education presentations
- Government agency-generated guidelines, such as Agency for Healthcare Research and Quality (AHRQ) guidelines

An NP who wishes to avoid breaching the standard of care will consult current books and journals on a day-to-day basis, will attend continuing education presentations regularly, will refer patients to specialists when necessary, and will seek consultation from attending or consulting physicians or from other NPs when necessary.

RISK OF BEING SUED FOR MALPRACTICE WHEN THERE WAS NO CLINICAL ERROR

Some patients sue health care providers when there was a poor outcome but no actual malpractice on the part of the provider. Whether a provider has, in fact, fulfilled the elements of malpractice is not determined until there is a trial on the matter or the matter is settled out of court.

NPs who have the opportunity to defuse a potential lawsuit through extra time spent with a dissatisfied patient should do so, even if they know that any threatened lawsuit is ultimately without merit. Therefore, risk management efforts aimed at avoiding lawsuits include keeping patients satisfied and appeasing dissatisfied patients. Patients are annoyed by long waits for appointments, by long waits in the office waiting room, by impersonal treatment, and by constant busy signals when trying to call the office. Keeping in mind the estimate that 90 percent of dissatisfied patients will not complain, it is wise to pay attention to patient complaints and to attempt to resolve problems with patients.

RISK OF PUBLIC PERCEPTION THAT THE INDIVIDUAL NP IS A POOR-QUALITY PROVIDER

The risk of being perceived as a poor-quality provider is perhaps more of a business than a legal risk. How could a nurse practitioner get a reputation as a poor provider? Like any other professional, an NP can get a poor reputation by failing to follow up with clients; by being inattentive, late, forgetful, or sloppy in appearance, demeanor, or intellect; by being unreliable; or by being unable to make a decision. Enough said.

RISK OF BREACHING PATIENT CONFIDENTIALITY

Patients have a right to confidentiality. Breach of privacy is an intentional tort and can be the basis for a lawsuit by a patient. Breach of privacy also can be malpractice, the basis for a disciplinary action by a state's board of nursing, and a violation of state and federal law. And, under new federal regulations, a patient who feels that his NP has violated his privacy rights can complain to the US Office of Civil Rights. The Office may investigate, and, if an NP has not complied with the government's recommendations aimed at protecting patient privacy, the government may fine the NP.

NPs can breach a patient's confidentiality in the following ways:

- Talking about a patient within earshot of others
- Releasing medical information about a patient without prior written permission
- Leaving a telephone message on a patient's answering machine
- Discussing a patient's condition with family members
- Leaving patient records within view
- Discarding unshredded duplicate records
- Giving a patient's name and address to a vendor

It is unusual for patients to sue for breach of confidentiality and difficult for patients to prove. The new federal regulations under which patients may complain to the Office of Civil Rights are untested, as of the publication date of this book. However, patient word of mouth about perceived breaches of confidentiality can harm community perception of a medical practice or provider. Therefore, NPs should seek private places to discuss patients, arrange for discarded records to be shredded, keep records out of view of others, and decline to discuss patient conditions or send written documents on a patient unless the NP has the patient's written permission. An example of an authorization form to use when it is necessary to disclose information about patients to third parties for reasons other than patient treatment, payment, or health care operations is found in Exhibit 8-1.

Exhibit 8-1 Sample Authorization Form

This form is used to allow a patient to authorize release of protected health care information for specified purposes other than treatment, payment, and operations, or to disclose protected health care information to a specified third party.

I authorize [Name of provider and/or class of person authorized to make the use or disclosure] to release my:

- ❑ Name
- ❑ Address
- ❑ Telephone number
- ❑ E-mail address
- ❑ Social security number
- ❑ Insurance policy information
- ❑ Diagnosis or health status
- ❑ Laboratory tests or results
- ❑ X-rays
- ❑ Immunization record
- ❑ Physical exam results

or

- ❑ Other information about my health status, described as follows:

____

____

To: [Name of authorized recipients or class of recipients to which information may be released]

via:

- ❑ Fax to [Name and number]
- ❑ Mail to [Name and address]
- ❑ Telephone to [Name and telephone number]
- ❑ Pick up in person

For the purposes of:

____

____

continues

Exhibit 8-1 *continued*

This authorization is effective on the date signed and continues until:

- ❑ Provide date

I understand the following:

a) If I refuse to authorize release of my health information, [Name of practice and provider] may not refuse to treat me.
b) I may revoke this authorization at any time by notifying [Name and contact information of privacy officer].
c) The information disclosed pursuant to this authorization may be re-disclosed by the recipient and therefore may be outside the protection of federal rules on privacy.
d) The health care provider named above:
   ❑ will
   ❑ will not
   receive remuneration for disclosing information about me.

____
Signature

____
Printed name

____
Date

RISK OF VIOLATING A PATIENT'S RIGHT TO INFORMED CONSENT

A patient has a right to consent to the care being given and a right to refuse care that is offered. An NP has a legal responsibility to give a patient enough information about risks and benefits of care being offered so that the patient can make an informed decision to accept the care.

Informed consent involves disclosure of material risks of care and requires that a patient be competent to understand the risks and make a judgment about accepting care. The doctrine of informed consent requires that there be no coercion in getting a patient to consent to care. The law of informed consent is physician oriented, but the doctrine can be expected to be upheld when an NP is the caregiver.

The doctrine of informed consent arose from a societal desire to discourage persons from unauthorized touching of others. That predisposition against nonconsensual touching became expanded when applied to the practice of medicine. In medicine, the requirement is that a physician must both inform a patient about what is to be done and obtain the patient's consent before treating. Even though the doctrine of informed consent is grounded in the law of battery, the objective of the courts in applying the doctrine of informed consent has been more involved than the simple avoidance of one person's unauthorized touching of another. The majority of courts have adopted a self-determination rationale for informed consent. That is, a person has a right to determine what shall be done with his or her body.[1]

Many cases where patients have complained that their right to informed consent was violated involve surgery. Of course, surgery is only one of many possible treatments, and physicians are only one of many possible health care providers. There are many decisions to be made when a person seeks medical attention, most of which are less dramatic than surgery. For example, prescription drugs have been known to have side effects not discovered until years after the drugs are in common use. Even when a treatment has been used for years with relatively few complications, patients subject to treatment may want to know that they are taking a risk and that there may be side effects.

An NP who is trying to minimize risk to a patient and to the NP will give as much information as possible to a patient contemplating any therapy. How much information does a patient need? Enough to formulate a reasonable decision.

If an NP failed to get informed consent from a patient before treating the patient, the patient could sue the NP, basing a suit on battery or on negligence. A patient who sued an NP for battery would claim that the patient had not authorized the NP to touch the patient. A patient who sued on the basis of negligence would claim that the NP had not given the patient enough information to consent, in an informed way, to the treatment. In either case, a patient could win monetary damages from an NP.

Does an NP need to get consent for everything? It is well established that before a surgeon performs surgery, he or she must obtain the informed consent of the patient. It is less clear whether an NP must get an informed consent before prescribing medication; whether minor but invasive procedures, such as blood transfusion, the starting of intravenous lines, and office incision and drainage, require informed consent; and whether noninvasive treatments carrying some risk, such as office psychotherapy, massage, or even an examination, require informed consent.

At least 25 states have legislation regarding informed consent.[2] An example of an informed-consent statute, one that is oriented toward the physician, is New York's (N.Y. PUB. HEALTH LAW § 2805-d). That law defines lack of informed consent as "failure of the provider of treatment or diagnosis to disclose alternative risks and benefits as a reasonable practitioner under similar circumstances would have disclosed, in a manner permitting the patient to make a knowledgeable evaluation." The law limits the right of action to nonemergent therapies and diagnostic procedures that involve invasion or disruption of the integrity of the body. The statute conforms with New York's case law, which limits the cause of action to procedures that are invasive. The law lists defenses.

Another example of a statute addressing informed consent is Washington's (WASH. REV. STAT. ANN. CODE § 7.70.050). That law states the elements of informed consent as: (1) failure to inform regarding a material fact; (2) patient consented without being aware of the facts; (3) a reasonably prudent patient would not have consented if the information had been adequately conveyed; and (4) injury to the patient.

In Maryland, a statute requires health care providers to give patients certain information, and obtain patient consent, prior to HIV testing (MD. CODE ANN., HEALTH-GEN. I § 18.336).[3] The provider must counsel the patient about HIV infection and methods of preventing transmission. Also, the provider must inform the patient that the provider has a duty to warn[4] and must assist the patient in finding sources of health care. The statutory law is silent regarding all other forms of medical treatment. Some other jurisdictions have statutes requiring that physicians generally get informed consent to their treatments (FLA. STAT. ANN. ch. 766.103).[5]

All states have case law requiring that physicians inform patients of the risks and benefits of surgery and obtain patient consent in writing before doing surgery.

Some courts have defined *treatment* broadly.[6] Among the nonsurgical treatments around which informed-consent issues have emerged are application of oxygen to a neonate [*Burton v. Brooklyn Doctor's Hosp.* 88 A.D.2d 217, 452 N.Y.S. 2d 875 (App. Div. 1982)],[7] radiation therapy [*Nelson v. Patrick,* 58 N.C. App. 546, 293 S.E.2d 829 (Ct. App. 1982)], *appeal after remand* [73 N.C. App. 1, 326 S.E.2d 45 (1985)], and gastroscopy [*Cooper v. Roberts,* 220 Pa. Super. 260, 286 A.2d 647 (Super. Ct. 1971)]. The courts found that the plaintiffs had causes of action. The Supreme Court of Pennsylvania stated that a physician's duty to disclose a collateral risk involved in treatment is the same "whether or not the treatment can be technically termed operative" (*Cooper v. Roberts,* 220 Pa. Super. 260, 2, 286 A.2d).

Other courts, while not *holding* that the doctrine of informed consent applies to nonsurgical treatments, have stated in an aside (dictum) that the term *treatment* can be broadly construed [*Pratt v. University of Minn. Affiliated Hosps. and Clinics,* 414 N.W.2d 399 (Minn. Ct. App. 1987)].[8] The state that defines treatment most broadly is Minnesota. According to the Minnesota Supreme Court, bed rest, when combined with special instructions, would constitute treatment [*Madsen v. Park Nicollet Med. Ctr.,* 431 N.W.2d 855 (Minn. 1988)]. At the opposite extreme is New York, where the need for informed consent is limited to invasive procedures [*Karlsons v. Guerinot,* 57 A.D.2d 73, 394 N.Y.S.2d 933 (App. Div. 1977)].[9]

At least one court has declined to find the need for informed consent in a common, minor, invasive procedure. Informed consent was not applicable to the giving of a flu shot in a Louisiana medical clinic. The court stated that "medical or surgical procedure" did not extend to a flu shot and that to hold otherwise would lead to results in the day-to-day practice of medicine never intended by the legislature [*Novak v. Texada, Miller, Masterson and Davis Med. Clinic,* 514 So. 2d 524, *writ denied,* 515 So. 2d 807 (La. 1987)].[10] That one court found bed rest a treatment but another found an injection not a medical or surgical procedure demonstrates the inconsistency of viewpoint among jurisdictions.

The Minnesota Supreme Court, going a step further than most other jurisdictions, stated, "[We] believe there may be some nontreatment situations where the doctrine should be applicable" [*Pratt v. University of Minn. Affiliated Hosps. and Clinics,* 414 N.W.2d 399 (Minn. Ct. App. 1987)]. In *Pratt v. University of Minnesota [Pratt v. University of Minn. Affiliated Hosps. and Clinics,* 414 N.W.2d 399 (Minn. Ct. App. 1987)], a case about genetic counseling, a plaintiff couple asserted that physicians had been negligent in not disclosing the risk of the couple's encountering a particular genetic abnormality in future children. The physicians, after interviewing the couple and obtaining the tests available, had rejected one possible diagnosis, autosomal recessive disorder, as highly unlikely. Therefore, they did not disclose to the parents the risks of that condition. A subsequent child of the couple was born with autosomal recessive disorder, the diagnosis thought unlikely by the physicians. The plaintiffs asked the Minnesota court to apply to genetic counseling a variation on the doctrine of informed consent [*Pratt v. University of Minn. Affiliated Hosps. and Clinics,* 414 N.W.2d 399 (Minn. Ct. App. 1987)]. Because diagnostic advice and counseling, not treatment, was the medical service involved, the term *negligent nondisclosure* was used. Negligent nondisclosure is discussed more fully below.

The court held that the mere diagnosis of a condition, where all appropriate tests have been performed, does not give rise to a duty to disclose risks inherent in conditions not diagnosed [*Pratt v. University of Minn. Affiliated Hosps. and Clinics,* 414 N.W.2d 399 (Minn. Ct. App. 1987)]. While negligent nondisclosure did not apply in this case, the court stated that the doctrine could be applicable in some other nontreatment situations [*Pratt v. University of Minn. Affiliated Hosps. and Clinics,* 414 N.W.2d 399 (Minn. Ct. App. 1987)].

In summary, there is wide disparity among the states regarding how the doctrine of informed consent may be applied. At one end of the continuum, informed consent is needed only for invasive procedures. At the other end, it is needed for counseling.

In *Canterbury v. Spence* [*Canterbury v. Spence,* 464 F.2d 777 (D.C. Cir. 1972)] [See also *Sard v. Hardy* (281 Md. 432, 379 A.2d 1014)], the US Court of Appeals for the District of Columbia Circuit gave some general advice to physicians that holds true today and can be applied to NPs. The court declined to adopt a standard of full disclosure, saying that it is prohibitive and unrealistic to expect physicians to discuss every risk of a proposed treatment and that such full information generally is unnecessary from a patient's viewpoint. However, the court listed physicians' responsibilities regarding disclosure:

1. Communicate information to the patient when the exigencies of reasonable care call for it.
2. Alert the patient to symptoms of bodily abnormality.
3. Inform the patient when the ailment does not respond to the physician's ministrations.
4. Instruct the patient as to any limitations to be observed for his or her own welfare.
5. Inform the patient about precautionary therapy that he or she should seek in the future.

6. Advise the patient of the need for or desirability of any alternative treatments promising greater benefit than that being pursued.
7. Advise the patient regarding risks to his or her well-being that the contemplated therapy may involve.

Citation: Canterbury v. Spence, 464 F.2d 772 (D.C. Cir. 1972).

Many practices cover the risk of a claim of battery by having each patient sign a consent to an examination at the time of registration. Most practices have informed-consent policies that address invasive procedures, such as endometrial biopsy, cervical biopsy, and incision and drainage.

NPs who want to avoid risk of violating the informed-consent doctrine should:

- Give patients information on risks, benefits, and alternatives to any invasive procedure, and obtain written consent to the procedure.
- Find out what state law requires in the way of informed consent for specific tests, treatments, and procedures.
- Give patients the risks, benefits, and alternatives to any treatment, including prescription medications, and ask for their agreement to the treatment.
- Document that risks, benefits, and alternatives of the treatment have been given to the patient and that the patient agrees to the treatment.

Does an NP Need To Get Consent in Writing?

Consent to surgery must be in writing. Consent for invasive procedures that could be considered surgery—endometrial biopsy, for example—should be in writing. If state law requires consent for specific testing, it must be in writing. In general, consent to medical treatment need not be in writing.

Special Cases

Emergency Situations

In an emergency, care may be given to save a patient's life, even if consent cannot be obtained prior to treatment.

Incompetency

A patient who is unconscious or mentally retarded, who has been adjudged insane, who cannot read, write, or hear, or who is under the influence of sedative drugs or alcohol is not competent to give consent. Unless it is an emergency situation, NPs should avoid treating such patients unless a parent or a court-appointed guardian is available to give consent.

Minors

Minor children cannot consent to treatment. Parental consent is necessary.

RISK OF NEGLIGENT NONDISCLOSURE

The doctrine of negligent nondisclosure emerged when a physician found an abnormality but failed to sufficiently alert the patient. For example, in *Cornfeldt v. Tongen* [262 N.W.2d 684 (Minn. 1977)] a physician failed to inform a patient of abnormalities in blood testing prior to surgery.

The Minnesota Supreme Court defined the elements of negligent nondisclosure as: (1) nondisclosure of a risk inherent in the treatment; (2) harm materialized from that risk; and (3) proximate causation. The elements of lack of informed consent are the same. The terms *lack of informed consent* and *negligent nondisclosure* refer to the same concept, though they are applicable in different situations. *Consent* is applicable when a treatment is proposed. *Nondisclosure* is applicable when an omission of information in itself leads to an injury.

Under the doctrine of negligent nondisclosure, a physician (or an NP), having examined a patient and having found an abnormality, has a duty to inform the patient of the abnormality so that the patient can choose whether to submit to further tests [*Gates v. Jensen,* 92 Wash. 2d 246, 595 P.2d (1979); *Canterbury v. Spence,* 464 F.2d 777 (D.C. Cir. 1972)].[11] All facts must be disclosed that the doctor (or, by inference, the NP) knows or should know the patient needs to make a decision. Some examples include *Truman v. Thomas,* 165 Cal. Rptr. 308, 611 P.2d 902 (Cal. 1980), where a patient sued a physician for failing to disclose the danger of refusing a Pap smear, and *Lauderdale v. United States,* 666 F. Supp. 1511 (D. Ala. 1987), where a physician was found liable when he did not inform a patient of a heart problem, the seriousness of the problem, and the necessity for a return visit.

In *Gates v. Jensen* (92 Wash. 2d 246, 595 P.2d 919 (1979),[12] a physician discovered an increased pressure in a patient's eyes. This suggested glaucoma, a treatable eye disease. The physician failed to inform the patient of the abnormality and of diagnostic procedures that could be undertaken to determine the significance of the abnormality. This resulted in a delay in the diagnosis and treatment of the glaucoma. By the time glaucoma was diagnosed, the patient was functionally blind. The Supreme Court of Washington found that the physician had a duty of disclosure. The court held that the doctrine of informed consent required that the ophthalmologist inform the patient of an abnormality discovered during a routine examination and of diagnostic procedures that could be taken to determine the significance of that abnormality. The court reasoned that a physician has a fiduciary duty to inform a patient of abnormalities in his or her body [*Gates v. Jensen,* 92 Wash. 2d 246, 595 P.2d 919 (1979)].[13]

In *Truman v. Thomas* [165 Cal. Rptr. 308, 611 P.2d 902 (Cal. 1980)], the issue was whether a physician should have disclosed to his patient the risks of refusing a test. There, a physician had advised his patient to have a Pap smear, a test that detects the presence of cervical cancer, but did not inform her of the risks of refusing the test [*Truman v. Thomas,* 165 Cal. Rptr. 308, 611 P.2d 902 (Cal. 1980)]. She refused to have the test. As a result, cancer of the cervix went undiscovered until it had become disseminated. The patient died at the age of 30 [*Truman v. Thomas,*

165 Cal. Rptr. 308, 611 P.2d 902 (Cal. 1980)]. The Supreme Court of California held that the trial judge should have given an instruction to the jury that would have allowed the jury to consider whether the physician breached a duty by not disclosing to the patient the danger of failing to undergo a Pap smear.

From a health care provider's point of view, there are few guidelines. To give too much detail could be uneconomical. To give too little could be negligent. From a patient's point of view, a requirement that more information be given can be only beneficial.

Right of Patients To Refuse Treatment

Patients may refuse treatment. NPs caring for patients who refuse treatment that the NP believes is necessary should inform such patients of the risks of refusing treatment. After that, it is the patient's right to decide. NPs should document that they have explained the risks, benefits, and alternatives of treatment and the risks of refusing treatment and that the patient nevertheless refuses treatment.

RISK OF POOR QUALITY RATINGS

Increasingly, consumer-oriented groups are compiling and reporting data on performance of health care providers, using various measures. The groups collect data from health plans, and health plans collect the data from medical practices. The National Committee on Quality Assurance's HEDIS (Health Plan Employer Data and Information Set) is currently the most commonly applied performance criterion. HEDIS data are gathered from patient surveys, patient charts, and billing forms. For more information or current HEDIS measures, visit www.ncqa.org.

An NP who wants to avoid the risk of poor quality ratings will:

- Understand what performance measures currently are being used.
- Develop personal or practicewide systems for complying with performance guidelines and monitoring his or her performance.
- Request and obtain feedback on performance.

For more information on measurement of performance, see Chapter 15.

RISK OF DISCIPLINARY ACTION

A state board of nursing approves an NP's right to practice in a state. A board of nursing can suspend or revoke an NP's license.

A court cannot revoke an NP's license. A court can find against an NP in a malpractice lawsuit and direct an NP to pay an injured patient monetary damages. If, on the basis of what a judge heard in a case, the judge believes an NP to be grossly negligent, the judge may report the nurse to the board of nursing. Gross negligence is indifference to duty or the intentional failure to perform a manifest duty in reckless disregard of the consequences as affecting the life of another.

A board of nursing will respond not only to reports of gross nursing negligence, but also to reports of impairment, fraud, or criminal activity by nurses. Impairment could be reported by a patient, coworker, or supervisor, based on observation of a nurse. Fraud might include falsifying the nurse's application to the board, falsifying medical records, or documenting that a patient has been seen when the patient has not been seen. A nurse convicted of a felony can expect to be investigated by the board of nursing.

In general, the disciplinary process is as follows:

1. The NP receives a letter stating that he or she is being investigated by the board and requesting that the NP call the board to arrange a meeting.
2. The NP meets with an investigator. The investigator will produce records or other evidence of questionable care given by the NP and ask the NP to respond. The NP may explain why the NP conducted the care or documented the care as the NP did.
3. The investigator will gather information from other sources. The investigator may talk with auditors, colleagues, patients, or administrators.
4. The investigator will recommend to the board that the investigation be dropped or will recommend a hearing.
5. An administrative hearing, resembling a trial, will be held. The NP should be represented by an attorney. The board of nursing will be represented by a state attorney. Evidence may be presented. Witnesses may testify. Sometimes, the board will give the nurse the option of a pre-hearing settlement conference. In that case, the nurse, his or her attorney, some board members, and some board staff meet around a conference table and discuss the matter. The board representatives may recommend a disposition of the matter without an evidentiary hearing.
6. A hearing officer (or board member present at the pre-hearing settlement conference) will make a recommendation to the board.
7. The board will decide to drop the matter or discipline the nurse.
8. Discipline may include probation, suspension of license, or revocation of license.
9. After the passage of a specified time period, the nurse whose license is revoked may reapply for licensure.

Only about 0.02 percent of registered nurses have been subject to disciplinary action by boards of nursing. The percentage of NPs subject to disciplinary action is probably even smaller. However, NPs are subject to discipline, and it is not unusual for an NP to be called before the board of nursing for an investigatory meeting. For example, an NP might be reported to the board of nursing after an audit of a hospital or nursing home turned up irregularities.

An NP who receives notice of investigation should be worried. Whether or not an investigator characterizes the meeting as nonadversarial and strictly information gathering, an investigation is in fact an adversarial situation where an NP has much to lose. NPs should know that state auditors of nursing homes are not NPs and may not be used to evaluating the work of NPs. Furthermore, board of nursing investigators usually are not NPs, though they are probably RNs. An RN investigator may ask such questions as, "This EKG reading says `abnormal EKG.' Why didn't you call in a cardiologist, or send the patient to the emergency room?" The answer may well be: "That abnormality is a left-axis deviation that was not clinically significant for that patient at that time. A cardiology consult or an emergency room visit was not clinically indicated." That response may end the inquiry about the abnormal EKG. The RN investigator may not know the nuances of EKG interpretation and may find that answer satisfactory. An NP who can explain all of his or her actions probably will find that the investigation ends with the meeting. However, an NP who is distraught by the nature of the investigation may not give clear explanations. An NP under the pressure and emotional upset of investigatory questioning may not be as assertive in defending his or her actions as is legally prudent.

An NP who receives a letter notifying the NP of an investigation by the board of nursing should retain an attorney immediately. The attorney should represent the NP at the initial meeting with the investigator for the board of nursing. Investigators may tell NPs that an attorney is not necessary. Investigators may tell NPs that attorneys are not allowed at the meeting. Nevertheless, the NP should engage an attorney, and the attorney can communicate with the investigator about attending the meeting. Attorneys are used to adversarial interactions, are used to advocating for clients, and are not likely to dissolve into tears when an investigator questions the NP's professional competency. Furthermore, an attorney will see that an NP's due-process rights are protected through the investigation and hearing.

RISK OF MEDICARE FRAUD

In the past few years, the US Justice Department has increased its investigative efforts into health care fraud and abuse. The level of fraudulent billing is such that an estimated 7 to 8 percent of total health care spending goes not for care given, but for care not given.[14]

NPs are responsible for ensuring that the billing for their services matches the level of care given and that their documentation matches the level of care billed. Upcoding is billing for a higher level of visit than actually was conducted. Upcoding is health care fraud.

Each Current Procedural Terminology (CPT) code has corresponding levels of required history taking, physical examination, and medical decision making, all of which must be supported in an NP's medical record documentation. For example, if an NP meets all of the criteria for a 99214 visit and bills for a 99214 visit but documents only the criteria for a 99213 visit, the NP is at risk of being charged with Medicare fraud. Fraud is intentional deception. Billing a higher code than is supported by documentation may be unintentional. However, NPs are expected to know how to bill correctly. Ignorance is a poor defense. Furthermore, if a provider pleads ignorance but auditors find that more errors were made in overcoding than undercoding visits, a court will find that the upcoding was intentional.

Consequences of selecting an inappropriate code are Medicare or Medicaid audit failure, loss of Medicare or Medicaid provider status, a fine, and loss or restriction of the NP's license by the board of nursing. Obviously, the consequences also include loss of one's job.

The Center for Medicare and Medicaid Services and the American Medical Association have agreed upon a set of documentation guidelines. These guidelines went into effect in July 1998. Revisions have been proposed since then, but as of the publication of this book, clinicians should abide by the 1995 or 1997 guidelines, whichever the clinician finds to be most useful. The guidelines appear in Appendix 4-A.

On the other hand, providers will not want to undercode. Undercoding will lead to low revenues for a practice.

BUSINESS RISK MANAGEMENT

An NP who starts a business risks business failure. If the NP has partners or fellow directors or stockholders in a corporation, the NP also risks failure of those relationships.

Who's the Boss?

Consider the following example: Nurse Practitioner Able and Nurse Practitioner Best have agreed to go into practice together. Able is an OB-GYN NP, and Best is a family NP. They are both very experienced. They have known each other for five years. They have never worked together, but each knows that the other is well respected in the community. They have carefully planned the business and have decided to be "equal partners."

Able and Best decided not to draw up a partnership agreement. A friend of Best's told Best that she should have a written agreement with Able. So, Best called Attorney Clodd, who told Best that Clodd charged $150 an hour and that a partnership agreement usually ran about $450. Clodd also told Best that Clodd would represent only Best and that Able should have her own attorney in the partnership-forming process. Able and Best wanted to forgo the expenses of attorneys at this stage.

The practice opened. Able and Best had no problem choosing the location for the practice, the furniture, or the equipment. They agreed on a receptionist.

After three months, Best noticed that half of Able's patients were without insurance and that many did not pay for service at the time of service and owed the practice money. Best's patients had insurance for the most part. Furthermore, the lab was billing the practice for Pap smears and other expensive gynecologic tests, and the lab's bills were mounting. Best had been telling her patients that if there was no insurance to cover the visit and any necessary laboratory work, the patient, not the practice, was responsible for the office visit and lab charges.

Best told Able about the bills and the accounts receivable on Able's patients. Able, who saw her patient roster growing, did not want to offend patients by pressing about the bills. Best wanted to press the patients with outstanding bills for payment. Best's husband was tiring of Best's being without a paycheck and was pressuring Best to be a better businessperson.

Who is the boss in this situation? Able and Best did not establish a method of resolving disagreements between them. Therefore, no one is the boss, and they could argue about this issue, or other issues, for years.

How To Avoid a Broken Partnership

When a practitioner starts a business alone, there is no confusion about who makes the administrative and business decisions. Whenever more than one person is involved, there will be more than one opinion on how the business should operate. Often, decisions must be made for which there is no "right" or "wrong" answer. Magazines on medical practice management, and the civil courts, are full of examples of partnerships gone sour. Often, the reasons for the breakup are differences of opinion on how practice collections are made and how practice money is spent. To avoid the risk of deadlocked disagreement, which can lead to hurt feelings, which in turn can lead to "wanting out," it is wise for the members of the group to agree upon a decision-making process.

Any private practice should have one of the following forms of business: sole proprietorship, partnership, or corporation. If the business is a corporation, the corporation's by-laws (or operating agreement, in the case of a limited liability corporation) describe the chain of command within the company. If the business is a partnership, the partners in the business should have an agreement among them specifying the decision-making process. Partners who fail to specify, early in the process of forming the practice, who is to make what decisions and how a deadlock will be resolved will be facing a short-lived association.

Drawing up an administrative chart should be one of the first tasks in the planning process. At minimum, all principal practitioners should agree to the administrative structure. It is prudent to consult an attorney.

DEALING WITH HIGH-RISK PATIENTS

Certain patient characteristics should alert an NP to be especially aware of risk management strategies. These characteristics are multisystem failure, low intelligence, polypharmacy, noncompliant behavior, positive review of systems, substance abuse, and litigiousness.

Multisystem Failure

Refer or work closely with a consultant when caring for patients with multisystem failure. The risk is of failure to refer when the standard of care would call for referral.

Low Intelligence

Have a guardian present when counseling or teaching a patient with low intelligence. The risk is failure to get informed consent to treatment. A patient who does not have the intellectual capability to process information and make decisions about his or her own care cannot be assumed to have consented to treatment.

Polypharmacy

When patients are on many medications, list the medications, side effects, cautions, and dosing instructions for the patient, or coordinate with a pharmacist who will run computer printouts with the information. Review the dosing schedule with the patient at every visit. Ascertain that the patient can read—that the patient is literate and has adequate eyesight.

Noncompliant Patients

Document attempts and strategies for increasing compliance in the noncompliant patient. Document the patient's verbal responses to the NP's questions about why the patient has not taken the recommended medication, controlled the diet, or changed the dressings.

Positive Review of Systems

When a patient has a generally positive review of systems, consider expanding the patient's problem list even further to include somatization, need for social support, inability to cope with life's pressures, and dependency issues. Consider repeating the review of systems on another visit to see whether the complaints persist. If so, an NP should be prepared to dissect each complaint, taking the more risky complaints first. Whether the problem list is long or short, there is no difference in the standard of care expected of an NP.

Substance Abuse

Do not be lured into becoming a source for a patient who is abusing substances. Patients have sued their health care providers for contributing to the patient's substance abuse by prescribing medication.

Litigiousness

Patients who bring up their ongoing lawsuits against another provider can be expected to repeat the performance by suing their current provider.

NOTES

1. The right to self-determination was explained by J. Cardozo in 1914: "Every human being of adult years and sound mind has a right to determine what shall be done with his own body; and a [physician who administers treatment] without his patient's consent commits an assault for which he is liable in damages." *Schloendorff v. Society of N.Y. Hospital*, 211 N.Y. 25, 105 N.E. 92 (1914).
2. Hospital Law Manual. Attorney's Vol. IIB. Gaithersburg, MD: Aspen Publishers; 1983.
3. The statute requires a health care provider to obtain written consent on a special form and to provide pretest counseling before obtaining a blood sample for HIV testing.
4. The statute leaves the decision about whether to inform partners to the physician. The physician may warn partners or may notify the health department, which will warn partners, or the physician may elect not to pass along information about a positive test. It is clear, however, that the patient has no choice about who is informed once the patient consents to testing.
5. This informed-consent statute states that it covers any medical treatment not covered by the Good Samaritan law.
6. For example, in *Head v. Colloton*, the court said, "Treatment is broad enough to embrace all steps in applying medical arts to a person." 331 N.W.2d 870, 875 (Iowa 1983). In *Patrich v. Menorah Med. Ctr.*, the Missouri Court of Appeals defined treatment as "measures necessary for physical well-being of the patient." 636 S.W.2d 134 (1982). *Black's Law Dictionary* defines treatment as including "examination and diagnosis as well as application of remedies" (6th ed., 1990, p. 1502).
7. In this case, administration of oxygen in high doses caused blindness in the infant.
8. The term *treatment* should be construed broadly for purposes of negligent nondisclosure.
9. "A cause of action based on this theory of liability exists only when the injury suffered arises from an affirmative violation of the patient's physical integrity."
10. Louisiana has an informed consent statute, LSA-R.S. 40:1299.40, that gives general requirements for informed consent. Id. at 528.
11. "Due care may require physician perceiving symptoms of bodily abnormality to alert patient to the condition."
12. The court used the doctrine of informed consent, even though the issue was not one of consent but of knowledge of an abnormality requiring further evaluation.
13. A duty arises whenever a doctor becomes aware of an abnormality that may indicate risk or danger. The facts that must be disclosed are all those facts that the physician knows or should know that the patient needs to make a decision about treatment. Id. at 923.
14. Sparrow, MK. License To Steal. Boulder, CO: Westview Press; 1996.

CHAPTER 9

Reimbursement for Nurse Practitioner Services

Except for a minority of patients who pay their own medical bills, every encounter between an NP and a patient has a third-party participant; the payer. Whether an NP is employed by a medical practice or self-employed, the reimbursement policies of third-party payers will determine whether an NP continues to provide care on a long-term basis.

PAYERS

There are five major categories of third-party payers:

1. Medicare
2. Medicaid
3. Indemnity insurance companies
4. Managed-care organizations (MCOs)
5. Businesses that contract for certain services

Each type of payer has its own reimbursement policies and fee schedules, and each operates under a separate body of law. Some payers have a history of reimbursing for NP services in the same manner as they reimburse for physician services. On the other hand, some payers recently have begun to reimburse NPs directly, separate from an employment relationship with a physician practice, and others have NP-specific rules and policies regarding reimbursement.

Each category of payer includes agencies or companies that reimburse NPs for medical services. However, not every company will pay every NP for every service.

MEDICARE

Medicare is a federal program, administered nationally by the Center for Medicare and Medicaid Services (CMS) and administered locally by Medicare carrier agencies. Medicare covers: (1) patients 65 years and older who have enrolled and pay premiums; and (2) disabled individuals who qualify for Social Security disability payments and benefits.

Medicare pays for the care of an enrolled patient under one of two arrangements. If a patient covered by Medicare is not enrolled with an MCO, Medicare reimburses the patient's health care provider on a fee-for-service basis through a local Medicare carrier agency. If a patient has enrolled in a managed-care health plan, there is an extra payment step between payer and provider. Medicare pays the health plan on a capitated basis, an all-inclusive lump sum per month for each patient. Health plans then pay providers on a fee-for-service or capitated basis.

Fee-for-Service Medicare

Fee-for-service reimbursement is payment for specific health care services under a fee schedule. A health service might be an office visit, surgery, ear irrigation, suturing of a wound, a Pap smear, or any one of thousands of other services. Fees are based on a complex variety of factors, including the number and type of services provided, the Current Procedural Terminology (CPT) and International Classification of Diseases, 9th revision (ICD-9) codes, the geographic area of service, and certain office and training expenses of the provider. All reimbursable services have a CPT code. CPT is a uniform coding system developed by the American Medical Association and adopted by third-party payers for use in claim submission. All CPT codes have a corresponding Medicare fee. All medical diagnoses have a six-digit ICD-9 code.

Fees for CPT codes may vary in different locations and for different providers depending upon a complex variety of factors, including the geographic area of service and certain office and training expenses of the provider. Under Medicare, NPs may be reimbursed at a rate of 85 percent of the physician fee schedule. Under a fee-for-service system of reimbursement, the more services an NP performs, the more money he or she will generate.

The physician fee schedule is determined using a system called a *resource-based relative value scale* (RBRVS). The RBRVS, developed by CMS, the federal agency charged with administering Medicare, is used to determine reimbursement for Medicare Part B services. The RBRVS assigns a relative value to each procedural code (CPT code). Under the RBRVS system, services are reimbursed on the basis of resources related to the procedure rather than simply on the basis of historical trends.

There are three components to a relative value: (1) a practice expense component; (2) a work component; and (3) a malpractice component. Each component is adjusted geographically, using three separate Geographic Practice Cost Indexes (GPCIs). The final formula to arrive at an area-specific relative value is:

(Practice Expense RV × Practice Expense GPCI) + (Work RV × Work GPCI) +
(Malpractice RV × Malpractice GPCI) = Relative Value

The relative value is then multiplied by a single "conversion factor" to arrive at the geographic-specific fee schedule allowable for a given area. The conversion factor is based on whether the service is surgical or medical. RBRVS affects payments made to physicians, NPs, and other providers entitled to Medicare and other forms of third-party reimbursement.

An NP wishing to provide service to a Medicare patient on a fee-for-service basis applies to be a Medicare provider. Once an NP has a provider number, the NP submits bills to the local Medicare carrier agency for each visit or procedure. A standard form, the CMS 1500, is used. NPs who are self-employed receive 85 percent of the physician charge for the billed procedure. When an NP is employed by physicians and can meet "incident to" requirements, the practice may receive 100 percent of the physician charge for the billed procedure, subject to the "incident to" rules.

"Incident to" Services

The full term for *incident to* is *incident to a physician's professional service. Incident to* is a term peculiar to Medicare. The legal definition of "incident to" services is services furnished as an "integral, although incidental, part of the physician's personal professional services in the course of diagnosis or treatment of an injury or illness."[1] To qualify under this definition, the services of nonphysicians must be rendered under a physician's "direct personal supervision." Nonphysicians must be employees of a physician or physician group or have an independent contractor relationship with the group. Services must be furnished during a course of treatment in which a physician performs an initial service and subsequent services of a frequency that reflects the physician's active participation in and management of the course of treatment. Direct personal supervision in the office setting does not mean that a physician must be in the same room. However, a physician must be present in the office suite and immediately available to provide assistance and direction throughout the time that an NP is performing services. *Incident to* may refer to the services of office nurses and technicians as well as NPs.

Capitated Medicare

Capitation is a fee paid by a managed care organization (MCO) to a health care provider, per patient, per month, for care of an MCO member. Capitated fees for primary care run between $5 and $35 per member per month, based on a patient's age and sex. Under a capitated system of reimbursement, NPs and physicians are paid a set fee per patient per month for all services agreed to by contract. If an NP has agreed to provide all primary care services for a patient, then the NP must provide an unlimited number of primary care visits. On the other hand, if a patient never visits, the NP operating under a capitated system of reimbursement still is paid.

An NP wishing to provide care for a Medicare patient who is enrolled in an MCO applies to the MCO for admission to the organization's provider panel. For information about how to apply for admission to managed-care provider panels, see Exhibit 9-1.

Exhibit 9-1 How To Apply for Provider Status

MEDICARE

1. Apply for a provider number by calling the Medicare carrier in the area and asking for an application.
2. Bill Medicare on a form called the CMS 1500, using the patient's name and identifying information, the diagnosis code (ICD-9), the procedure code (CPT), the charge, and the NP's provider number. CMS 1500 forms are sold by the American Medical Association (AMA) and are ordered by calling the AMA in Chicago. Some bookstores also sell the forms.
3. If a Medicare patient is enrolled in managed care, see "Managed Care Organizations," in this box.

MEDICAID

1. Apply for a provider number through the state Medicaid agency. Ask for Provider Relations, and ask for a provider application as an NP. Fill out the application, return it, and receive a Medicaid provider number.
2. Bill the state Medicaid agency on a CMS 1500 form, using the patient's name and identifying information, the ICD-9 code, the CPT code, the charge, and the NP's name, provider number, and location.
3. If a Medicaid patient is enrolled in managed care, see "Managed Care Organizations," in this box.

INDEMNITY INSURER

1. Call the company to inquire whether a provider number is required. If so, apply for a provider number. If not, submit a CMS 1500 form to the company for the services rendered.
2. If the company rejects a bill, the company will return the CMS 1500 with a short explanation about why it is being rejected. If the rejection is erroneous, write a letter to the company protesting the rejection and explaining the error, if possible, or supply whatever further information is needed. Sometimes several letters will be necessary before a bill is paid. Sometimes it will be necessary to include a copy of appropriate law with correspondence. Occasionally, intervention by a practice's attorney is necessary. Occasionally, a company will persist in refusing to pay. If so, the patient is liable for the bill.

MANAGED CARE ORGANIZATIONS

1. Call Provider Relations for each MCO for which admission is needed, and request an application for admission to the panel of providers.
2. If rejected, note the reason for rejection and, if applicable, consult state insurance law. In some states, an HMO or MCO cannot discriminate among providers on the basis of class of license. In other states, HMOs can accept or reject any provider. Ask for an opportunity to present the case for admitting NPs to the provider panel. Pursue a company through letters, presentations, meetings, and telephone calls, going up the supervisory line if necessary.

Source: Reprinted with permission from Buppert C. Reimbursement for Nurse Practitioner Services, In: The Nurse Practitioner, Vol. 23, No. 1, pp. 67-81, © 1998, Springhouse Corporation.

Individuals covered by Medicare may choose between traditional fee-for-service coverage and managed care. The advantage of managed care to the patient is that pharmaceutical products usually are covered. Under traditional Medicare coverage, pharmaceuticals are not covered. There are Congressional proposals to cover pharmaceuticals for Medicare beneficiaries, but none had been passed at the time of publication of this book.

MEDICAID

Medicaid is a federal program, administered by the states, for mothers and children who qualify on the basis of poverty and for adults who are disabled for the short term—for one year or less—and who qualify on the basis of poverty.

Like patients covered by Medicare, some patients covered by Medicaid are enrolled in MCOs, and others are not. To serve a Medicaid patient not enrolled in an MCO, an NP must apply and be accepted as a Medicaid provider by the state Medicaid agency. To serve a Medicaid patient enrolled in an MCO, an NP must apply and be admitted to the provider panel of the MCO in which the patient is enrolled.

Medicaid pays NPs 70 to 100 percent of the fee-for-service rates set for physicians by state Medicaid agencies. State law controls the rate. Medicaid reimbursement generally is lower than the rates paid by commercial insurers. For information on rates, contact the state Medicaid agency.

Many states have applied to the federal government for "Medicaid waivers." A Medicaid waiver is permission to a state from CMS to administer Medicaid in ways that differ from the federal laws and regulations; specifically, to enroll patients covered by Medicaid in MCOs. Once a state has received a Medicaid waiver, NPs can expect that most, if not all, patients covered by Medicaid will enroll in MCOs or other managed-care plans. NPs who have served Medicaid patients on a fee-for-service basis must apply for admission to the appropriate managed-care provider panels to maintain reimbursement.

INDEMNITY INSURERS

An indemnity insurer is an insurance company that pays for the medical care of its insured but does not deliver health care. Indemnity insurers pay health care providers on a per-visit, per-procedure basis. To obtain reimbursement, an NP submits a billing form to the insurance company (see "Billing" later in this chapter).

Indemnity insurers have fee schedules based on "usual and customary" charges. *Usual and customary* is an insurance industry term for a charge that is (1) usual and customary when compared with the charges made for similar services and supplies; and (2) made to persons having similar medical conditions in the county of the policyholder or such larger area than a county as is needed to secure a representative cross section of fees. "Usual and customary" may be figured differently from insurer to insurer. Therefore, some insurers pay more than others for the same procedure.

If a provider charges more than what an insurer considers to be "usual and customary," the insurer pays only the usual and customary charge. In that case, the patient may be responsible for the difference between what a provider charges and what an insurer pays. It is up to the provider to collect the difference from the patient. Some providers agree to accept the "usual and customary" payment and will not pursue patients for the difference. Other providers pursue patients for the provider's full charge, no matter what portion is paid by an insurer.

MANAGED-CARE ORGANIZATIONS

An MCO is an insurer that provides both health care services and payment for the services. *MCO* is an umbrella term that may include HMOs, provider-sponsored organizations (PSOs), or physician-hospital organizations (PHOs). An HMO is a prepaid, comprehensive system of health benefits that combines the financing and delivery of health services to subscribers. A PSO is a group of providers that has organized for the purpose of taking on managed-care contracts. A PHO is a legal or informal organization that bonds hospitals and attending medical staff, frequently developed for the purpose of taking on managed-care contracts. In this chapter, the umbrella term MCO will be used to refer to HMOs, PSOs, and PHOs.

NPs are gaining admission to MCO provider panels. With panel membership comes the designation *primary care provider* (PCP), a contract for providing care, credentialing, directory listing, and reimbursement.

A PCP has full responsibility for a patient's primary care, including: (1) complying with the MCO's quality, utilization, and patient satisfaction standards; (2) coordinating care with specialists, hospitals, or long-term care facilities; (3) approving or disapproving referrals for specialty care; (4) keeping costs as low as possible while maintaining quality; and (5) providing a system for 24-hour access to care.

MCOs reimburse PCPs on a fee-for-service basis, a capitated basis, or a combination of fee-for-service and capitation. Each MCO negotiates a payment arrangement with each group, practice, or provider on its panel. See the section "Negotiating an MCO Contract" in this chapter.

How MCOs Work

MCOs sell a priced package of health services to their clients, who may be employers, individuals, or government agencies, such as the state Medicaid agency or Medicare. A client signs up for a particular plan and offers that plan to patients, or "members," who often share in the cost of the plan. Each MCO has a panel of health care providers who may or may not be employed by the MCO.

Group-Model versus Practice-Model MCOs

There are two types of affiliation between MCO and provider. The first type is an employer-employee arrangement, called the *group-model MCO*. The best known group-model MCO is Kaiser Permanente. A group-model MCO pays a provider a set salary in return for taking care of a panel of patients. In the second type of affiliation, called the *practice-model MCO,* the MCO contracts with independent providers, group practices, or practice associations for a "product line" of services. Contracts between MCO and a practice govern the relationship. See the section "Negotiating an MCO Contract" in this chapter.

Both group-model and practice-model MCOs are allowing patients the option of choosing NPs as PCPs. Not all MCOs currently recognize NPs as PCPs, however.

Applying for MCO Provider Panel Membership

NPs should determine which MCOs are prevalent in the geographic area of practice and prevalent among the practice's patients. Once the NP has compiled a short list of MCOs, it is wise to do some research on the MCOs.

Ask other providers who have done business with the MCO, or the state agency that oversees MCOs, the following questions:

- Have other providers been paid promptly?
- Who are the specialists on the MCO's referral network? Are you familiar with them?
- Does the MCO have a strong presence in the community?
- Is the MCO financially sound?
- Is the MCO's record with the Insurance Division relatively free of complaints?
- Does the company have decent quality data?

Then apply to the MCOs for which the above answers are "yes."

NPs who have been admitted to MCO provider panels are: (1) those whose practice is in a geographic area of interest to an MCO; (2) those who have large numbers of patients who are attractive to the MCO; (3) those who offer a service unavailable elsewhere; or (4) those who have been endorsed and supported by the physicians in a large group practice. In general, these are the same characteristics distinguishing physicians who have been admitted to MCO provider panels.

In brief, the application process is: (1) call Provider Relations at an MCO and request an application; (2) apply for admission; and (3) follow up by telephone or letter.

Provider Credentialing

MCOs "credential" providers, meaning that they collect educational, license, malpractice, employment, and certification data on each provider and make a judgment that a provider is adequately prepared to care for the MCO's patients. For the information commonly required of applicants to provider panels, see Appendix 9-A.

An MCO that is interested in an NP as a panel member will verify data submitted on the application and make a site visit. A site visitor will be looking for a clean office, safe access, sufficient parking, adequate staffing, and other signs of a well-organized practice. In the case of an NP practice, a site visitor may ask about systems for admitting patients and access to a physician consultant. With an offer of admission to a provider panel will come a contract, to be signed by the NP and MCO.

Negotiating an MCO Contract

Contractual relationships with MCOs cover not only compensation, but also many other issues concerning practice. Some attorneys specialize in assisting providers to negotiate contracts with MCOs, and NPs are encouraged to seek counsel of an attorney experienced in these matters. A detailed explanation of the terms below is beyond the scope of this book. There are books devoted entirely to negotiating managed-care contracts.

Contract issues to be negotiated include:

- What is included? What is excluded?
- What are the carve outs; that is, what patients are treated in special programs because of special needs?
- What is the process for transferring the care of a patient who becomes eligible for a carve out?
- What is the fee schedule or capitation schedule?
- What are the stop-loss provisions?
- Are there withholds?
- Are there referral pools?
- What is the level of distributions from withhold and referral pools to PCPs during the last five years?
- What is the bonus system?
- What are the provisions for closing the practice to additional patients from the MCO?
- Is claims processing done in house or contracted out?
- Who does the lab work?
- What will the MCO base renewal upon? What is its renewal rate with providers?
- What is the procedure for the MCO's review of office practices?
- How will the directory listing read?
- Is there any prohibition on joining other MCOs?
- How does the MCO define *experimental, emergency,* and *preexisting condition?*
- Who bears the brunt of a mistake in eligibility or coverage determination?
- Can preadmission or referral approval be rescinded retroactively?
- What is in the formulary?
- What are the requirements for:

1. Utilization management
2. Quality assurance
3. Credentialing
4. Member grievance
5. Record keeping
6. Claims submission
7. Hours of operation
8. Appointment response times
9. On-call coverage
10. Employing other providers
11. Arranging backup with other groups
12. Minimum/maximum numbers of patients
13. Antidisparagement
14. Business confidentiality

- What is the system for verifying member eligibility? How often is the provider notified of members who have selected him or her? When in the month is this done?
- What are the provisions for dispute resolution?
- What are the provisions for member grievance?
- What marketing is provided by the MCO?
- Who owns the records/data?

If an NP is an employee of a group practice, then someone within the group will have responsibility for negotiating the terms of the MCO contract for the group. An NP who owns a practice will need to negotiate the above points individually or join a practice association in which there will be a designated negotiator.

Some providers are joining provider groups for the express purpose of collectively negotiating contract terms and rates. While some providers enter into a contract with an HMO without experienced legal counsel, it is unwise to do so.

Steps for Dealing with Denial of Provider Status

Gather Information

An NP who is denied a request for an application should ask the following questions of an MCO representative:

1. Does the MCO admit NPs to provider panels?
2. If not, why not?
3. If it is a policy matter, who is the decision maker in the company who could change the policy?
4. If state law is given as a reason for denial, ask: Which law precludes NPs' being PCPs?

Strategize

Enlist the help of the state NP organization to hire an attorney to analyze an alleged legal barrier and to determine whether, in fact, there is a true legal barrier. If there are legal barriers to NPs' becoming panel members or PCPs, hire a lobbyist who will work to change the law.

Research options for using existing state law to encourage MCOs to admit NPs to provider panels. For example, some state laws preclude discrimination by HMOs against classes of health care providers who are legally authorized to provide health care services. NPs or their attorneys will want to cite such laws when making presentations to MCO executives.

Take Action

If an MCO has a policy against admitting NPs as PCPs, NPs may employ the following actions to effect a policy change.

1. Write letters to MCO presidents, stating how NPs can satisfy the business needs of the MCO (see Chapter 13, especially Exhibit 13-1). Ask for an informational meeting, and present information on NP scope of practice, sources of third-party reimbursement, and arguments supporting NPs as PCPs, backed up by supporting data.
2. Ask patients to request, through their employer's benefits office and through their MCO, the services of an NP as PCP.
3. Ask colleague physicians to support NP admission to provider panels.
4. Testify at hearings and speak at community meetings about the advantages of NPs as providers.
5. Ask for language changes from businesses that use the following message: "Ask your doctor." Ask that the language be changed to "Ask your doctor or NP" or "Ask your health care provider."
6. In six months, request an application, and try again.

Carrying Out an MCO Contract

NPs who are admitted to MCO provider panels will want regular periodic analysis of the income and expense associated with each MCO contract. Such an analysis might reveal that a practice is losing money on one contract while breaking even on another and making a profit on yet another. If there is a discrepancy between reimbursement from various MCO contracts, an NP will want to determine the reason for the unprofitability of certain contracts, and either negotiate a different arrangement when the contract expires or cease to deal with an MCO.

NPs also will want to evaluate MCO contracts regarding the effect of the contract on staff and providers. For example, is one MCO's paperwork or procedures for reimbursement overwhelmingly more complicated than another's? If so, then whatever reimbursement is being reaped may be offset by costly staff services. Is the lag time between services and payment greater than 120 days? If so, the practice manager will need to insist upon prompt payment or cease to deal with the offending MCO.

DIRECT CONTRACTS FOR HEALTH SERVICES

There are no barriers to the NP who wishes to contract directly with businesses or agencies that need health services. For example, NPs are contracting directly with colleges to provide college health services, with businesses to provide occupational health services, and with government agencies to provide school-based health services.

BILLING THIRD-PARTY PAYERS

Billing third-party payers includes filing the proper forms, including the appropriate diagnostic and procedure codes, and documenting encounters in the medical record in a manner that justifies a bill.

Standard Form

The standard billing form is the CMS 1500. It can be purchased from the American Medical Association and from other commercial suppliers such as bookstores. The CMS 1500 form asks for ICD-9 codes, CPT codes, date of service, patient identifying information, and provider identifying information. A bill submitted without a CPT or ICD-9 code will be rejected.

Coding

The most frequently used procedure codes in primary care are the Evaluation and Management (E&M) Services (CPT codes 99201 through 99456). Specialty practices use the E&M codes as well. E&M codes represent a health care provider's cognitive services, such as office or clinic visits, consultations, preventive medicine examinations, and critical care services. In addition to E&M codes, a primary care practice will use other CPT codes to bill for such procedures as suturing and irrigation of ears.

E&M codes require providers to bill on the basis of the extent and complexity of history taking, physical exam, and medical decision making. For an example of E&M code requirements for a routine visit, see Exhibit 9-2.

A typical bill for an office visit could list one or more CPT codes and one or more ICD-9 codes. For example, a bill for a routine annual gynecologic exam would include ICD-9 code V72.3 for a diagnosis of routine annual exam and CPT codes 99213 or 99214 for an office visit for an established patient, 87210 for a wet mount, and 87205 for a Pap smear.

CMS has developed "Guidelines for Evaluation and Management Coding" that NPs and other Medicare providers will be expected to follow in coding patient visits. See Appendix 4-A for these guidelines. NPs can expect that other insurers will expect the same attention to coding and documentation as CMS.

Exhibit 9-2 Selecting an E&M Code

A 99213 visit, the most common E&M code for an established patient, includes:

- An expanded problem-focused history
- An expanded problem-focused examination
- Medical decision making of low complexity
- Counseling and coordination of care consistent with the nature of the problem and the patient's needs
- 15 minutes of face-to-face time

Examples are office visits with:

- A 55-year-old male established patient for management of hypertension and mild fatigue, on hydrochlorothiazide and a beta blocker
- A 50-year-old female established patient with insulin-dependent diabetes mellitus and stable coronary artery disease, for monitoring

Source: CPT five-digit codes, nomenclature and other data are copyright 2003 American Medical Association. All Rights Reserved. No fee schedules, basic unit, relative values or related listing are included in CPT. The AMA assumes no liability for the data contained herein. CPT only © 2003 American Medical Association.

General guidelines for legal coding are as follows:

1. A billable visit is a face-to-face contact between the patient and an NP, physician assistant, or physician. An encounter may occur in the provider's office, an inpatient setting, or the patient's home. Each billable visit must be a diagnostic visit, identified with an ICD-9 code.
2. If care is given in an office, an NP must distinguish between a new patient and an established patient, and then select the proper E&M CPT code for the visit. A new patient is one who has not received professional services within the past three years from a provider in the same specialty in the same practice. Telephone communication is considered a professional service.
3. History taking, examination, and medical decision making are the key components in determining code selection. Time is the least important factor. In ambulatory care, only face-to-face time is to be considered in selecting an appropriate CPT code. Other components to be considered when selecting a code are counseling, coordination of care, and the nature of the presenting problem. These last three components are considered contributory components and are more important than time but less important than history taking, examination, and medical decision making.
4. Medical record documentation must support the level of care billed. Underdocumentation can lead to charges of fraudulent billing or "false claims."
5. A practice's billing naturally will include a variety of E&M codes because patient encounters vary in amount of attention required. A provider with a pattern of coding all visits with one of the higher level codes is likely to be identified by the Medicare carrier as an "upcoder"; that is, a provider

who bills for a higher level of service than actually provided in order to get a higher fee. Upcoding is false claims. A normal distribution of E&M codes for established patients (99211 through 99215) is a bell-shaped curve, with most visits being 99213.

6. Failing to bill for all billable services rendered can mean unnecessarily low revenues for a practice. Consistent overcoding without medical record documentation that supports the level of visit billed can mean an audit by the Medicare carrier, fines, criminal prosecution for Medicare fraud, loss of Medicare provider status, and loss of license.

Table 9-1 shows a comparison for the five levels of visit (99211 through 99215) for an established patient. For a complete discussion of choice of code, see *Current Procedural Terminology* for the current year, published by the American Medical Association. For the CMS guidelines on documentation for evaluation and management visits, see Appendix 4-A. These guidelines will be revised from time to time. At press time, a current copy of the guidelines is posted on the CMS Web site, www.cms.gov.

In general, the appropriate documentation for the codes for an established patient visit, mid-level visit (99213), is as follows. Under the documentation guidelines released on the CMS's Internet Web site in November 1997 and posted as of June 2003, a bill for a 99213 visit (established patient, mid-level office visit) will have to be backed up by a medical record entry that includes certain elements of history taking, physical examination, and medical decision making.

For example, *CPT 2003* requires a clinician to document, in detail, two of the three key aspects of a visit. Key aspects of an office visit, according to CMS, are history, examination, and medical decision making. The guidelines also address documentation of three other elements of a medical visit, time spent, counseling, and coordination of services. The November 1997 guidelines' requirements to satisfy documentation requirements for history taking, examination, and medical decision making for a 99213 visit are given below, along with the guidelines' discussion of documenting time, counseling, and coordination of services. The November 1997 guidelines are the most current guidelines, as of June 2003.

History Taking

Clinicians must document:

- At least one of the symptom descriptors (location, quality, severity, duration, timing, context, modifying factors, and associated symptoms)
- A review of systems for at least one pertinent body area or system; the acceptable body areas and systems are constitutional, eyes-ears-nose-throat/mouth, cardiovascular, respiratory, gastrointestinal, genitourinary, musculoskeletal, skin/breasts, neurologic, psychiatric, endocrine, hematologic, or immunologic

No past, family, or social history is required.

TABLE 9-1

A Comparison of Requirements for the Five Levels of Visit for an Established Patient

Level of Visit	*History*	*Exam*	*Need Two of These Three Components*		
			Diagnoses	*Data Reviewed*	*Risk*
99211	None required	None required	None required	None required	None
99212	1 descriptor	1	1 minor or established	Order or study 1 lab	1 minor problem, noninvasive labs, home-based management
99213	1 descriptor 1 ROS	6	2 minor or established, or 1 new	Order or study 2 labs, or summarize old records or personally view tracing	2 minor problems or 1 chronic stable problem or 1 acute problem; management is minor surgery, OTC drugs, or physical therapy
99214	4 descriptors 1 PSFH 2 ROS	12	1 new or 1 worse and 1 minor	Order or study 3 labs, or order 1 lab and summarize old records or personally view tracing	1 chronic problem, worse, or 1 chronic problem, stable, or 1 acute systemic problem; invasive diagnostic procedures needed; prescription drugs indicated
99215	4 descriptors 2 PSFH 10 ROS	18	1 new problem needing workup, or 1 new, stable and 1 minor	Order or study 4 labs, or order/study 2 labs and summarize old records or personally view tracing	1 severe chronic problem, 1 life-threatening chronic problem, 1 acute life-threatening problem or acute mental status change; contrast studies or endoscopy with risk factors as indicated; parenteral therapies, fracture treatment, major surgery or monitoring is indicated

Abbreviations: ROS, review of systems; PFSH, past, family, or social history; OTC, over the counter.
Source: CPT five-digit codes, nomenclature and other data are copyright 2003 American Medical Association. All Rights Reserved. No fee schedules, basic unit, relative values or related listing are included in CPT. The AMA assumes no liability for the data contained herein. CPT only © 2003 American Medical Association.

Examination

Clinicians must document at least six elements from a body system or area. Acceptable systems or body areas include constitutional, eyes-ears-nose-throat, neck, respiratory, cardiovascular, breasts, abdomen, genital, lymphatic, musculoskeletal, skin, neurologic, or psychiatric.

Medical Decision Making

According to the guidelines, medical decision making has three components; making a diagnosis, choosing treatment options, and reviewing data. Clinicians are to consider one additional factor when choosing a code and documenting the risk of complications and/or morbidity or mortality. For a 99213 visit, medical decision making is "low complexity" under the guidelines.

According to the guidelines, the diagnostic component of medical decision making is fulfilled by documenting a "limited" number of diagnoses or management options. Carole Guillaume, a physician writing for *Family Practice Management*, published by the American Academy of Family Physicians, consulted "score sheets" to be used by CMS in auditing compliance with the guidelines and noted that auditors verifying a 99213 visit will be looking for diagnoses for at least two minor problems, or two established stable problems, or one established problem that is documented as worse and one minor problem, or one new problem that is stable or in need of workup.

As for the component of medical decision making that consists of reviewing data, the guidelines give examples of what indicates increased complexity in a visit—a personal review of an electrocardiogram tracing, for example—but the guidelines do not list what documentation is needed to justify a particular level of visit. According to Guillaume, the score sheets require, for a 99213 visit, that a clinician document that two types of diagnostic tests have been ordered or reviewed or that an X-ray, tracing, or slide interpreted by another clinician has been reviewed, or that old history has been summarized.

Unlike the guidelines, which appear on the CMS Web site on the Internet (www.cms.gov; use the search engine to find "Evaluation and Management Guidelines"), the score sheets are not widely available to clinicians.

As for the final component of medical decision making, the risk of complications and/or morbidity or mortality, the guidelines are more specific. For a 99213 visit, the risk is "low." Examples of "low" risk for complications are visits where there are two or more self-limited or minor problems, a stable chronic illness, or an acute uncomplicated illness or injury. Diagnostic procedures that might be ordered during such a visit are physiologic tests not under stress, such as pulmonary function tests, clinical laboratory tests requiring arterial puncture, or skin biopsies. According to the guidelines, management options could include over-the-counter drugs, minor surgery, or physical therapy.

Time

Time is a minor consideration in determining the level of visit to bill, according to the guidelines, if a clinician is billing an office visit for evaluation and management (99211–99215 for an established patient and 99201–99205 for a new patient). If a visit is primarily counseling, however, time matters and should be documented. The visit is billed as a counseling visit, not an evaluation and management visit.

Counseling and Coordination of Services

While clinicians are expected to document patient counseling and coordination of services, there are no specific guidelines for this documentation. The guidelines state that it is expected that documentation will reflect the appropriate level of counseling and coordination based on patient needs.

Rejected Bills

If a bill is rejected by a payer, a member of the medical practice's staff should ask the following questions of the payer, document responses, and follow up by letter:

1. Why was this bill rejected?
2. Is more information needed about the procedure? About the diagnosis? About the documentation? About NP practice?

Every practice should have copies of relevant law regarding NP reimbursement. Relevant law includes the state regulation or statute that gives NPs the authority to provide care, the section of the Medicaid and Medicare regulations that apply to NP reimbursement, and any parts of the state insurance law that mandate payment for services provided by NPs. If bills are rejected for reasons related to NPs as a profession, the practice should send copies of relevant laws to insurers, along with any other information the payer requests.

BILLING SELF-PAYING PATIENTS

Though patients who pay their bills themselves are not, by definition, third-party payers, they deserve mention as a source of reimbursement.

Cash at time of service works only when patients are aware of what the bill will be before they arrive for their visit. Many practices are unable to give patients that information, but some can.

Some practitioners take credit cards. Some allow patients to run a balance with the practice and pay a monthly installment. Many practitioners who extend credit to patients have found it necessary to establish a relationship with a collection agency.

CONCLUSION

Reimbursement is a high-stakes issue for any practice, for without steady income, no practice will survive. Each of the topics discussed in this chapter deserves a book's worth of discussion. In fact, there are publications available on every topic. For sources of more information, see the section "Resources" below.

NOTE

1. Medicare Carriers Manual, Part 3, § 2050.

RESOURCES

Medicare

Health Law Digest. Published monthly. Washington, DC: American Health Lawyers Association.

Modern Healthcare. Business news. Published weekly. Chicago, IL: Crain Communications, Inc.

Managed-Care Quality Standards

HEDIS. National Committee on Quality Assurance. (www.NCQA.org/Programs/HEDIS. Accessed September 2003).

Diagnostic Coding

International Classification of Diseases, 9th Revision. Chicago, IL: American Medical Association; 2003.

Procedural Coding

Buppert C. The Primary Care Provider's Guide to Compensation and Quality. Sudbury, MA: Jones and Bartlett Publishers; 2000.

Buppert C. Safe, Smart Billing and Coding for Evaluation and Management. An Instructional CD. Law office of Carolyn Buppert; 2003. www.buppert.com. Accessed July 2003.

Physicians' Current Procedural Terminology: CPT 98. Chicago, IL: American Medical Association; 2003.

Reimbursement for Nurse Practitioner Services. *The Green Sheet*, newsletter from the law office of Carolyn Buppert. www.buppert.com.

APPENDIX 9-A

Credentialing Information

A typical credentialing application will ask for:

- The NP's name, and other names used in past licensure and certification
- States of licensure
- Type of license
- Specialty
- Subspecialty
- UPIN number
- Social Security number
- Birth date
- US citizenship
- Place of birth
- Home address and telephone
- Practice status (individual, partnership, or group)
- Practice name, address, telephone, tax identification number, and office manager
- Dates at this practice
- Undergraduate and graduate education: institution, address, dates attended, degrees conferred
- Postgraduate training: institution, address, dates attended, type of training, name of program director, specialty
- Fellowship training: institution, address, dates attended, type of training, name of program director, leadership positions held, reason for leaving, type of facility
- Employment history/professional affiliations: institution, address, dates of privileges, position title, leadership positions held, name of department chair, type of facility, reason for leaving
- Current admitting privileges: primary admitting hospital, address, date received privileges, staff category, leadership positions held, name of department chair

- Military service: branch, period of enlistment, discharge status, rank
- Specialty board certification:
  - Board, year certified or recertified, expiration date
  - If you are not certified, whether you have taken the certification examination
  - Number of times you have taken the examination
  - Date that your eligibility to take the examination expires
  - Whether you intend to apply for the certification examination
  - Whether you have been accepted to take the certification examination
  - Date of next certification examination
- Licensure:
  - States, license number, expiration date, current status
  - DEA license number, expiration date, current status
  - State controlled-substance license number, expiration date, current status
- Professional liability coverage:
  - Proof of current coverage, name of previous carrier, period of coverage, limits of coverage, type of coverage, reason for discontinuance
  - Whether you have maintained continuous professional liability coverage since first obtaining coverage
  - Whether you have been subject to a professional liability suit, including but not limited to malpractice claims, in the past five years
  - Whether there are any restrictions, limitations, or exclusions in your current professional liability coverage
  - Whether your professional liability insurance coverage has ever been denied, limited, reduced, interrupted, terminated, or not renewed
- Personal information:
  - Date of last physical examination
  - Whether you are currently suffering from, or receiving treatment for, any physical or mental disability or illness, including drug or alcohol abuse, that would impair the proper performance of your essential functions and responsibilities as a health care provider
  - Whether you have ever been convicted of, or pleaded guilty to or nolo contendere to, any crime other than traffic violations
- Professional sanctions:
  - Whether your license to practice any health occupation in any jurisdiction has ever been limited, suspended, denied, subjected to any conditions, terms of probation, or formal reprimand, not renewed, or revoked
  - Whether you have surrendered your license to practice any health occupation in any jurisdiction
  - Whether your request for any specific clinical privilege has ever been denied or granted with stated limitations
  - Whether you have ever been denied membership on a hospital medical staff
  - Whether your staff privileges, appointment, and/or delineation of privileges at any hospital or other health care institution has ever been suspended,

revoked, limited, reduced, denied, or subject to any conditions or not renewed

- Whether your DEA or other controlled-substance authorization has ever been limited, suspended, denied, reduced, subject to any conditions, terms of probation, not renewed, or revoked
- Whether proceedings toward any of these ends have ever been initiated
- Whether your controlled-substance authorization has ever been voluntarily or involuntarily relinquished
- Whether you have ever been subject to disciplinary action in any medical organization or professional society
- Whether there are any disciplinary actions pending against you
- Whether you have resigned from any hospital or health care institution or professional academic appointment
- Whether you have ever been placed on probation, suspended, asked to resign, or been terminated while in a training program
- Whether you have ever been placed on probation, suspended, or asked to resign or been terminated while in a hospital program
- Whether you have ever withdrawn your application for appointment, reappointment, or clinical privileges or resigned before a decision was made by a hospital's or health care facility's governing board
- Whether you have ever been denied certification or recertification by a specialty board or received a letter of admonition from such a board or committee
- Whether you have ever been investigated by any private, federal, or state agency concerning your participation in any private, federal, or state health insurance program
- Whether you have ever been subject to probation proceedings or suspended, sanctioned, or otherwise restricted from participating in any private, federal, or state health insurance program
- Whether you have received a determination from any professional review organization indicating a "final severity level 3" or a "gross and flagrant" quality concern

- Professional references: List names and addresses of four persons who have worked extensively with you or have been responsible for professionally observing you. Do not list more than two current partners or associates in practice, relatives by blood or marriage, the chief of service to whom you are applying, any person in current or past training programs with you (unless he or she is now a colleague), or persons who cannot attest to your current level of clinical competency, technical skill, and medical knowledge.

CHAPTER 10

The Employed Nurse Practitioner

The majority of NPs are employed by others, rather than self-employed. The advantages of employment are:

- A built-in collaborative agreement
- No struggles for reimbursement from third-party payers who may balk at paying NPs directly

WHAT RIGHTS DOES AN EMPLOYED NP HAVE?

At Will Employment

In most states, employment is "at will." "At will" employment means the employment continues at the will of the parties. Unless an employee has a contract for a specified term of employment, an employee has no legal right to a job. An employer may end employment at any time. Likewise, an employee may end the employment at any time, barring a contract for a specified term. The only protections for an employee are those offered by the equal opportunity and disability laws; that is, an employee cannot be terminated solely on the basis of age, gender, race, or disability.

An NP who is employed but has no contract must negotiate terms of employment on a piecemeal basis, relying on the ability of the NP and the other party to reach agreement as issues arise. If an employer changes the pay scale or work responsibilities for the better, the NP benefits. If the employer reduces the pay scale or unreasonably increases responsibilities, the NP has no recourse but to keep working under the new conditions or to leave.

Employment by Contract

Many NPs seeking employment are being offered employment contracts. An employment contract is a written agreement under which the employee and employer agree on the terms and conditions of a working relationship.

Employment contracts can be complex and lengthy, and require careful analysis. Some of the issues often addressed in an employment contract are:

- Scope of services to be performed
- Compensation
- Duration of employment
- How the agreement can be altered or updated
- Responsibility to maintain credentials
- Terms of on-call responsibilities
- Benefits
- Time off and expenses for continuing education
- Vacation time
- Number of office hours per week
- Restriction on competition
- Bonuses
- Reasons for termination
- Assistance with continuing education

Some issues that often are not addressed but can be dealt with in an employment contract are:

- Extent of support service to be offered the NP
- Expectations regarding the number of patients seen per day
- Expectations regarding nonclinical (administrative) work to be done by the NP
- Listing of the NP on the door, in directories, and in advertisements
- Use of the NP's name when the office telephone is answered
- On-call responsibilities and backup
- Release to the NP of the NP's quality performance as measured by health plan auditors

An employment agreement can include anything the parties wish to address. Often, agreements are written by attorneys for the practice and therefore are oriented to the needs of the employer.

DOES AN NP NEED A CONTRACT?

Many NPs practiced for many years without employment contracts. In the past, an employer called to offer a job, and the employer and employee then negotiated salary, benefits, and hours of employment. The arrangement was sealed with a handshake. Details were handled as issues arose, but NPs sometimes were unhappy with how the details were handled.

Contracts have certain advantages over the informal employment arrangement. First, contract negotiation forces parties to discuss issues. When the parties agree to terms, there is a document that records the agreement and can be referred to as necessary to refresh memories about details of the agreement. In most cases, an employment agreement is protective to both employer and employee.

For an employee, a contract ensures some degree of job security. In most states, unless there is a written contract defining the duration of employment, employment is "at will." This means that either party may terminate the employment without cause at any time. For example, a practice that hires an NP and then loses a lucrative patient care contract can terminate an NP who is employed "at will" with no severance pay, even though the NP is not at fault. "At will" employees are often surprised to learn that they have no legal rights to their jobs. An NP who has a contract, however, has an agreement for work during the duration of the contract, unless a clause in the contract states otherwise. An employer who wants to end the employment of the NP must wait until the contract terminates or attempt to settle the matter with the NP, possibly by offering severance terms.

For an employer, an employment agreement can afford protection against competition from an employee who leaves the practice and takes patients to another practice. An employer wants to avoid a situation where a departing NP who has built a patient following takes patients to the next NP position. An employer can restrict a departing NP from competing with a practice. The method of restricting competition is a "restrictive covenant" in an employment agreement.

A multitude of lifestyle-affecting and work style-affecting issues can arise among coworker health care providers. An employment contract can delineate the expectations of employer and employee before such problems arise. A contract also can specify problem-solving procedures.

THREE DIFFICULT CLAUSES

Three clauses commonly found in employment agreements offered by medical practices to NPs are especially difficult for NPs to interpret and can have profound effects on an NP's life, restrictive covenants, bonus formulas, and termination clauses. It is these clauses that often bring NPs to attorneys for advice. Restrictive covenants require an NP to promise, up front, not to compete with an employer when the present employment ends. Bonus formulas specify conditions under which an employer rewards an NP for superior performance. Termination clauses specify that an employer may end the agreement, without cause, with 30 days' notice.

Restrictive Covenants

A restrictive covenant is a promise not to compete. Specifically, a restrictive covenant is a clause that restricts an employee from practicing within a set number of miles from an employer's business for a set period of time after the employee leaves the employer's business.

Employers are insisting on restrictive covenants. An employer wants to avoid a situation where a departing NP who has built a patient following takes patients to the next NP position.

Restrictive covenants are legal in many states and enforceable as long as they are reasonable. If a former employee challenges the validity of a restrictive covenant by taking the matter to court, a judge will determine whether a restrictive covenant is reasonable. A judge will balance the needs of the employer against the harm to the employee. A judge will decide whether the geographic restriction and the time restriction are appropriate to accomplish the employer's needs, but no more. Further, a judge will consider whether there is any potential injury to the public if a restrictive covenant is enforced.

A judge will analyze the past court decisions in the state and compare the facts of those cases with the current case. Such facts include: what size city or town the practice is in; the severity of the geographic and time restrictions in the clause; what the practice is like; the availability of other health care providers; and what the employment climate is like for health care providers.

Judges have found restrictive covenants unreasonable when the restraint is greater than necessary to protect the legitimate business interests of the employer. Judges also have found restrictive covenants unreasonable when the restraint is not greater than necessary to protect the business interests but when the employer's need for protection is outweighed by the hardship to the employee. Occasionally, judges have found restrictive covenants to be unreasonable when there is neither excessive restraint nor excessive hardship, but there is a likely injury to the public. For example, a covenant restricting an oral surgeon from practicing in a particular city for three years after termination from a practice was found to be unreasonable. The restraint was greater than necessary. However, a covenant restricting a veterinarian from practicing in a different city for three years after termination was found to be reasonable. In that case, the restraint was not greater than necessary. In yet another case, a covenant restricting a physician from practicing in a rural town for three years after termination was found to be unreasonable. In that case, there was a potential injury to the public. The injury to the public was a potential shortage of physicians if one of the two town physicians could no longer practice there. The difference in outcome in these three cases can be reconciled only by comparing the factual details of the cases. A decision that one clause was reasonable while a seemingly identical clause was unreasonable was due to differences in profession, practice, city, availability of other providers, and many other factors.

When negotiating the terms of a restrictive covenant, an NP needs to consider the circumstances of the job offer, the severity of the restriction, the potential hardship imposed on the NP by the covenant, the availability of health care providers in the area, and the availability of other practice opportunities.

In agreeing to a restrictive covenant, an NP is giving up something of value; the ability to take any other NP job that is offered. However, an NP who refuses to sign a reasonable restrictive covenant may be seen by an employer as someone who is looking to start a competing practice nearby. The best advice on restrictive covenants is to negotiate one the NP can live with, one that seems reasonable for all concerned under the particular circumstances of the practice and the NP. Examples of more reasonable and less reasonable restrictive covenants are provided in Exhibit 10-1.

Bonus Formulas

Some employers offer NPs the opportunity for bonuses. The criteria for bonuses vary greatly. The two most important criteria for bonuses are that both employer and employee understand the formula and that it be consistent with good patient care.

The most common problem with bonus formulas is vague language. If a formula is vague, it is sure to be interpreted in different ways by different individuals. There could be disagreements and disappointments at distribution time.

Productivity-Based Formulas

Many formulas are based on the number of patient visits per year. This makes good business sense under a fee-for-service system of reimbursement. If a prac-

Exhibit 10-1 Restrictive Covenants

Restrictive covenants are enforceable if they balance:

- The employer's need for protection
- Hardship to the employee
- Likelihood of injury to the public

Example 1: "Upon termination of employment for any reason, NP agrees not to practice in any location within 25 miles of any present or future office of this practice for a period of five years."

Analysis: Accomplishes employer's need for protection, but may be broader than necessary to accomplish employer's need and may put excessive hardship on employee to find alternative work 25 miles away.

Example 2: "Upon termination of employment for any reason, NP agrees not to practice in any location within one mile of the Jones Road office of this practice for a period of one year."

Analysis: Not a hardship on employee but may not accomplish employer's need for protection, as patients may be willing to travel one mile to see the NP.

Source: Reprinted with permission from Buppert C. Employment agreements. Nurse Pract 1998; 22:108–119. © 1998, Springhouse Corporation.

tice is at least half fee-for-service, patient visit-based formulas can be a reasonable choice. Tracking patient visits is uncomplicated and is not usually susceptible to vagueness. Generally, an NP who sees large numbers of patients is a productive employee who deserves a bonus.

Bonus formulas based on numbers of patient visits make less sense when reimbursement to the practice is capitated. Under a capitated system of reimbursement, a practice is paid a set fee per patient per month, regardless of the number of patient visits. Under capitated reimbursement, the ultimate goal is not a high number of visits from each patient but good patient care in as few visits as possible. Under capitated reimbursement, bonuses should be given to those providers who demonstrate high-quality care as evidenced by some documented quality measurement tool. Numbers of patient visits should not be relevant when a practice's patients are capitated. Employers have to be careful not to give providers bonuses for withholding care. Aside from the moral and ethical problems involved, there are federal laws that prohibit health care providers from profiting by delivering inadequate or inappropriate care.

Many practices are in transition from fee-for-service to capitated care. Many practices have a mix of fee arrangements with patients and payers. Employer and employee should plan for such transitions and mixes when devising a bonus formula. A bonus formula should fit the practice's payer mix.

Quality-Based Bonuses

When more than half of the patients are covered by some form of managed-care plan, NP performance can be rewarded on the basis of meeting or exceeding quality standards set by the health plan. For example, bonuses could be awarded when the percentage of patients who have met health maintenance criteria—such as childhood immunizations or mammograms for women over 50—exceeds 80 percent. Or bonuses could be awarded if emergency department visits declined in the past year.

While performance measures are more difficult to track than patient visits, they are more suited to managed care. Some health plans supply performance data to practices, and these data could be used to determine bonuses.

To track this kind of performance data and apportion bonuses based on performance, patients and primary providers will have to be paired. NPs will need to have their own panels of patients and be designated as primary care provider for that panel. Or NP-physician teams will have to work together and share bonuses.

Profit-Based Formulas

Some employers share profits with NPs. This can be satisfying to both employer and employee as long as the method for determining profits is clear.

NPs should be aware that there are accounting methods that can maximize or minimize profits and that *profit* is a word that has modifiers, such as *gross* and *net,* that can mean the difference between a bonus and no bonus. NPs who agree to profit-based formulas should negotiate for the right to audit financial records. NPs also should negotiate for a process by which a dispute about profits could be resolved.

Patient Satisfaction-Based Formulas

Patient satisfaction is a measure that employers and employees often suggest as a basis for awarding bonuses to providers. Patient satisfaction is subjective, difficult to measure, and open to conflicting interpretations. On the other hand, there is a multitude of patient satisfaction tools available, and if employer and employee can agree upon a method of measurement, patient satisfaction certainly can be part of the bonus formula.

Bonus formulas are one of the most controversial aspects of provider relationships. Many practices are struggling with this issue. One approach being taken by employers is to implement a bonus formula with the understanding that it will be altered and improved upon from year to year.

See Exhibit 10-2 for some examples of bonus formulas that have been offered to NPs.

Termination without Cause

Typically, the "Termination" section of an employment agreement will list events that are a basis for termination of the employee "with cause." These events often include conviction of a felony, loss of license, loss of hospital privileges, and gross negligence that compromises patient safety.

In addition to termination-with-cause provisions, some employment agreements include a "termination-without-cause" clause, which states that employer can terminate employee at any time, without cause, with 30 days' notice (see examples in Exhibit 10-3).

Exhibit 10-2 Examples of Bonus Formulas from NPs' Contracts

- Up to 15 percent of base salary: 5 percent if practice is profitable, 5 percent based on meeting a threshold of patient visits, and 5 percent based on patient satisfaction, staff satisfaction, and citizenship.
- The product of "collected billings" multiplied by "total employee billings" divided by "total practice billings," with a cap.
- A figure determined by a committee, based on meeting criteria for (1) financial performance; (2) quality of medical services determined by outcomes, medical appropriateness, and extent of health promotion services provided; and (3) level of patient satisfaction.

Source: Reprinted with permission from Buppert C. Employment agreements. Nurse Pract 1998; 22:108–119. © 1998, Springhouse Corporation.

Exhibit 10-3 Examples of Termination Clauses

A Termination-with-Cause Clause

The employer may terminate this agreement at the sole discretion of the employer, by written notice to the NP upon the occurrence of any of the following:

a. The NP dies or becomes disabled. . . .
b. The NP loses his or her professional license. . . .
c. The NP is limited or restricted by any governmental authority having jurisdiction over the NP to the extent that the NP cannot render the required professional services. . . .

A Termination-without-Cause Clause [Not Recommended for NPs]

The employer may terminate this agreement at any time, for any reason, after thirty (30) days' notice to NP.

Source: Reprinted with permission from Buppert C. Employment agreements, Nurse Pract 1998; 22:108–119, © 1998, Springhouse Corporation.

A termination-without-cause clause effectively defeats the purpose of a contract for an employee. An employee who can be terminated at any time for any reason or for no reason not only has no job security but also will think twice about pressing for performance of any of the other provisions in the employment agreement. For example, an NP may believe that a bonus was due, while the employer may believe that no bonus was due. If the NP protests too much, an employer can simply terminate the NP. If, on the other hand, an NP can be terminated only "for cause," the NP will feel freer to be assertive about the other provisions of the contract.

There are reasons to agree to a "termination-without-cause" clause, however. If an NP cannot commit to a full year's employment, it may be best to agree to the "without-cause" clause. Most employers will not agree to delete a "without-cause" clause unless the employee also gives up the right to leave with just 30 days' notice.

HOW TO NEGOTIATE A REASONABLE AGREEMENT

Preparing To Negotiate

NPs who have worked for years without contracts are being offered contracts. NPs who are working without contracts, who foresee an offer in the future, and who want to negotiate a satisfying contract will lay the groundwork a year ahead.

First, an NP should be able to state clearly what he or she has contributed to the practice in the past year and have data to prove it. Specifically, have at hand the total number of patient visits and the dollars billed and received as a result of those visits. If an NP does administrative work, he or she should make a list of administrative projects and determine the dollar worth of the projects to the practice. Contrast the revenues brought in by the NP with the NP's expenses to the practice, including salary, benefits, and continuing education. If there are patient satisfaction surveys or quality-of-care data that support the NP, have those data at hand. While new NPs will not have the option of collecting data in preparation for negotiating first contracts, they should find out everything they can about the practice with which they plan to negotiate. Once employed, new NPs should begin to collect data for future contract negotiations.

First, an NP needs to make the following assessments about his or her speed and comfort level:

1. How many patients can I see per hour, day, month, and year?
2. How much physician consultation time will I need; a ten-minute consultation on every patient, a five-minute consultation once a day, or a five-minute consultation once a year?

Second, an NP should gather basic information on how the practice gets its revenues. Know which insurers pay for NP services and how much. If the payer mix is likely to change in the coming year, be ready to explain how the NP's value to the practice will continue to increase in the coming year. Propose ways in which the practice can increase its efficiency and revenues in the coming year, and offer to help implement plans. An NP embarking on a salary negotiation needs to gather the following data from the employer:

1. What is the most frequently billed CPT code for the practice? What amount does the practice bill and receive, on average, for that CPT code?
2. What percentage of practice income goes to cover practice expenses? If the employer will not reveal that information, ask how many providers share practice overhead expenses. A solo practitioner pays 43 percent of income for office expenses, whereas a practice of 10 to 24 doctors pays 23.5 percent for office expenses. Determine the appropriate rate to deduct for practice expenses.
3. What is the collection rate for the practice? Remember, 90 percent is good.

Third, decide which terms of employment are essential and which can be given up. An NP should ask for everything the NP wants but be ready to back down on nonessential terms.

Fourth, anticipate any drawbacks that an employer might raise in negotiations and prepare to defend or minimize those drawbacks.

Negotiating

Generally, it is best to negotiate individually rather than as a member of a group. For a variety of reasons, some NPs will be more valuable than others to an employer. A more valuable NP should get better offers. On the other hand, some employers have a standard NP offer and will not deviate for the individual NP. In that case, NPs need to negotiate as a group.

Whether negotiating individually or as a group, read a proposed contract carefully, note areas that are confusing, and get clarification. Remember that everything is negotiable. While a contract may look intimidating, it was typed on a word processor and can be changed.

Seek legal counsel to review a proposed contract.

Getting Help: What To Look for in a Lawyer

While the negotiating is best done by the NP employee, contract review is best done by an attorney. An attorney who is familiar with NP contracts and business issues is a good first choice. Second choice would be an attorney who reviews contracts of other health care providers—physicians in particular.

Avoid the attorney who needs to research the law regarding NPs. One NP spent $1,500 for an attorney to research the law on NPs, only to find that she knew the answers to the questions he was looking up.

Attorneys charge between $75 and $400 an hour. Many will negotiate a flat fee for reviewing a contract. It is worth spending $400 (though not $400 an hour) for review of a contract that is worth between $60,000 and $100,000 per year to the NP. If an attorney finds vague wording that needs to be made more specific, the investment in the attorney will be repaid in the long run.

Understanding Business

If an employer has a well-run, profitable practice to which an NP contributes significantly, the NP should expect to be rewarded well under an employment agreement. If a practice is losing money, no NP will be able to negotiate a satisfying agreement, no matter how excellent the NP.

NPs are clinicians by nature rather than businesspeople. However, all types of clinicians are finding that they need to understand more about the business of health care. An NP who understands the financial base for a practice is in a better position to negotiate a satisfactory employment agreement than an NP who knows only the clinical side of practice. An employer will respect an NP who approaches negotiations with attention to both business principles and patient care concerns.

*Negotiating Salary**

New NPs are notorious for asking only two questions of a new employer: What does it pay, and what are the benefits?

Source: Portions of this section have been reprinted with permission from NP Communications Group, Inc., from an article that appeared in July–August 1997, in *NP World News.*

Four methods of payment are currently being used to pay employed NPs:

1. Straight salary
2. Percentage of net receipts
3. Base salary plus percentage
4. Hourly rate

In a *straight salary* arrangement, an NP is paid a set amount to perform according to a job description. In a *percentage salary* arrangement, an NP is paid the amount the NP bills minus accounts receivable, minus the NP's portion of practice expenses (which includes the expense of physician consultation). In a *base salary plus percentage* arrangement, an NP is guaranteed a set salary but can make additional salary if the NP generates practice income over some set amount. NPs working on an *hourly* basis are paid only for the hours worked.

Straight salary and hourly are more commonly encountered arrangements than percentage or set salary plus percentage. The advantage of percentage-based salaries is the opportunity for productive NPs to have some control over their earnings. The disadvantage is that the method sets up fellow providers in a practice as competitors for patients.

No matter what arrangement an NP chooses, it is wise to focus on hard figures that document an NP's monetary contribution to a practice and the costs of an NP to a practice.

NPs bring in income on a fee-for-service basis or a per-member-per-month basis. Figuring an NP's share of income for a fee-for-service practice is done by multiplying the number of visits by the collected fee per visit. When a practice's patients are capitated, an NP's share of income is figured by multiplying the number of patients on an NP's panel by the per-member-per-month fee coming into the practice.

The cost of maintaining an NP is figured by adding practice expenses and the cost of physician consultation. Practice expenses can be estimated or calculated for a particular practice. For a solo practice, expenses can be 40 to 50 percent of the income. For a large practice, expenses are lower, 20 to 30 percent of income. Practice expenses include rent, salaries, taxes and benefits of support staff, taxes and benefits of NPs, supplies, laboratory expenses, depreciation, car, continuing education, and insurance (malpractice, workers' compensation, and premises insurance).

An NP who needs a great deal of physician consultation should expect to compensate the NP's employer physicians for their time. An NP who needs little consultation should command a higher salary because he or she needs little of a physician's time. Until NPs no longer need a physician on written agreement, all NPs should expect to pay something for physician consultation. Experienced NPs often pay physician employers/consultants 10 to 15 percent of their net income brought to the practice.

Most employers will want a percentage of an NP's earnings as profit. An experienced NP who needs little consultation from an employer physician might consider his or her contribution to profit to be the 10 to 15 percent of net income paid for consultation, as noted in the paragraph above. A newer NP should expect to contribute 10 to 15 percent of net earnings to an employer as profit in addition to 15 to 25 percent of net earnings for physician consultation.

To project an appropriate salary for a particular NP:

1. Calculate income to the practice based on NP billings
2. Subtract 10 percent for unpaid bills
3. Subtract
   a. The calculated figure for practice expenses (20 to 50 percent of earnings)
   b. The cost of physician consultation (10 to 20 percent of net earnings)
   c. A percentage for employer profit

Fee-for-Service Practices. For example, an NP who sees 15 patients per day at $35 per patient visit, on average, brings in $525 per day. Allowing one week off for continuing education, one week off for illness, and four weeks off for vacation, this NP will bring in $120,750 a year, potentially. However, not all bills are paid. With a 90 percent collection rate—a reasonable collection rate for an efficient practice—this NP actually will bring in $108,675 per year. An NP who sees 24 patients per day will bring in $840 per day, or $193,200 per year in accounts receivable. With a 90 percent collection rate, this NP will bring $173,880 to the practice.

Deducting 40 percent of the NP's gross generated income for overhead expenses (rent, benefits, continuing education, supplies, malpractice, lab expenses, and depreciation of equipment) leaves $65,205 for the 15-patient-per-day NP and $104,328 for the 24-patient-per-day NP. Further deducting 15 percent of that figure to pay a physician for consultation services leaves $55,425 in salary for the 15-patient-per-day NP and $88,679 in salary for the 24-patient-per-day NP. Deducting 10 percent for employer profit leaves $49,882 in salary for the 15-patient-per-day NP and $79,811 for the 24-patient-per-day NP.

Capitated Practices. In a fully capitated practice, an NP who has a panel of 1,000 patients at an average fee per member per month of $10 will bring in $120,000 annually. There should be a 100 percent collection rate under a capitated system of reimbursement.

Applying 40 percent to overhead leaves $72,000, and paying 15 percent for physician consultation and 10 percent for employer profit leaves $55,080 for NP salary. An NP with a larger panel will make more.

The New NP. A newly graduated NP without experience may be able to see only ten patients a day, with four or five ten-minute physician consultations per day, for the first six months. Plugging in the figures as in the examples above, the NP will bill 2,400 visits per year (two weeks' vacation for the new grad) at $35 per visit to total $84,000 in accounts receivable. With a 90 percent collection rate, the new NP will bring in $75,600.

Deducting 40 percent for practice expenses brings the net income to $45,360. Because a new NP often requires significant consultation time with a physician (or experienced NP), deduct 25 percent ($11,340) for payment for consultation, bringing the NP salary down to $34,020. With a contribution to employer profit, this new NP's appropriate salary is down to $30,618.

After six months, when the same NP becomes more comfortable and more efficient, the income numbers should double and consultation requirements should decrease, so that the appropriate salary will more closely approximate the salary of the 15-patient-per-day NP and eventually the 24-patient-per-day NP in the examples above. Many employers start a new NP at a salary significantly higher than $30,618, expecting that low productivity in the first six months will be balanced by high productivity in the second six months.

Experienced NPs who are seeing more than 15 patients per day at CPT code level 99213 or higher should be making at least $50,000 per year. If not, there are inefficiencies in the practice, or the NP is not getting a share of his or her profits.

Are These Projections Accurate? One could argue about whether the percentages used above are correct. In fact, some practices have poor rates of collections, some practices have higher overhead expenses, some physicians want more payment for consultation than $9,780 per year for a 15-patient-per-day NP or $15,649 per year for a 24-patient-per-day NP, and some employers want more profit than projected here. However, an NP should not be subsidizing a poorly run practice and should not be overcompensating a physician or employer. Many practices receive more than $35 per NP visit on average. In these practices, an NP's salary should be proportionately higher.

Reported Median NP Salaries. Comparing these calculated NP salaries with some of the recently reported median salaries for NP salaries is an interesting exercise. Some medical groups use the Medical Group Management Association's (MGMA) median salary data. Those data are available to the group's members. The median salary reported by MGMA often is lower than other surveys. As reported in the February 2002 issue of *Advance for Nurse Practitioners,* the median NP salary for 2001 was about $63,000. The median primary care physician salary was approximately $130,000.

NPs should keep in mind that salary averages are based on mail-in surveys. There is no way of knowing whether the respondents were representative of NPs. NPs who believe they are worthy of higher salaries than surveys suggest should present all of the reasons why they deserve the figure they are seeking.

As in all negotiating, there are three things to remember:

1. One who does not ask will not receive.
2. One who does not deserve will not receive.
3. Even when one asks and deserves, one will need to do some selling to get what one wants.

Negotiating Benefits

There are three yardsticks by which to evaluate a benefits package:

1. What benefits does the NP need?
2. What is reasonable?
3. What are other NPs getting?

Only numbers 1 and 2 count.

An NP in the late stages of job interviewing should ask a prospective employer:

- What benefits usually are offered?
- Does the employer pay for continuing education?
- Is time away for continuing education paid time?
- What is the retirement plan?
- What are the basics of the health plan? Is dental included? Vision coverage included?
- If call is required, are a cellular telephone, beeper, and car allowance included?
- What vacation time is being offered?
- How is sick time handled?
- Is malpractice insurance paid by the employer? If so, will a separate attorney for the NP be covered? Is the policy occurrence or claims made? (See Chapter 7 for the distinction.)
- Are relocation expenses paid?
- Is there a sign-on bonus?
- Are expenses of travel for the interview to be paid?
- Does the employer pay for professional dues? If so, how much?
- Does the employer pay for reference books and subscriptions to professional journals? If so, how much?
- Are there any tuition reimbursement benefits for NP or for dependents?
- Is there a short- or long-term disability insurance benefit?
- If travel to various sites is necessary, are automobile expenses reimbursed?

Negotiating a Working Environment

Of course, many nonmonetary aspects of an NP's working life affect job satisfaction. An NP contemplating a new job is advised to spend some time thinking about and perhaps listing the aspects of former jobs that have been most satisfying and most frustrating. Then the NP can briefly summarize the best and the worst of former jobs with the prospective employer and try to maximize the positive in the new position. Ask such questions as:

- Is call required? If so, how is call shared? What backup will an NP have if consultation is needed for a call?

- What kind of and how many support staff will the practice provide?
- What will support staff do for the NP? What will support staff expect the NP to do for them?
- To whom will the NP report about medical issues? Administrative issues? Payment issues?
- What continuous quality improvement methods does the practice use?
- If the NP finds some aspect of practice organization that he or she would like to change, what will the process be?
- Is the NP expected to build a panel of patients or cover for overbookings of the other providers, or both?

INTERVIEWING

A physician or administrator who is interested in hiring an NP may have significant, little, or no experience working with NPs. Therefore, NPs should be prepared to define NP scope of practice, list state requirements for collaboration or supervision, if any, and identify the sources of reimbursement for NP services.

In an interview for employment as an NP, be prepared to answer the following questions:

- Why should I hire an NP?
- Why should I hire you?
- How many patients are you used to seeing in a day?
- Do you have a DEA number?
- How independently are you used to practicing?
- What can you bring to the practice?
- What is your greatest job strength? Weakness?
- What can an NP legally do in this state?
- What do you want to be doing in five years? In two years? In ten years?
- Does working evenings and/or weekends bother you?

RESPONSIBILITIES OF AN NP EMPLOYEE

Whether or not an NP has a contract, an NP has certain ethical responsibilities to an employer. These include responsibilities to:

- Add to the good will an employer has built in the community by promoting the practice to the public
- Protect the employer's "trade secrets," such as patient mailing lists
- Provide one's best customer service to patients of the employer
- Remain unimpaired by alcohol or drugs
- Maintain one's credentials, knowledge of standard of care, and continuing education
- Maintain patient confidentiality

EMPLOYER'S EVALUATION OF THE NP'S PERFORMANCE

Some employers evaluate NP performance in highly structured ways—number of patients seen per month or quarter, income generated, detailed evaluation tools—and others use either no measure or very subjective measures.

An NP is advised to ask, in the interview stages, about the employer's expectations for productivity, measures of quality, and other performance measures. If an NP knows how the NP's work will be evaluated, the NP has a better chance of meeting expectations. If there are no set methods of evaluation, an NP may want to offer to develop some standards.

MALPRACTICE INSURANCE

The best malpractice policy for an NP is an occurrence policy, for at least $1 million per claim and $3 million aggregate, which covers an attorney for the NP as an individual rather than as a member of a group. If an NP must purchase an individual policy to obtain this coverage, the NP should do so.

COLLABORATIVE PRACTICE AGREEMENTS

In states where a collaborative agreement is required by law, the NP or the physician or both are legally responsible for drafting and filing the agreement with the appropriate agency. The most prudent process for drafting a collaborative agreement is as follows:

- Collect information:
  1. Review the state law regarding NP scope of practice. Questions to be answered are: Must the practice agreement be approved by the board of nursing and/or board of medicine prior to beginning practice? Are there qualifications for the collaborating physician? Are there limitations on the collaborating physician (such as a limit on the number of NPs who may collaborate with the physician)? Is the practice agreement required solely for prescriptive authority or for any form of advanced practice?
  2. Determine the functions that the NP will supply to the proposed collaborative practice. Will there be in-hospital care? Suturing? Surgical assistance? Prescription of controlled substances? Nursing home practice?
  3. Determine whether the physician collaborator's area of specialty matches the NP's. Interview the physician collaborator much as you would conduct a job interview, and check references. Ask whether there are any current or past malpractice cases against the physician or practice. Ask whether there has been any loss of hospital privileges or loss of Medicare participation.
- Draft an agreement for the collaborator's review. Often, the board of nursing will have sample written agreements upon which an NP can base the draft.

- Finalize and submit the agreement. Sometimes the board of nursing will return an agreement with a request for more information. If so, simply redraft and resubmit.

An example of a practice agreement is given in Appendix 10-A and a sample employment agreement is provided in Appendix 10-B.

APPENDIX 10-A

Sample Nurse Practitioner Collaborative Practice Agreement

I. GENERAL INFORMATION

A. Nurse Practitioner

Name Jane Doe Md. License Certification 00000000 CRNP-Adult

Date Designated 2003 Certifying Organization ANCC

B. Licensed Physician

Name Gregory James License/Certification 00000000

C. Description of Setting of Practice

1. Type of setting: The setting is Dr. James's internal medicine office at 600 Ridgely Avenue in Annapolis, Maryland.
2. Type and expected volume of patients: Patients are adult outpatients. Volume will vary—two to four per hour—and is expected to be similar to other internal medicine practices in the area.

II. NURSE PRACTITIONER FUNCTIONS

The nurse practitioner will provide general preventive care and diagnosis and treatment of episodic, short-term, and stable chronic health problems. Provisions for referring patients with unstable or acute life-threatening conditions are detailed below. Such care will include, but not be limited to, the following functions.

A. Perform Comprehensive Physical Assessments of Patients as Needed

The nurse practitioner will perform pertinent history and physical examination of any patient to establish a database and identify the patient's immediate and comprehensive health care needs.

B. Establish Medical Diagnosis for Common Short-Term or Chronic Stable Health Problems

The scope of practice of the nurse practitioner will depend upon the category of problem and will become clear by the delineation of the following categories of problems:

- For common acute, chronic stable conditions, the nurse practitioner will diagnose, manage, and treat, including prevention and patient education. Examples of these would be upper respiratory infections, pharyngitis, otitis media, common skin lesions, and management of chronic problems such as asthma and diabetes mellitus uncomplicated.
- For uncommon or unstable conditions, the nurse practitioner will participate in the diagnosis with consultation and either refer to a specialist or participate in the dual management and treatment with a consultant. Examples of these would be fractures and acute severe abdominal pain.
- For acute life-threatening conditions, the nurse practitioner would provide a working diagnosis, institute emergency management, and immediately refer to a secondary care center. Examples of these would be status asthmaticus, airway obstruction, and cardiac arrest.

C. Order, Perform, and Interpret Laboratory Tests (Including Diagnostic and Invasive Procedures)

The nurse practitioner will order and interpret any test necessary to the medical evaluation. Examples of laboratory and diagnostic tests that the nurse practitioner orders, performs, and/or interprets:

- Orders and interprets: Complete blood count, serum chemistry, thyroid function tests, EKG
- Performs: EKG
- Orders: Chest X-ray

The nurse practitioner has 12 years of experience in ordering, performing, and interpreting diagnostic tests and has had didactic training in a baccalaureate nursing program, in intensive care unit training, and through continuing medical education in interpreting laboratory data.

D. Prescribe Drugs

The nurse practitioner will prescribe drugs as necessary and appropriate for an internal medicine office, in accordance with state and federal law. Examples of classes of drugs to be prescribed are antihypertensives, antianginals, antibiotics, bronchodilators, diuretics, and analgesics, including controlled dangerous substances (CDSs). The nurse practitioner may order any CDS covered by the nurse practitioner's DEA permit. This includes all classes applied for, that is, all but experimental drugs. Specifically, the nurse practitioner prescribes analgesics, such as Tylenol with codeine, benzodiazepines, and certain weight reduction medications that include amphetamines. CDSs will be limited to short-term, acute episodes, such as migraine headache.

E. Perform Therapeutic and Corrective Measures

The nurse practitioner will order and may perform such therapeutic measures as are appropriate for an internal medicine practice, for example, patient education, cleaning and dressing of superficial wounds, splinting, and irrigation of ears and eyes.

F. Emergency Care

The nurse practitioner will perform cardiopulmonary resuscitation as necessary until emergency vehicles arrive. The nurse practitioner successfully completed the national cognitive and skills examination in accordance with the Standards of the American Heart Association for Course C, Basic Life Support, in November 1997.

III. NURSE PRACTITIONER/PHYSICIAN RELATIONSHIP

A. Referrals

The nurse practitioner will evaluate, diagnose, manage, and treat common acute and chronic stable conditions as described in Section II.B. above, seeking consultation as she deems necessary.

In dealing with uncommon or unstable conditions as described in Section II.B, the nurse practitioner will take the history, do the physical exam, obtain laboratory and other necessary data, participate in the diagnosis with consultation, and either refer to the physician consultant or to a specialty clinic or secondary treatment center or participate in dual management and treatment with a physician consultant or specialty clinic.

In dealing with acute life-threatening conditions as described in Section II.B. above, the nurse practitioner will take a history, do the necessary initial physical exam, make a working diagnosis, institute emergency management, and immediately refer to the nearest emergency department.

B. Drug and Medical Guidelines

The nurse practitioner will collaborate with the physician in establishing and reviewing drug and other medical guidelines. Review of guidelines will be done in a continuing manner, but no less frequently than annually.

C. Schedule for Review

The nurse practitioner will review and discuss medical diagnoses and therapeutic or corrective measures employed in a continuing manner when the dual management method of care is employed. The nurse practitioner and physician will review and discuss patient care management no less than monthly.

D. Schedule for Consultation, Record Review, Cosigning of Records

The physician will be in attendance at the practice daily, except when on leave, and generally be available for consultation, record review, and cosigning of records as needed in the discretion of the nurse practitioner.

E. Availability of Physician for Consultation

The physician consultant will be available in person or by telephone on an as-needed basis in order to consult with the nurse practitioner on diagnosis and treatment of medical problems. In the event that he is on leave, the physician will designate another physician who will be available to consult with the nurse practitioner as needed.

IV. AUTHORIZATION

The nurse practitioner shall immediately notify the Nursing Board if this written agreement is ended by either party. The physician shall immediately notify the Medical Board if this written agreement is ended by either party.

The nurse practitioner shall submit a new or amended written agreement for approval before altering the practice setting or modifying or expanding the medical functions that the nurse practitioner is authorized to perform.

______________________________ ____________

Nurse Practitioner Date

______________________________ ____________

Physician Date

APPENDIX 10-B

Sample Employment Agreement

Note: The following contract is suited for a particular NP and a particular medical practice. Other NPs and practices may need different or additional provisions. NPs and employers each should seek the counsel of an attorney for drafting a contract suitable to the needs of the particular parties.

EMPLOYMENT AGREEMENT

THIS PROFESSIONAL SERVICES EMPLOYMENT AGREEMENT (the Agreement) made this ____ day of __________, 2003, by and between Jones Medical Clinic, a professional corporation in the State of Maryland, hereinafter referred to as "the Corporation," and Jane Doe, MS, CRNP, an individual, hereinafter referred to as "the Nurse Practitioner."

RECITALS

The Corporation is a professional association formed in Maryland and engaged in the practice of medicine. The services rendered by and on behalf of the Corporation are referred to as the Practice.

The Nurse Practitioner is licensed to practice in Maryland.

The Corporation desires to employ the Nurse Practitioner upon the terms and conditions hereinafter set forth, and the Nurse Practitioner desires to accept such employment.

ARTICLE I—EMPLOYMENT

1.1. Professional Services. The Corporation agrees to employ the Nurse Practitioner under this Agreement. The Nurse Practitioner agrees to render professional services for individuals who present themselves as patients of the Practice and to carry out the duties described in Schedule A, which is attached to and made as a part of this Agreement. In performing such services, the Nurse

Practitioner shall comply with policies and procedures established by the Corporation, including participation in quality assurance and utilization review activities. The Nurse Practitioner shall render professional services at the Jamestown location.

1.2. Full-Time Employment. The Nurse Practitioner agrees to devote her full time and best efforts to the performance of the duties outlined in Schedule A attached to this Agreement.

1.3. Standards. The Nurse Practitioner shall exercise independent professional judgment with respect to the care and treatment of all patients. The Nurse Practitioner agrees that the patient care services will be provided promptly, efficiently, and in strict accordance with the ethical and professional standards for the provision of health care services adopted by the Practice. The Nurse Practitioner agrees that her patient care efficiency and productivity (i.e., number of outpatient visits per week, etc.) will be consistent with or better than past experience.

1.4. Authorization for Exchange of Information. The Nurse Practitioner authorizes the Corporation to obtain credentialing information from any necessary source. Credentialing information includes all information related to the Nurse Practitioner's education, training, qualifications, character, and experience, including patient care, quality assurance, utilization review, and risk management records.

1.5. Charges and Accounts Receivable. The Nurse Practitioner assigns to the Corporation the full right to bill for all professional, administrative, and clinical services performed by the Nurse Practitioner. The Nurse Practitioner agrees that all fees, when accrued or paid, are the sole property of the Corporation and that the Nurse Practitioner has no direct interest in any of these fees. All fee schedules shall be established by the Corporation.

1.6. Medical Records. All medical records of the Practice shall be the property of the Corporation, subject to applicable provisions of the medical records law of Maryland.

ARTICLE II—COMPENSATION, BENEFITS, DISABILITY, AND INSURANCE

2.1. Nurse Practitioner Compensation. In consideration of the Nurse Practitioner rendering services under this Agreement, the Corporation will pay the Nurse Practitioner the compensation as set forth on Schedule B.

2.2. Vacation and Employee Benefits. In addition to the monetary compensation, the Corporation shall provide the Nurse Practitioner with the vacation and employment benefits listed on Schedule C.

2.3. Termination of Disability. If the Agreement is terminated because of the Nurse Practitioner's disability pursuant to Subsection 3.2.1, the Nurse Practitioner's compensation shall terminate after the twenty-six week determination period, but the Nurse Practitioner shall have the right to claim benefits under the long-term disability insurance policy provided as an employee benefit.

2.4. Professional Liability Insurance. During the term of this Agreement and thereafter, the Corporation shall continuously maintain in effect professional liability malpractice insurance for the Nurse Practitioner in the amount of $1,000,000 per occurrence/$3,000,000 annual aggregate coverage.

2.5. General Liability. During the term of this Agreement, the Corporation shall include the Nurse Practitioner as a covered employee under the Corporation's general liability insurance policy.

ARTICLE III—TERM AND TERMINATION

3.1. Term. The term of this Agreement shall be one year beginning __________, 2003, and, if not sooner terminated as provided below, ending ____________, 2004. Thereafter, this Agreement shall automatically renew on a year-to-year basis, unless sooner terminated as provided below.

3.2. Termination by Corporation—Without Cure Period. The Corporation may terminate this Agreement at the sole discretion of the Corporation by written notice to the Nurse Practitioner (or representative) upon the occurrence of any of the following:

3.2.1. The Nurse Practitioner dies or becomes disabled. As used in this Agreement, *disabled* means the Nurse Practitioner's inability to perform the material and essential functions of clinical care for patients, despite reasonable accommodations by the Corporation, by reason of any medically determinable physical or mental impairment that has been determined to be terminal or that has lasted or can be expected to last for a period of not less than twenty-six weeks, based on an examination by an independent physician selected by the Corporation.

3.2.2. The revocation, suspension, or cancellation of the Nurse Practitioner's professional license.

3.2.3. The imposition of any restriction or limitation on the Nurse Practitioner by any governmental authority having jurisdiction over the Nurse Practitioner to the extent that the Nurse Practitioner cannot render the required professional services.

3.2.4. A final determination by any board, hospital, or other organization having jurisdiction over the Nurse Practitioner's right to practice that the Nurse Practitioner has engaged in unprofessional or unethical conduct.

3.2.5. The Nurse Practitioner's clinical privileges at a hospital are involuntarily reduced, suspended, or revoked by final action of the hospital board under the bylaws, rules, or regulations of the hospital.

3.2.6. The Nurse Practitioner is convicted in a criminal or civil proceeding of fraud, misappropriation, embezzlement, or Medicare or Medicaid fraud and abuse.

3.2.7. The Nurse Practitioner is excluded from participation in the Medicare or Medicaid program by reason of fraud and/or abuse.

3.2.8. The Nurse Practitioner has misused assets of the Corporation by fraud.

3.3. Termination by Corporation—With Cure Period. The Corporation may terminate this Agreement based upon a failure of the Nurse Practitioner to comply with the terms and provisions of the Agreement after giving the Nurse Practitioner a notice of the alleged deficiency and allowing the Nurse Practitioner thirty (30) days to cure the alleged deficiency. The following are examples of deficiencies subject to the provisions of this Section:

3.3.1. The failure or refusal of the Nurse Practitioner to comply with the reasonable policies, work requirements, standards and regulations of the Corporation that may be established from time to time.

3.3.2. The Nurse Practitioner breaches any obligation, covenant, or warranty under this Agreement, or the Nurse Practitioner fails to faithfully and diligently perform the services required by the provisions of this Agreement.

3.3.3. Notwithstanding the above, a thirty (30)-day notice shall not be required if the same deficiency has occurred more than twice in any eighteen (18)-month period and written notice to cure was provided with respect to the previous occurrences, or if the deficiency is material and is incapable of being cured.

3.4. Termination by Nurse Practitioner. The Nurse Practitioner may terminate this Agreement:

3.4.1. Based upon a breach by the Corporation for failure to pay the compensation payable under the Agreement or failure to fulfill any other obligations under this Agreement, provided that the Corporation was given written notice of default and thirty (30) days to cure the specified breach.

3.4.2. The physicians of the Corporation are convicted in a criminal or civil proceeding of fraud, misappropriation, embezzlement, or Medicare or Medicaid fraud and abuse.

3.4.3. The physicians of the Corporation are excluded from participation in the Medicare or Medicaid program by reason of fraud and/or abuse.

3.4.4. The Nurse Practitioner moves out of the State of Maryland and gives thirty (30) days notice.

3.5. Effect of Termination. Upon termination of this Agreement as provided in this Article III, neither party shall have any further rights, duties, or obligations under this Agreement, except as otherwise provided herein. The termination or expiration shall not affect any liability or other obligation of either party that accrued prior to the termination or expiration.

ARTICLE IV—MANAGEMENT SUPPORT SYSTEMS AND PERSONNEL

4.1. The Corporation shall provide for or secure nonphysician personnel (including administrative, nursing, and other medical support personnel) and services that are reasonably needed by the Practice consistent with sound management standards for similar practices in the community. These services shall include administration, marketing and financial services, computerized management information systems, and computerized billing systems.

4.2. The Corporation shall provide the Nurse Practitioner with monthly statements of billings, collections, and accounts receivables attributable to the Nurse Practitioner. Should the Nurse Practitioner have questions about the data supplied, the Corporation shall provide access to the Corporation's accounting records and a clerk who keeps these records and who will answer the Nurse Practitioner's questions or supply further information as needed.

4.3. If the Nurse Practitioner's own records of patient visits and billings differ from the records of the Corporation, and the discrepancy cannot be resolved by the information seeking covered by Section 4.2, the Corporation agrees to designate one representative to negotiate a settlement acceptable to both parties within 30 days. If no settlement can be reached internally, the Corporation agrees to submit any unresolved dispute to third-party arbitration, with the arbitrator selected from a list provided by the American Arbitration Association. The Corporation agrees to share equally with the Nurse Practitioner the expenses of arbitration.

4.4. The Corporation shall assign one physician to sign the Nurse Practitioner's written agreement, as required by Maryland law. The physician assigned shall be available or shall appoint a designate who will be available for consultation with the Nurse Practitioner when needed.

ARTICLE V—NOTICES

All notices shall be in writing and personally delivered or sent by certified or registered mail, postage prepaid, return receipt requested, addressed to the Corporation and the Nurse Practitioner at the addresses shown below. Any and all notices or other communication given pursuant to this Agreement shall be deemed duly given on the date personally delivered or on the date deposited in the US Postal Service. The parties may change its or his or her address by specifying the change in a written notice to the other:

If to the Nurse Practitioner:

Jane Doe, CRNP
98 Merit Drive
Jamestown, MD 20000-3000

If to the Corporation:

Jack Frost, MD
201 Medical Drive, Suite 100
Jamestown, MD 20000

ARTICLE VI—MISCELLANEOUS

6.1. Entire Agreement. This Agreement embodies the entire agreement between the parties and supersedes all prior agreements, letters of intent, or understandings of any nature whatsoever between the parties with respect to the matters covered herein.

6.2. Amendment: Nonwaiver. Except as otherwise specifically provided, no amendment or modification of this Agreement shall be valid unless it is in writing and signed by the Nurse Practitioner and the designee of the Corporation as named in Article 5. No waiver of any of the provisions of this Agreement shall be valid unless it is in writing and signed by the party against whom it is sought to be enforced. Any waiver of breach of this Agreement shall not be considered to be a continuing waiver or consent to any subsequent breach on the part of either the Corporation or the Nurse Practitioner.

6.3. Counterparts. This Agreement may be executed in counterparts, and each counterpart shall be deemed an original.

6.4. Assignment. This Agreement may not be assigned by the Corporation to any entity without the prior written consent of the Nurse Practitioner. This Agreement is personal to the Nurse Practitioner and is not assignable by the Nurse Practitioner, in whole or in part, without the prior written consent of the Corporation. This Agreement is binding upon and inures to the benefit of the parties respective permitted successors and permitted assigns.

6.5. Governing Law. This Agreement shall be construed in accordance with and governed by the laws of the State of Maryland.

6.6. Governmental Requirements. This Agreement is subject to the requirements of all applicable laws and regulations and any government agency having jurisdiction. The parties agree to negotiate in good faith to amend this Agreement to comply with any governmental requirements affecting the Agreement or either party, including, without limitation, requirements affecting reimbursement for health care services. If the parties are unable to negotiate a mutually acceptable amendment to comply with any provision of law, regulation, or ruling, either party may initiate a voluntary termination of this Agreement on thirty (30) days' notice.

6.7. Confidentiality. The parties agree not to disclose this Agreement or its contents to any person, firm, or entity, except the agents or representatives of the parties, and except as required by law.

6.8. Further Assurances. The Nurse Practitioner agrees to execute, acknowledge, seal, and deliver further assurances, instruments, and documents and to take such further actions as the Corporation may reasonably request in order to fulfill the intent of this Agreement.

IN WITNESS WHEREOF, the parties have caused this Agreement to be executed as of the day and year first above written, with the intent that this be a sealed instrument.

WITNESS/ATTEST: Jones Medical Clinic, PC

By: ______________________ Date________

__________________________ Date________

Jane Doe, MS, CRNP

SCHEDULE A—DUTIES

1. The Nurse Practitioner shall provide clinical and professional medical services to patients within the scope of Nurse Practitioner's qualifications and consistent with accepted standards of medical practice and consistent with the reasonable productivity standards adopted by the Corporation and the Nurse Practitioner.

2. The Nurse Practitioner shall provide general patient care at the site specified by performance of accepted procedures and commonly used therapies and provision of appropriate support services. The Nurse Practitioner's duties shall include, but not be limited to, keeping and maintaining (or causing to be kept and maintained) appropriate records relating to all professional services rendered by Nurse Practitioner under this Agreement and preparing and attending to, in connection with such services, all reports, claims, and correspondence necessary and appropriate in the circumstances, all of which records, reports, claims, and correspondence shall belong to the Corporation. The Nurse Practitioner shall do all things reasonably desirable to maintain and improve her professional skills, including attendance at professional, postgraduate seminars and participation in professional societies. In addition, the Nurse Practitioner shall perform the following administrative, teaching, or professional services for the Corporation:

   a. Order medical supplies for the office.
   b. Review lab and radiology reports of office patients, and take appropriate follow-up action.
   c. Precept students from Johns Hopkins University.

3. The Nurse Practitioner shall be responsible for the quality of medical care rendered by Nurse Practitioner to the patients of the Practice and for ensuring that such care meets or exceeds currently accepted standards of medical competence.

4. The Nurse Practitioner shall participate in the quality assurance and risk management program.

5. The Nurse Practitioner shall assist in the recruitment and hiring of professional personnel and support staff to work in the practice.

6. The Nurse Practitioner will relate to colleagues, staff, patients, and the public in a collegial manner and will abide by standards of conduct appropriate to the workplace.

7. The Nurse Practitioner shall assist in the marketing of the Practice and participate in the professional activities that promote the Practice.

SCHEDULE B—COMPENSATION

1. During the year of this Agreement (__________, 2003, to ____________, 2004), the Nurse Practitioner shall be paid a salary of $75,000, payable in biweekly installments. Salary is understood to include the Nurse Practitioner's share of collected billings, as determined in Paragraph 2 below, and the Nurse Practitioner's performance of administrative, teaching, and other professional duties as specified in Schedule A, Paragraph 2, above.

2. Billings shall be apportioned as the Nurse Practitioner's share as follows:
   a. The Corporation and the Nurse Practitioner agree that efficiency at collections is outside of the control of the Nurse Practitioner, but within the control of the Corporation. Therefore, the Corporation and the Nurse Practitioner agree to apply a 75 percent collection rate (percentage of billings collected, as of 120 days after billing) for the purposes of determining the Nurse Practitioner's collected billings. The Corporation agrees to take responsibility for maintaining a 75 percent rate of billings collected. In the event that the Corporation does not collect 75 percent of its billings during the term of this Agreement, Corporation agrees to pay the Nurse Practitioner salary as if the Corporation had maintained a 75 percent collections rate.
   b. The Corporation and the Nurse Practitioner agree to a fee schedule for the Nurse Practitioner's services, which is attached.

3. The Nurse Practitioner agrees to bill a minimum of $200,000 per year.
   a. Billings shall include self-paying patients, third-party payers, and internal billings, which shall include surgical follow-up visits handled by the Nurse Practitioner for the Corporation.
   b. Surgical follow-up visits are assigned a value of $55.00.

4. The Corporation shall retain all but $75,000 of collected revenues from the first $200,000 of billings generated by the Nurse Practitioner.

5. The Nurse Practitioner shall receive bonus payments to be determined as follows:
   a. If the Nurse Practitioner's billings exceed $50,000 in any quarter, collected revenues exceeding $50,000 per quarter shall be shared jointly and equally by the Nurse Practitioner and the Corporation, and the Corporation shall pay the Nurse Practitioner's 50 percent share to the Nurse Practitioner as a bonus within 30 days of the last day of the quarter.
   b. If the Nurse Practitioner bills less than $50,000 in any quarter, the Nurse Practitioner shall receive no bonus for that quarter, and the difference between the amount billed by the Nurse Practitioner in the deficient quarter, and $50,000 shall be deducted from any bonus the Nurse Practitioner shall receive in a future quarter. There shall be no deduction from the Nurse Practitioner's salary.

c. In the event that this Agreement is terminated prior to receipt of any bonus payment due the Nurse Practitioner, the Corporation agrees to pay the Nurse Practitioner the bonus earned within 15 days of termination. In the event that termination occurs mid-quarter, both parties agree that neither bonus nor deficiency will apply for the final quarter.

SCHEDULE C—BENEFITS

1. The Nurse Practitioner shall be entitled to the following benefits:
   a. Health insurance: The Corporation shall pay directly to the health insurance company up to $4,000.00 per year for premiums for health insurance.
   b. Malpractice insurance: The Corporation shall pay the malpractice insurance premiums for the Nurse Practitioner.
   c. Pension benefits: The Corporation will fund the Nurse Practitioner's pension benefits.
   d. Vacation: Four (4) weeks per year.
   e. Continuing medical education time: One (1) week.
   f. Continuing medical education expenses: Up to $1,500.00 per year, paid for by the Corporation.
   g. Life insurance: In an amount equal to annual base salary.
   h. Salary continuation plan: Short-term disability—Full pay continuation until Long-Term Disability coverage begins at 90 days.
   i. Sick leave: Ten (10) days per year.
   j. Professional fees and medical staff dues: Professional journals in the amount of $350 per year, medical staff dues at hospitals where the Nurse Practitioner attends patients of the Practice, state license fee, state Controlled Dangerous Substances and DEA license fees, and Basic Cardiac Life Support/Advanced Cardiac Life Support recertification fees.

CHAPTER 11

Practice Ownership: Legal and Business Considerations for the Nurse Practitioner Owner

Some state law is more conducive to NP practice ownership than others because of collaboration requirements, or lack thereof, and because of laws concerning reimbursement. Nevertheless, NPs are starting their own practices, and others have owned their own practices for over 20 years, hiring physicians where necessary to conform to the law.

The NPs who have been in practice for more than a decade often bought an existing practice from a physician. In such cases, the NP was initially an employee or partner of the physician, and the physician opted to leave the area and sold the practice to the NP. In that situation, the NP was faced with many adjustments but did not have to start from scratch.

In the past ten years, NPs serving Medicaid enrollees have started practices from the ground up. Some of these have started faculty practices, associated with nursing schools. Others have been strictly private entrepreneurs.

ADVANTAGES OF PRACTICE OWNERSHIP

Even without a general redesign of primary care, NPs who wish to run their own practices have been able to do so in many states. The advantages to an NP of practice ownership are:

1. The NP decides upon the length of patient visits.
2. The NP decides how the practice is run.
3. The NP chooses employees.
4. The NP controls quality.
5. The NP controls referrals.
6. The NP may titrate workload to income.
7. The NP keeps profits.

The advantages to the public of NP practice ownership are:

1. The patient gets the benefit of combined nursing and medicine.
2. The patient reaps the benefit when the patient gets more face time with the provider.

3. The patient may pay less or get more for the same money.
4. The patient may have better access to health care.

In an NP practice, physicians are called in when necessary, but not all patients have to pay for a physician visit or wait for physician availability when a nurse could fulfill the patient's needs. Physicians see patients who have multisystem disease or unstable, life-threatening illness.

Examples of NP Practices

NPs own the following types of practices:

- Travel medicine clinic
- Pediatric primary care
- Wound care consultations
- Home visits
- Family health center
- Urgent care

Barriers

It is true that NPs have more obstacles to overcome than physicians when starting a practice. These include:

1. Getting on managed care provider panels.
2. Getting and keeping a collaborating physician, if required by state law or if billing Medicare.
3. Getting referrals from hospital emergency rooms.
4. Getting privileges at hospitals.
5. Lack of legal authority to admit patients to nursing homes, to order home care, or to direct hospice services.

Physicians have no legal barriers. As for "support," it is unclear whether NPs as a group need more encouragement than other entrepreneurs or whether the combination of a lack of business training among NPs, physician resistance to the idea of independent NP practice, and legal and reimbursement barriers combine to give NPs a negative impression of starting a practice.

This chapter is for the NP who has started a practice or has considered, is considering, or might think of considering opening an NP practice if only he or she had the support, legal leeway, and knowledge of the details involved. Appendix 11-A offers a checklist of considerations relevant to opening a practice.

DECISIONS BEFORE STARTING A PRACTICE

There are eight major business considerations in starting a practice:

1. Whom will I practice with?
2. Where will reimbursement come from?

3. Will reimbursement cover expenses?
4. How will we get patients to come?
5. Where will the practice be located?
6. If the state requires a collaborative agreement, how will that be handled?
7. What sort of quality measures will we institute?
8. How will patient flow be handled?

Also important, though somewhat less important than the eight major considerations, are:

9. What form will the business take?
10. What systems need to be set up for getting supplies, equipment and repairs, depositing cash, and disposing of hazardous waste?
11. Whom will we hire to help?

Whom Will I Practice With?

There are advantages to solo practice and to group practice. Advantages to solo practice are:

- Autonomy
- Efficiency of one-person decision making
- Less income necessary to support one person than multiples
- No chance that another person's lack of productivity will affect one's business

Advantages to group practice are:

- Possible greater access to capital
- Possible shared call and office coverage
- Another source of expertise
- Social support
- Possible economies of scale

There are many potential partners for NPs and many ways of aligning practices. In addition to the traditional solo practitioner or group practice of professionals, where patients come to the office and providers collect from insurance companies, there are hospital-affiliated practices, nursing home-based practices, employer-affiliated practices, and agency-affiliated practices.

Where Will Reimbursement Come From?

Reimbursement might come from any or all of four sources:

1. Government payers: Medicaid and Medicare
2. Private insurers: HMOs and indemnity
3. Patients who pay their own bills
4. Contracts

For details on reimbursement for NP services, see Chapter 9.

A practice owner will be interested in looking into any and all sources of reimbursement. For example, some government and private agencies will contract with health care providers for health services. A pediatric NP might contract with the county school system to do immunizations or school physicals. Certain procedures and diagnostic testing can be billed separately from visits, and a potential practice owner will want to see what opportunities there are for getting that income.

Will Reimbursement Cover Expenses?

Practice Expenses: Crunching the Numbers

Many an employed NP has thought, "If I ran this practice, I would never run it like this." Before going too far down this line of thought, an NP considering opening a practice, and even an NP who expects to remain employed, needs to know how the numbers crunch in the business of primary care. Simply put, it takes a large number of patient visits to support a practice.

Using established numbers from physician practices, one can plug in the numbers for NPs and compare various patient loads. It costs about $200,000 a year to run a primary care physician practice, not including physician compensation.[1] Expenses include:

- Rent
- Payroll
- Quarterly state and federal taxes
- Office expenses
- Utilities
- Answering service
- Supplies
- Hazardous waste disposal
- Payment on start-up loan
- Professional dues and subscriptions
- Fee to register lab with federal and state governments
- Accounting fees
- Attorney fees
- Business travel (to nursing homes, patients' homes, educational seminars, etc.)
- Gifts to staff
- Cleaning
- Insurance (professional liability, workers' compensation, fire, etc.)
- Application fee for hospital privileges
- Beeper and cellular telephone
- Advertising

Office Expenses. Payroll costs for nonphysician employees averaged $93,000, office rent $20,700, malpractice insurance premium $6,000, business supplies $8,300, lab expenses $7,900, medical supplies $17,000, car $2,000, depreciation of equipment $3,400, equipment rental $3,500, equipment maintenance $2,300, and continuing education $1,600. These data are from a 2001 survey by *Medical Economics.*

Figures for internists, family practitioners, and pediatricians are comparable. Expenses are 20 to 66 percent of gross receipts, depending on practice size. Per-practitioner expenses go down as practice size rises. A solo practitioner pays 40 to 60 percent of income for office expenses, whereas a practice of 10 to 24 doctors pays 25 percent for office expenses.

Compensation and Charges. Primary care physicians earn, on average, $150,000 annually in compensation, according to *Medical Economics* magazine data for 2001. Keep in mind that physicians in private practice take as compensation the difference between income and expenses. How they apportion this compensation—retirement, health insurance, vacation pay—is up to them.

For the sake of illustration, let's consider the average cost of running a solo primary care physician practice to be $350,000: $200,000 in expenses and $150,000 in physician compensation. To cover salary and expenses, a physician has to see 4,700 patients a year at a rate of 20 per day, 5 days a week, 47 weeks a year at a charge of $74.46 per visit. If the physician can get only $50, on average, per visit, the physician must see 7,000 patients per year, or 29 to 30 patients per day. This assumes that payment is received for each visit. In reality, not all bills are paid.

If a physician has contracts to see patients on a capitated-payment basis, the physician has to have 2,916 members at an average fee per member per month of $10.00. If $10.00 per member per month is not attainable, then the physician has to have more than 2,916 members on the panel.

NP Practice Compared

Now let's run the numbers for a practice where the owner-provider is an NP. Assume that the NP pays a physician to be the collaborator on a written agreement required by state law.

An NP practice will have all of the same office expenses, plus the expense of paying a physician who signs the NP's written agreement. However, malpractice insurance costs considerably less than $6,000 for an NP: it's more like $500 for an adult NP. For the sake of this illustration, let's call the expenses equal for an NP and an MD.

Reasonable NP compensation, considering the responsibility of a private practice, would be $90,000. Total expense of running an NP practice, using these projections, would be $284,500.

Assume 4,700 patient visits a year, which translates to a daily load of 20 patients, 5 days a week, 47 weeks a year. An NP could charge $60.50, on average, per visit, and make the salary and expenses listed above. If an NP charged less than $60 per visit, he or she would have to: (1) take less compensation; (2) pay less for office, supplies, and so on; (3) have fewer office personnel than the average MD; (4) see more than 20 patients per day, 5 days a week; or (5) work more than 5 days a week, 47 weeks a year.

Twenty patients a day is a reasonable load, but $60.50 per visit may be unattainable. An NP willing to see 21 patients per day—three an hour for seven hours a day—could charge $57.64 per visit, if all visits were collected upon, and support a practice. More than twenty patients a day, every day, is a taxing patient load. That is not counting return telephone calls, personnel problems, payroll, and so on.

Still, the economics are favorable for NPs who want to be their own bosses. They may not be working any harder than employee NPs. Those NPs who work for someone else are going to be expected to see about 20 patients a day, but it will be someone else's decision that they do so, and employed NPs probably will not make $90,000 per year.

For examples of practice expenses and revenues of a physician practice and an NP practice compared, see Exhibits 11-1 and 11-2. Exhibit 11-1 demonstrates that an NP practice could be run on approximately $100,000 less per year than a physician practice, due largely to the differential in salary between NPs and physicians.

Looking at expenses as a percentage of collections, one author calculates that a physician's salary is generally 41 percent of collections.[2] Borglum advises practices to count on paying 26.2 percent of revenue for nonprovider staff salaries, 7.3 percent for rent, 5.9 percent for supplies, 1.8 percent for insurance, 0.9 percent for outside professional fees, and 0.4 percent for marketing. An NP who practices in a state that requires physician collaboration will have to add the cost of physician consultation to the cost of doing business.

How Will We Get Patients To Come?

An NP who starts a new practice, as opposed to buying an established practice, will need to bring in patients with whom the NP has already established a relationship or bring in new patients. Either way, there are costs involved.

If an NP has signed an employment contract with a previous employer in which the NP has agreed not to compete with the previous practice under specified conditions, the NP must honor the agreement or face the possibility of a lawsuit. If the NP has not signed such a "noncompetition" clause, then the NP is legally free to take established patients to the NP's own practice. However, the previous employer who has lost patients is quite likely to be upset, and this nonmonetary "cost" is certainly worth considering.

Whether the NP is seeking new or old patients, some marketing efforts will be necessary. Marketing can take the form of word of mouth, letters, flyers, advertisements, health fair appearances, speaking engagements, television appearances, radio announcements or talk shows, or newspaper articles.

Through marketing the practice, potential patients learn what services the practice provides and the advantages of visiting the practice. Advantages of a particular practice to a patient may be convenient location, ease of getting an appointment, acceptance of the patient's insurance, an especially personable provider, extraordinary personal attention, or a reduced fee for cash-paying patients.

Exhibit 11-1 Primary Care Practice Expenses (in $), NP versus MD

NP Practice Expenses		**MD Practice Expenses**	
Rent	20,700	Rent	20,700
Utilities	7,400	Utilities	7,400
Supplies	25,300	Supplies	25,300
Depreciation	3,400	Depreciation	3,400
Equipment rental	3,500	Equipment rental	3,500
Equipment maintenance	2,300	Equipment maintenance	2,300
Continuing education	1,600	Continuing education	1,600
Advertising/promotion	1,700	Advertising/promotion	1,700
Cleaning	10,000	Cleaning	10,000
Insurance	1,500	Insurance	9,000
Answering service	4,500	Answering service	4,500
Licenses	1,200	Licenses	1,200
Car	2,000	Car	2,000
Legal	1,000	Legal	1,000
Lab	7,900	Lab	7,900
Dues	600	Dues	2,000
Taxes	14,000	Taxes	15,700
Other expenses	3,000	Other expenses	5,000
	111,600		124,200
NP Practice Salaries		**MD Practice Salaries**	
NP, 1.2 FTE	102,600	MD, 1.0 FTE	150,000
RN, 1.0 FTE	45,000	NPs, 1.2 FTE	80,000
Business manager, 1.0 FTE	45,000	RN, 1.0 FTE	40,000
Receptionist, 1.2 FTE	25,000	Receptionist, 1.2 FTE	25,000
MD consultant	5,000	Clerks	10,000
	222,600		305,000
Benefits at 25%	55,600	Benefits at 25%	76,250
Total personnel	278,250	Total personnel	381,250
Total yearly expenses	389,850	Total yearly expenses	505,450

Note: FTE, full-time employee. Projections based on real practices in 2002.

Some general principles of practice marketing are:

- The marketing message must be repeated many times—some say 12, some say 27 times—before a person learns it.
- Create a sense of affiliation with the practice.
- Create an image for the practice and a marketing message.
- Strive to exceed the patient's expectations, and the patient not only will stay with the practice but also will tell others about it.
- A new patient is worth the price of a visit; a patient kept is worth thousands of dollars.

Exhibit 11-2 Primary Care Practice Revenues, NP or MD*

Assumptions:
Practice size: 3,000
Office hours: 48 hours per week
Number of visits/year: 7,488

Included Services:
Health care maintenance and preventive care, all episodic visits including primary care gyn, primary care, mental health care, suturing, nebulization of asthmatics, skin biopsies and I&Ds, outpatient detoxification, hospital medical visits, home visits, 24-hour on-call, venipuncture, lab services as allowed under CLIA exemption.

Excluded Services:
Diagnostic labs other than CLIA-exempt, pharmacy, emergency department visits, physical therapy, obstetrics, emergency transport, patient transportation, hospitalization, medical specialist care, surgery, chemotherapy, sigmoidoscopy, fracture repair.

Excluded Patients:
Pregnant, AIDS, ALS, MS, paraplegics, quadriplegics, spina bifida, chronic nursing home, hospitalized mentally ill.

Capitation and Patient Mix:#

Age	*%*	*N*	*Rate*	*Income/Mo.*
0–2	5	150	29.09	4,362
2–4	5	150	10.75	1,612
5–11	10	300	8.46	2,538
12–20	10	300	7.08	2,124
21–64	60	1,800	11.67	21,006
65+	10	300	29.00	8,700
				$40,342

Yearly income: $484,110

* Projections based on real practices in 2002.
\# Based on one MCO's rates, as of 2002, for commercially insured patients.

Where Will the Practice Be Located?

The location of the practice will determine how easy or difficult it is for patients to come. If the patient base that the NP is looking for is using public transportation or foot transportation, then the practice must be on a bus line or in a neighborhood. If it is an inner-city practice but the patients are coming by car, then convenient and inexpensive parking is a consideration. If a practice is looking for walk-in traffic, then a storefront location would be better than a second-story office in a large building.

Location also can have implications for practice income. In rural areas, there could be more opportunity due to less competition. On the other hand, there could be too few patients to support a practice. In certain urban areas, there is actually a dearth of health care providers, while in other urban and suburban areas, there is an oversupply of providers. A study of locations of other providers is a prerequisite for choice of practice location.

If the State Requires a Collaborative Agreement, How Will That Be Handled?

If a collaborative agreement is required by state law, a practice will need to find a collaborator before opening.

The first step is to find out what the state law requires in the way of physician collaboration. Is it a signature on a written agreement and an agreement to consult when necessary, or is it more involved, such as quarterly review of charts, cosignatures on charts and prescriptions, and monthly meetings?

The second step is to make a list of possible collaborators. NPs will want to look for a collaborator who is competent, has a similar philosophy of patient care, will be accessible when necessary, and will do what is needed for a reasonable price.

The third step is to discuss the NP's needs, the state requirements, and fees with the potential collaborators. Many potential collaborators are worried about increasing their liability for malpractice suits if they collaborate with an NP. Therefore, an NP may want to suggest that potential collaborators inquire about any such increased liability from their malpractice insurer. If a physician's premiums will go up, then that cost will have to be borne by the NP. It is unlikely that an insurer will raise a physician's premium for collaborating with an NP, however.

The fourth step is to weigh the potential contributions and expense of various possible collaborators.

The fifth step is to draft, or have an attorney draft, a professional services contract between the physician collaborator and the NP. If there are few willing collaborating physicians, then a practice's longevity is threatened if a collaborator bows out after the practice has opened. Therefore, it is wise to hire a collaborator and seal the arrangement with a written contract with a term of at least one year and 60 days' notice before the collaborator terminates the relationship. See Appendix 11-D for an example of an NP-collaborator agreement.

Finally, draft the written agreement as required by state law. If written practice protocols or guidelines are required by law, obviously those must be drafted also.

What Sort of Quality Measures Will We Institute?

If quality measures and systems to collect data on performance are set up at the time a practice opens, then data collection will proceed from day 1, and attention to demonstration of quality will be built into the structure of the practice.

What sort of quality measures should a practice look at? In short, quantity and quality are most important. Practices will be interested in quantity—productivity—because the practice must do enough business to cover costs. Practices will be interested in high-quality clinical care, so that the practice can build a reputation for quality to satisfy patients and to avoid medical errors.

Productivity

Productivity directly affects income. In a fee-for-service system of reimbursement, the more visits made and billed, the more a practice makes. In a capitated system of reimbursement, the more patients enrolled with a practice, the more monthly fees the practice receives, and the more patients potentially will need attention. Providers and staff who generate lots of work should be rewarded accordingly, and providers and staff who generate little work should be encouraged to be more productive.

Therefore, a prudent practice owner will build systems for tracking productivity into a practice from day 1. Most software systems for practice track provider productivity. As for office staff productivity, measures should be agreed to by staff members and practice administration at the time of hiring, with periodic review and revision, if necessary, of standards that are set.

Clinical Performance

A good start when attempting to measure clinical performance is the Healthplan Employer Data and Information Set (HEDIS) put out by the National Committee on Quality Assurance (NCQA). Because NCQA audits health plans, and health plans audit practices to collect data to submit to HEDIS, the HEDIS measures are becoming the industrywide standards for comparing quality among providers. For more about HEDIS, see Chapters 14 and 15.

How Will Patient Flow Be Handled?

From day 1, there must be an agreed-upon way of setting up appointments, greeting patients, getting insurance or other payment information, obtaining clinical intake information (history, old records, chief complaint, vital signs), visiting the provider or providers, and arranging follow-up as needed.

Appointments

Appointment-making software is available. Appointment books from office supply stores and a pencil also work fine.

Payment Intake Information

For each patient, the intake staff person will need to obtain:

- Name
- Address
- Telephone number
- Social Security number
- Date of birth
- Method of payment: insurance, cash, credit card
- Insurance company name, address, and telephone number
- Copy of insurance card
- Emergency contact name, address, and telephone number

Clinical Intake Information

A practice should have a clinical intake form—a history and physical form—suited to the patient. An example of such a form for the college-aged patient is included as Exhibit 11-3.

Provider Visits

A system for dealing with patient flow would address the following questions:

- Does the provider see one patient at a time or work multiple rooms?
- Does the provider get the patient from the waiting room, or does an assistant get the patient into the examination room?
- Does the provider talk to the patient while the patient is dressed, or does an assistant get the patient into a gown prior to the arrival of the provider?
- Does the provider chart and make telephone calls in a separate office, or is the provider's office space within the exam rooms?
- When the provider is finished, who takes care of ordering referrals and laboratory tests?
- Does the provider do all of the history taking and teaching, or will registered nurses do these things?

Follow-up

Review and follow-up of laboratory testing, telephone calls to patients who need follow-up contact, and telephone calls to other providers about patient issues all are tasks that providers or some staff member who is integrally involved in patient care must do. If a provider is to do these things, there must be time built into the schedule. If another staff member is to do these things, there must be systems for communications among provider, helper, and patient and documentation in medical records.

What Form Will the Business Take?

There are four options for the business structure of a practice: sole proprietorship, partnership, corporation, and limited liability company (LLC).

Exhibit 11-3 History—New Patient

Family history

	Age	Health	Occupation	Alive?	Age and Cause of Death
Father					
Mother					
Brothers					
Sisters					

State any blood relative, including parents, grandparents, and siblings, who have/had any of the following:

Alcoholism ____________	Diabetes ____________
Asthma ____________	Tuberculosis ____________
Cancer or leukemia ____________	Stroke ____________
Infectious disease ____________	Epilepsy/seizure ____________
State disease: ____________	Bleeding disorder ____________
High blood pressure ____________	Psychiatric illness ____________
Kidney disease ____________	Other familial disease: ____________
Heart disease ____________	____________

Personal health history:

Give the approximate age at which you had any of the following:

Chicken pox	Pneumonia	Attention deficit disorder
German measles	Pleurisy	High cholesterol
Measles	HIV infection	Diarrhea, chronic
Hepatitis	Tonsillitis	Hernia
Mononucleosis	Diabetes	Overweight
Malaria	Kidney disease	Joint injury/disease
Mumps	Thyroid disease	Gonorrhea
Rheumatic fever	Concussion	Syphilis
Meningitis	Seizures	Herpes
Tuberculosis	Bleeding disorder	Other infectious disease
Asthma	Fainting	Heart murmur
Allergies	Migraine	Heart disease
Hay fever	Mental illness	Circulatory problems

Hospitalizations for injury, illness, surgery, or diagnostic testing:

____________________________ Age ____________

____________________________ Age ____________

____________________________ Age ____________

continues

Exhibit 11-3 *continued*

Females:
Menstrual history:
Age of onset _______ Interval _______ Duration ____________________
Current menstrual problems____________________________________
Contraceptive method, if any___________________________________
Date of most recent Pap smear________ Normal? ______ Yes ______ No
Date of most recent mammogram______ Normal? ______ Yes ______ No

Please rank the following by circling severity in last 3 years:
0 for absent, 1, 2, 3 for increasing severity or frequency.

Acne	0 1 2 3	Fatigue	0 1 2 3
Allergy injection	0 1 2 3	Frequent urination	0 1 2 3
Anxiety	0 1 2 3	Headaches	0 1 2 3
Back trouble	0 1 2 3	Health worries	0 1 2 3
Blood in urine	0 1 2 3	Heart racing	0 1 2 3
Blurred vision	0 1 2 3	Indigestion	0 1 2 3
Boils	0 1 2 3	Lack of energy	0 1 2 3
Chest pain	0 1 2 3	Loss of hearing	0 1 2 3
Chronic cough	0 1 2 3	Nausea	0 1 2 3
Constipation	0 1 2 3	Nightmares	0 1 2 3
Depression	0 1 2 3	Sexual abuse	0 1 2 3
Diarrhea	0 1 2 3	Sexual problems	0 1 2 3
Difficulty concentrating	0 1 2 3	Short of breath	0 1 2 3
Difficulty or pain		Sinus trouble	0 1 2 3
swallowing	0 1 2 3	Skin problems	0 1 2 3
Difficulty making friends	0 1 2 3	Sleeplessness	0 1 2 3
Discord with parents,		Sleepwalking	0 1 2 3
spouse	0 1 2 3	Sore throat	0 1 2 3
Dizziness	0 1 2 3	Stuttering	0 1 2 3
Domestic violence	0 1 2 3	Suicidal thoughts	0 1 2 3
Earaches	0 1 2 3	Tension	0 1 2 3
Fainting spells	0 1 2 3	Trouble falling asleep	0 1 2 3
		Use of laxatives	0 1 2 3

When did you last see your dentist for an oral exam? __________________
Do you smoke?_____ If so, what and how much? ______________________
How much alcohol do you drink? ______________________________
Have people annoyed you by criticizing your drinking? ________________
Have you ever felt bad or guilty about your drinking? ________________
Have you ever had a drink first thing in the morning to steady your nerves or to get rid of a hangover? ______________________________

continues

Exhibit 11-3 *continued*

Are you using street drugs?____ If yes, drug? ____________________

Have you used street drugs in the past two years?____________________

If yes, drug? ____________________

A positive answer to any of the previous five questions is highly indicative of having an alcohol or drug problem. You are invited to discuss your answers with the nurse practitioner or physician.

Do you have an eating disorder? ________ Type? ____________________

Are you allergic to cats, dust, trees, grass, or other substances in the environment? If so, what? ____________________

If you are ALLERGIC TO ANY MEDICINE, please list here____________________

Has your physical activity been restricted during the past five years?_____ Give reason and explanation ____________________

Do you have any physical or emotional disability that interferes with your daily activities? If so, detail ____________________

Have you been physically violent with yourself or others? _____ Yes _____ No If so, detail ____________________

Have you consulted a primary care provider recently for any illness or health problem? _______ If so, detail ____________________

Have you consulted a psychiatrist or psychologist in the last two years? If yes, for how long? _______ Please provide the name, address, and telephone number of your therapist ____________________

Previous primary care provider's name, address, and telephone number

____

Do you take any medication regularly? _______ If so, what? ____________________

IMMUNIZATION RECORD

Tetanus booster within 10 years. Date__/__/__

Measles vaccine, two doses required after 12 months of age.

Dose 1, date __/__/__ Dose 2, date__/__/__

Mumps, one dose required. Date__/__/__

Rubella, one dose required. Date__/__/__

Polio Date__/__/__

How would you usually rate your health?

Excellent ____ Average ____ Poor ____

continues

Exhibit 11-3 *continued*

Would you estimate that health problems keep you from your day's work or activities ____ Never ____ Occasionally ____ Sometimes ____ Often

If health problems keep you from your daily activities, what health problem bothers you the most? ____________________

____

Would you say that your health in the past six weeks has ____ improved

____ stayed the same ____ declined.

Date __________ Signed ____________________

Sole Proprietor

In a sole proprietorship, the business and the individual are one and the same. Any debts or legal liability belong to the individual owner. The owner files tax information on a Schedule C, along with the individual's tax return. Year-end losses can be deducted from the individual's taxable income. Year-end profits are added to other income the individual may have and are taxed accordingly.

Advantages of a sole proprietorship are: (1) the owner makes all decisions; (2) losses can be deducted from personal/family income; (3) there is no potential liability for purchases, mistakes, or bad judgment of a partner; and (4) there is no double taxation as is possible with a corporation. Disadvantages of a sole proprietorship are: (1) there is no one to help with expenses of start-up and maintenance, and (2) ups and downs are dealt with alone.

Partnership

A partnership is a business relationship involving two or more individuals or business entities. Most partnerships spell out the relationships between or among the parties in a partnership agreement. If there is no partnership agreement, state law of partnerships governs the relationships.

Partners are liable for the debts and legal liabilities of the other partners. Partners share profits, decision making, administration, and workload in some way agreeable to all partners.

Profits and losses in a partnership are divided and deducted or added to the individual's tax forms. The partnership has a tax form, and the partnership's distributions of profits or losses to the individuals involved appear on the individuals' tax forms.

A lawsuit against the partnership implies liability for all partners. A debt incurred by one partner is a debt shared by all partners.

The major decisions to be made by partners are:

1. What happens if one partner wants out?
2. Who inherits if one partner dies?
3. How will profits and losses be divided?
4. What contribution to start-up expenses will each partner make?
5. How will duties be carried out?
6. How will decisions be made?
7. How will disputes be settled?

Advantages of a partnership include: (1) risk is shared; (2) success and failure are shared; (3) losses can be deducted from individual partners' taxable income; and (4) there is backup for individual partners in the practice. Disadvantages of a partnership include: (1) the debts incurred by one partner are the debts of the partnership; (2) a partner may be liable for another partner's mistakes; (3) there are many opportunities for dispute among partners; and (4) a less productive partner will affect all other partners.

Limited Liability Company

An LLC combines some of the best attributes of partnership with the best attributes of a corporation. State laws vary regarding the specifics of LLCs. The general provisions, however, are:

1. Income passes through to the individual members of an LLC, as in a partnership.
2. Losses pass through to the individuals, as in a partnership.
3. Individual members are liable for the debts of the company only up to a limit.
4. Members agree on operational matters through a written document. If there is no written agreement, differences are settled according to state law regarding LLCs.
5. Professionals may form LLCs.

The main advantage of an LLC is that this business form combines the best of partnerships and corporations. The disadvantages of an LLC include: (1) a state may not include the LLC in its legal forms of business entity; (2) because the LLC is a relatively new business form, the law is not as extensive addressing this form as the other forms; and (3) states may have specific conditions that must be met before forming an LLC.

A professional forming an LLC is still liable for professional malpractice. However, in other forms of lawsuits against an LLC, the business entity affords protection against individual liability as in corporations.

Corporation

A corporation is a business entity with its own identity. Although one individual may be the sole stockholder, director, and officer—the owner—the corporation is nevertheless a separate legal entity.

Under state law, professionals often must form a specific form of corporation with specific laws. Called a *professional corporation* or *professional association,* this form of company resembles a general corporation in many ways. The corporation has its own identifying number and tax return with the Internal Revenue Service. Decisions are made by officers, a board of directors, and stockholders. In some states stockholders must be like-licensed professionals.

Advantages of a corporation are: (1) when several individuals have ownership interest in the business, there are mechanisms for decision making and dispute resolution; (2) there are mechanisms set for dividing profits and losses, based on capital contribution and professional work done; (3) many corporations like to deal with other corporations; (4) expenses of doing business are taken from a central pool before distribution of profits to stockholders; and (5) there are legal limits on the personal liability of individuals. Disadvantages are: (1) much paperwork is required by state and federal governments; and (2) corporate profits are taxed, and, thus, an owner could pay tax on corporate profits and pay again on a distribution of profits.

Liability Ramifications. A corporation is often liable for corporate debts, rather than each individual stockholder. Professionals are not shielded from malpractice liability, however.

Professional Corporations. Some states' laws prohibit the forming of a professional corporation by professionals with differing forms of licenses—for example, nurses and physicians. Before an NP attempts to form a corporation with a physician, he or she should consult state law.

Choice of Corporate Structure. State laws governing partnerships, corporations, and LLCs differ. Consult a local attorney about choosing a business form and drafting the necessary legal documents.

Corporate Practice of Medicine Doctrine. This doctrine is based on a tradition that medicine and business do not mix. Some states have ignored or dispensed with this doctrine. In other states, it is still on the legal books. Nevertheless, professional corporations are an option in every state.

What Systems Need To Be Set Up?

In addition to systems for tracking quality and quantity of care provided, systems will be necessary for:

- Tracking inventory of supplies.
- Purchasing supplies.
- Purchasing equipment.
- Getting equipment repaired.
- Depositing cash at day's end.
- Disposing of hazardous waste.

There will be vendors locally with whom accounts can be opened and arrangements made for each of these tasks.

Whom Will We Hire To Help?

An early decision to be made is: How many staff will be needed? What kind of talents and skills will be needed? Where can these employees be found?

New practice owners are likely to use past experience to judge how much employed help will be needed. Minimum services include:

- Reception/appointment making
- Billing
- Cleaning
- Accounting
- Payroll
- Legal
- Medical assistance

Many of these services can be obtained on an as-needed basis as opposed to hiring employees. In many communities, medical billing is done by billing services, as is payroll. Reception and appointment making, however, are almost always done by employees of the practice.

BUSINESS PLANNING

The success of a practice is closely related to several factors that can be researched prior to opening the business. Those factors include:

- The need for the services in the community
- Community interest in the services to be provided
- Size of the potential patient pool in the community
- Willingness of the community to use the services of an NP
- Willingness of third-party payers to reimburse NPs for services

The best way to plan for a practice is to produce a business plan for the practice. A business plan is a written document that answers the questions:

- What do you plan to offer?
- How will you market the services?
- Who will purchase the services?
- Where will the business be located?
- How big will the practice be?
- How will the practice's activities, policies, and procedures be organized?
- How will expenses be covered?
- What are the potential problems with the business?
- How will those problems be dealt with?
- What start-up money is needed, if any?
- What form will start-up funds take: equity, debt?
- How will start-up costs be repaid?

Often used to convince investors to invest or lenders to lend money to get the business started, a business plan also is an exercise that forces someone who is considering starting a business to research the feasibility of the business and organize a plan for carrying out the business goals.

Writing a Business Plan for an NP Practice

A business plan can run 25 to 40 pages and can cost thousands of dollars in consulting fees. A short version may be satisfactory if a business owner is looking for a rather small start-up loan and few investors are needed. Some NPs who have started practices have enlisted students in graduate business programs to do business plans for them as part of a class project. In these cases, the NPs have gotten a business plan for a much lower rate than is often commanded. For the do-it-yourself enthusiast, there are business plan software programs that an NP can adapt to suit the NP's purposes.

At a minimum, a business plan for an NP practice would include:

- A list of services provided to patients
- Evidence of the need for those services
- Projections for the practice's income compared with expenses
- A description of the principal movers who are starting the business, including relevant experience and skills
- An organizational plan
- A plan for managing the day-to-day operations
- Investment needs
- Potential problems and critical risks

A sample business plan is given in Appendix 11-C.

Services Provided

In a business plan, an NP contemplating a practice venture lists the services to be offered. For example, in a primary care practice, the likely services might include:

- Health assessment (histories and physicals)
- Management and treatment of acute episodic illnesses and chronic stable illnesses
- Preventive education and counseling
- Screening for health maintenance
- Urgent care, such as stitching of lacerations and incision and drainage of certain lesions

Evidence of the Need for Those Services

If a proposed location for the practice is in a community that has been documented as underserved for the services listed above, the business plan should include citations of the documents evidencing lack of primary care services. On the other hand, if the location is adequately served but the practice is offering some more attractive way of providing the service, the business plan should describe how the new practice will participate in the current market.

Projections for the Practice's Income Compared with Expenses

This part of a business plan requires the writer to estimate. Some knowledge of the economics of private practice will be necessary to complete this section. In the case of an NP practice, one would need to know the number of people in the community who are potential patients, the income that could be expected per enrolled patient or per patient visit, the going rate of collected billings in a similar practice, and the projected expenses of the practice. Expenses such as rent would be documented by citation to classified ads for business space or by an oral quotation given by a commercial realtor based on number of square feet needed and location.

Description of the Principal Movers Who Are Starting the Business

This section is résumé material. It answers the question: Do these potential business owners have the relevant experience and skills to make a go of the business?

Organizational Plan

If there is to be more than one owner/director, the principal movers should draw up an organizational chart that shows how authority will be distributed.

Plan for Managing the Day-to-Day Operations

Practice owners who also are providers may want to have a nonprovider—an office manager—handle the day-to-day operations.

Investment Needs

If outside funds are needed for start-up, the business plan should include an estimate of what is needed. If partners or corporate codirectors are contributing start-up funds, the business plan should state who is contributing and how much and should state a plan for return on or repayment of investment.

Potential Problems and Critical Risks

If there are known risks to the business, the owners should state these risks in the business plan and state a plan for addressing these risks. For example, if an NP knows that MCOs are reluctant to admit NPs to provider panels, thereby contributing to a risk of inability to collect reimbursement, the NP should include this risk in the business plan and give a plan for addressing or minimizing the risk. An example would be meeting, prior to the opening of the practice, with MCO executives and obtaining a letter that one or more MCOs are willing to admit NPs as providers.

A Business Plan's Top 20 Questions

Usually a business plan answers 20 questions, the questions that most people will ask about the business. The 20 questions that are most asked of owners of new businesses and that an NP thinking of opening a practice should be prepared to answer are:

1. What type of business do you have?
2. What is the purpose of this business?
3. What is the key message or phrase to describe your business in one sentence?
4. What is your reason for starting your own business?
5. What is your product or service?
6. Can you list three unique benefits of your product?
7. Do you have data sheets, brochures, diagrams, sketches, photographs, related press releases, or other documentation about your product/service?
8. What is the product?
9. What led you to develop your product?
10. Is this product or service used in connection with other products?
11. What are the top three objections to buying your product/service immediately?
12. When will your product be available?
13. Who is your target audience?
14. Who is your competition?
15. How is your product differentiated from that of your competition?
16. What is the pricing of your product versus your competition?
17. Are you making any special offers?
18. What plans do you have for advertising and promotions?
19. How will you finance company growth?
20. Do you have the management team needed to achieve your goals?

Sections of a Business Plan

The following are the customary sections of a business plan:

- Executive summary
- Vision/mission statement
- Background information on the business
- Objectives
- Capital requirements
- Management team (in-house and outsourced)
- Product strategy

- Current product/service
- Research and development
- Key factors in delivery of service
- Analysis of the market
- Definition of the market
- Profile of clients
- Competition
- Business risks
- Plan for marketing the practice
- Marketing strategy
- Advertising and promotion
- Publicity strategies
- Financial plan
- Repayment plan for loans/dividends to investors

A typical way to begin is to answer the top 20 questions. From the answers, one can develop the executive summary, then work on the details of the sections one by one.

An NP entrepreneur (or any entrepreneur) is not expected to be an expert on writing a business plan. An entrepreneur should be prepared to answer these 20 questions, however, so that a business consultant will have some substance to use as the framework for developing the plan.

It is common for someone with an idea for a business to give it up after considering all of the questions brought up by a business plan. If this happens, the exercise of producing a business plan will have served to save a wealth of lost time and money.

Getting a Business Loan

A prospective practice owner may want a bank loan or a venture capitalist's investment to cover the expenses of start-up. A business plan will set out the start-up costs and a plan for repayment.

Multiple Uses of a Business Plan

In addition to helping a practice owner decide whether a practice will be profitable and helping lenders decide whether to participate, a business plan can be used to orient employees, suppliers, and other people whom the business will deal with. A strong business plan points out to the practice owner potential adversities and weak areas, giving an opportunity to respond before there is a business failure.

Resources for Getting Help with a Business Plan

Among the resources for more information on business plans are the Small Business Administration and the Service Corps of Retired Executives, both of which may be listed in the telephone book. Other possible resources are business consultants, business-oriented community groups, professional organizations and professional journals, business consultants, and public libraries. Every local library will have at least one book on writing a business plan.

Looking at the Big Picture

An NP planning to start a practice will need to take a look at the health care industry in general, and particularly the climate in the NP's geographic area. Whether there is a need for the NP in practice to fill, whether there will be enough business to support the practice, and whether there are any barriers to overcome are three questions that an assessment of "the big picture" can answer. The big picture includes the business climate, the competition, the law regarding NPs, and patient and public perceptions of NPs. All of these considerations will affect how the practice does and whether it will survive. An investor or lender reviewing a business plan will be impressed by a plan that takes the big picture into account. For a sense of "big picture" implications for the small NP practice, see Chapters 12 and 13.

Looking at the Smaller Picture

An NP considering starting a practice also will need to consider how entrepreneurship and business ownership will affect the NP's life. Possible effects of small business ownership on an individual include:

- Lack of a separation between work life and personal life
- Necessity of an investment of time and money in start-up
- Inconsistent income while practice is growing
- Uncertainty about success of the business
- Anxiety about ability of partners or coworkers to hold up their end

DOING BUSINESS

Several responsibilities come with being a practice owner. They include:

- Protecting the confidentiality of and storage of patient records
- Carrying out the responsibilities of an employer (see below)
- Registering the practice name with local government
- Disposing of hazardous waste produced in the course of business
- Complying with fire marshall inspections and building codes
- Maintaining the laboratory facilities in accordance with federal and state law
- Credentialing providers
- Ensuring that hiring and firing are done in accordance with the nondiscrimination provisions of law
- Providing malpractice coverage for the providers or company
- Providing general liability for the practice (against slip-and-fall or other injuries to patients)

Responsibilities of an Employer

Employers have legal and practical responsibilities. Legal responsibilities include:

- Withholding and paying employment taxes
- Ascertaining that a hiree is an American citizen or legal immigrant
- Paying workers' compensation and unemployment insurance premiums for employees
- Ensuring that employees actually have the credentials and licenses that they say they have
- Training employees to provide safe care or ensuring that hired employees are already adequately trained
- Ensuring that employees have a safe working environment
- Complying with the provisions of the Americans with Disabilities Act, which prohibits discrimination against a prospective hiree with a disability who needs only "reasonable accommodation" to do the proposed job

Practically, employers want to hire employees who have social skills, are motivated to perform, and will either make decisions or take direction, depending on the need.

Employment Agreements

In most states, employment is "at will." "At will" employment means that an employee has a job at the will of the employer. In an "at will" state, an employer may end an employee's job at any time. Likewise, an employee may leave a job at any time. Good public relations dictates reasonable notice, but there is no legal requirement of notice. Except for a few protections provided by federal law—protection against firing on the basis of race, age, gender, or exercise of free speech—employees are employees at the will of the employer. Therefore, an employer who wants to ensure that an employee will stay with the practice for a specified length of time will want to have employment agreements with employees. Employees will find employment agreements useful as well.

Employee Rights

The rights of an employee include coverage by workers' compensation and unemployment insurance, safe working environment to the extent specified by the Occupational Safety and Health Act, and freedom from discrimination on the basis of race, age, or disability. An employee has a right to health insurance according to some state laws, under certain conditions. A new employer should check the laws of the state regarding employer responsibilities.

Employer Rights

An employer has no legal rights.

Independent Contractors

A practice owner may want to have an independent contractor, rather than employee, relationship with some staff. An independent contractor is not an employee. An employer's responsibilities to independent contractors are only as specified by a contract between practice owner and independent contractor. An independent contractor is responsible for his or her own taxes, insurance, health benefits, tools, and possibly supplies and workspace.

An employer must withhold payroll taxes—income, Medicare, Social Security, and unemployment—for employees. An employer is responsible for paying workers' compensation of an employee injured on the job. In some states, small businesses must offer health benefits to employees. An employer may be held responsible for the malpractice of an employee and therefore should have professional liability insurance covering employees. All of these employer responsibilities are expensive to maintain.

An employer cannot avoid the legal responsibilities connected with being an employer by calling an employee an independent contractor. The Internal Revenue Service and other governmental agencies may investigate an employer who appears to be avoiding insurance and taxes by claiming that workers are independent contractors. To minimize unpleasant contact with the Internal Revenue Service, an employer should know the important, but subtle, legal distinctions between employees and independent contractors.

Employee versus Independent Contractor

In determining whether an individual acting for another is an employee or independent contractor, the following matters are considered:

- The extent of control that, by agreement, the employer may exercise over the details of the work.
- Whether the one employed is engaged in a distinct occupation or business.
- The kind of occupation, with reference to whether, in the locality, the work is usually done under the direction of the employer or by a specialist without supervision.
- The skill required in a particular occupation.
- Whether the employer or the worker supplies the instruments, tools, and place of work for the person doing the work.
- The length of time for which the person is employed.
- The method of payment, whether by the time spent or by the job.
- Whether the work is a part of the regular business of the employer.

- Whether the parties believe they are creating the relationship of employer and employee.
- Whether the principal is or is not in business.

What Is an Employee?

NP Jones, after working for Physician Smith for five years, noticed that a nearby town, growing in size, was lacking a health care provider. NP Jones, familiar with the current sources of reimbursement for NPs, did a business plan and determined that he could in fact support himself if he left the employ of the physician and set up a private practice.

NP Jones asked Dr. Smith to supply, for a fee, medical backup for his practice and to collaborate on a written agreement. Dr. Smith agreed to provide those things and offered to cover one session a week at the new practice for a percentage of the reimbursed charges.

Is Dr. Smith an employee? Can NP Jones avoid the responsibilities of being an employer?

Under the circumstances described above, Dr. Smith is an employee of NP Jones. The factors that make Dr. Smith an employee are:

1. NP Jones will control when the job is done and the place where it is done.
2. NP Jones will hire the medical assistant with whom Dr. Smith will work.
3. NP Jones will supply the equipment necessary to do the job.
4. NP Jones, not Dr. Smith, will suffer financial losses if the work does not produce income for the practice.

Clearly, an independent contractor will be less expensive for the NP. A physician who provided consultation as needed, at an hourly rate, over the telephone, would be an independent contractor. To ensure that the Internal Revenue Service (IRS) will view the physician as an independent contractor, the NP should have the physician:

1. Bill the NP periodically on the physician's stationery for work done.
2. Bill the NP varying amounts. A standard weekly or monthly fee will sound like salary to the IRS.
3. Not work at the NP's place of business.

See Appendix 11-D for a sample contract between an NP and a physician for consultation services.

Some business owners have attempted to make employees independent contractors by writing a contract stating that the arrangement is one of independent contractors, not employer-employee. The IRS is unimpressed with this maneuver. The IRS, if it determines that the NP was an employer and did not provide proper coverage for employees, could fine the NP and create other business headaches.

Furthermore, if Dr. Smith suffers a needle stick at NP Jones's place of business, Dr. Smith will want workers' compensation. The Workers' Compensation Commission is likely to find that Dr. Smith was an employee, and NP Jones will be liable for compensating Dr. Smith for his or her injuries and lost wages.

Employment Contracts and Independent Contractor Contracts

Prospective practice owners should consult attorneys when drafting employment or independent contractor agreements. They are different contracts. A contract for an independent contractor should not only state that the relationship is one of independent contractor but also show how the relationship fits the definition of independent contractor. An employer who attempts to avoid employer responsibilities by calling an arrangement an independent contractor arrangement when it actually fits the definition of employment will find the need for an attorney for representation before the Internal Revenue Service.

Evaluating Performance

An employer will want to evaluate the performance of all employees on a regular basis. Employees who are adding value to a practice should be rewarded, and employees who are not worth the money paid to them should be encouraged to improve performance or leave. To approach performance evaluation rationally, a set of expectations should be drafted and agreed upon by both employer and employee. In some organizations, a new employee has an evaluation at 90 and 180 days and then yearly. In other organizations, a yearly performance review is the standard.

Terminating Personnel Legally

An employer who wants to terminate a staff member should consider legal necessities and public relations realities. Legally, an employer may not terminate an employee solely on the basis of race, age, gender, or disability. That is not to say that an employer may never terminate a minority or older employee. The law simply requires that termination not be made solely on that basis. Independent contractors, on the other hand, can be terminated for any reason, pursuant to the conditions of a contract between contractor and contractee.

Getting Paid for Services

Practices have three general sources of income: (1) patients who self-pay for services; (2) insurance; and (3) contracts.

Self-Paying Patients

Patients who pay their own bills are in the minority. However, patients who either are uninsured (estimated at 17 percent of the population of the United

States) or prefer to go to a provider who is out of their plan but attractive for reasons of convenience or service would appreciate a provider who could offer medical services at a reasonable rate. An NP may want to market to such patients.

For convenience to both the patient and the practice owner, a practice may want to set up a charge account with a major credit card company. A practice owner also must decide whether to extend credit to patients and if so, how to deal with delinquent payments.

Insurers

Insurers fall into two categories: managed-care organizations (MCOs) and indemnity insurers. MCOs contract with an employer to provide, for a set sum, all health services, with some exceptions, needed by employees for a year. MCOs contract with practices or groups to provide health services on a capitated or fee-for-service basis. A practice must be admitted to panels of MCO providers and have a contract that contains the details of the arrangement between the provider and the MCO. Indemnity insurers likewise contract with employers to provide health services, with exceptions, for employees. Indemnity insurers pay providers' bills, according to a fee schedule, on a fee-for-service basis. Indemnity insurers have no relationship with providers other than to pay bills presented by the provider to the insurer for the care of a covered patient.

Obtaining payments from third-party payers is not necessarily any easier than obtaining payment from patients directly. It can be three months between the time the provider bills the insurer and insurer payment. When payment is capitated, practices sometimes have trouble establishing that a patient is, in fact, enrolled with the individual provider and with the MCO at the time the care was given.

Contracts

Practices may contract with businesses to provide certain health services, under any sort of arrangement that is agreed upon by both parties. For more about the specifics of reimbursement, see Chapter 9.

Applying for Provider Status*

Health care industry watchers are predicting that managed care will become universal and that care in the future will be capitated. If predictions hold, a practice that

---

**Source:* Portions of this section have been reprinted with permission from NP Communications Group, Inc., from an article that appeared in the November–December 1997 issue of *NP World News.*

survives will be a practice that is admitted as a provider with dominant MCOs. NPs have identified panel admission as a significant barrier to starting a practice.[3]

It is important for NPs opening a practice to gain admission to some managed-care provider panels for the following reasons:

1. If NPs do appear in MCO directories of providers, and if an NP's name is not on the patients' cards as the primary care provider (PCP), patients are going to think that the NP is some sort of assistant provider. They will not take the NP's advice as seriously as they would take advice from a "real provider."
2. It is necessary to get paid.

There are other sources of direct reimbursement: Medicare, Medicaid, indemnity insurers, and direct payments from patients or companies. However, many patients covered by Medicare and Medicaid and more and more patients previously covered by indemnity insurers are now enrolling in MCOs.

If NPs do not become providers for those MCOs, the NPs will not have access to a large portion of the patient population. Of course, NPs with their own practices can see the patients under the auspices of a physician practice. But with the competition high for patients, physicians who will agree to such an arrangement are few and far between. The goal of NPs realistically should be to see patients as full-fledged providers, not under the auspices of physicians. The relationship should be one of consultation, not supervision.

Attaining the designation of PCP from MCOs, with all of its attendant authority and responsibilities, is now the most important professional goal facing NPs. Some NPs have attained the goal. Others are still trying, and meanwhile are working on NP-MD teams where an MD is the designated PCP. Some NPs do not want the responsibilities attached to being a PCP and are content to assist a physician or other NP.

The argument that NPs should be admitted to MCO panels as PCPs can be tailored to the target of the persuasion. Here are some of the arguments supporting NP admission to provider panels as PCPs. There are specific arguments to make to physicians, MCOs, practice managers, and other NPs.

Arguments to Physicians

The following points may be helpful to raise with physicians:

1. If an NP works under a written agreement with a physician, but only the physician may be a PCP, then the physician will have to sign all of the referral forms for the NP's patients. It is unwise for a physician to sign a referral unless he or she has reviewed the patient's chart. Chart review for every referral written by an NP will require a significant time investment. On the other hand, if the NP is a PCP, then the NP can make referrals without investment of physician time.

2. If an NP with whom a physician is associated is a heavy referrer, and if all of the NP's referrals are attributed to the physician (because the physician is the PCP), that will reflect poorly on the physician's utilization rates with an MCO. An NP should be responsible for the NP's referrals and a physician for the physician's referrals.
3. If an NP does not make a necessary referral on a patient or misdiagnoses a problem, a physician who is the PCP for the patient involved bears ultimate responsibility and is much more likely to be liable in any future malpractice case than if the NP were the PCP for the NP's patients. If the NP is the PCP, then it is far less likely that a physician will be found liable for any errors made by the NP.

Arguments to MCOs

Perhaps the toughest audience is the MCOs, whose executives may have little experience with NPs and are used to dealing with physicians. When attempting to convince MCOs of the need to admit NPs to provider panels, consider using the following arguments:

1. NPs fill MCOs needs of getting the job of patient care done in a high-quality manner and cost-effectively. NPs are the appropriate providers of first-level care: that is, primary care. They are educated specifically for this role, enjoy this role, and are well accepted by patients. The top ten reasons for "visits to the doctor" are: (1) hypertension, (2) diabetes, (3) acute upper respiratory infection, (4) bronchitis, (5) chronic sinusitis, (6) acute pharyngitis, (7) routine medical exam, (8) inner ear infection, (9) depressive disorder, and (10) urinary tract infection.[4] All of these illnesses are appropriate for NP management. It makes no sense to use a physician when an NP is perfectly suited for this role.
2. In virtually every study done on the matter, NPs have been found to be high-quality providers, at least as safe and effective as physicians.
3. In virtually every study done on the matter, NPs have been found to be cost-effective—more cost-effective than physicians.
4. Patients are highly satisfied with NPs.
5. NPs focus on the kind of care that the agencies that accredit MCOs are looking for. For example, NCQA has a set of standards for measuring clinical performance in primary care: HEDIS. HEDIS measures include:
   - Keeping childhood and adolescent immunizations current
   - Advising smokers to quit
   - Giving annual flu shots to older patients
   - Screening appropriately for cervical cancer
   - Screening appropriately for breast cancer
   - Giving prenatal care in the first trimester
   - Checking on postpartum women within six weeks of delivery
   - Maintaining patients who have had myocardial infarctions with beta blockers[5]

The only HEDIS measure that NPs cannot accomplish is eye exams for people with diabetes. (Neither can internists, pediatricians, and family physicians perform diabetic eye exams; they must be performed by an ophthalmologist.)

6. Use physicians where necessary. Have NPs take care of patients where it makes sense to use NPs.

Many studies are done by researchers who are not nurses and therefore should be unbiased bolster the arguments given above. For example, Salkever found in 1982 that per-episode costs with NPs as the initial providers are approximately 20 percent below the cost of episodes in which physicians are the initial providers.[6]

A 1991 study by Avorn et al.[7] gave 799 physicians and NPs the following case in a telephone interview:

> A man you have never seen before comes to your office seeking help for intermittent sharp epigastric pains that are relieved by meals but are worse on an empty stomach. The patient has just moved from out of state and brings along a report of an endoscopy performed a month ago showing diffuse gastritis of moderate severity, but not ulcer. Is there a particular therapy you would use at this point, or would you need additional information?

The results of the study showed that the majority of physicians put the patient on a prescription antacid and did not want more information from the patient. The majority of NPs wanted to know more about the man's intake of caffeine, medications, alcohol, and cigarettes and wanted to know the level of stress in his life. The researchers revealed that the man was a heavy drinker, was on high doses of aspirin, had just lost a son, and smoked. NPs said they would counsel the patient about these issues and put him on a less expensive form of antacid.[7] This study shows the differences in approach between many NPs and many physicians and shows how NPs are cost-effective. MCO executives can understand this example.

A 1990 study compared performance of primary care by physicians and NPs on eight tasks. Comparisons were made according to gender and type of provider. There were not enough physician assistants (PAs) to make the study of PAs valid, nor enough male NPs. Tasks included:

- Cancer screening (breast exam and Pap smear)
- Follow-up of high serum glucose
- Monitoring of patients on digoxin
- Compliance with American Academy of Pediatrics standards for well-child care
- Follow-up of children with otitis media

The study found that NPs were comparable or superior in all but one of eight tasks.[8]

A 2000 study by Mundinger et al. showed that in "an ambulatory care situation in which patients were randomly assigned to either nurse practitioners or physicians, and where nurse practitioners had the same authority, responsibilities, productivity and administrative requirements, and patient populations as primary care physicians, patients' outcomes were comparable."[9]

Certain arguments can backfire, for example, the argument that NPs can provide care for a lower fee-for-service than physicians. NPs in private practice do not want to undercut physician charges because they have to pay physicians to be their collaborators as is required by the law of most states and by Medicare. If the NP is earning less than a PCP earns to care for a patient, where is the NP going to find the money to pay the physician collaborator?

Another thorny argument is that NPs have less malpractice litigation than physicians. It is true that claims against NPs are minuscule compared with claims against physicians. To be fair, there are many reasons to explain that observation. Yes, NPs have good relationships with their patients and are very conscientious; but NPs are not perceived by the public to be wealthy. Further, the reporting requirements are somewhat different for NPs, so the data may be misleading.

Arguments to Practice Managers

The following points may be persuasive with practice managers:

1. It is unreasonable for an NP to stop in the middle of clinical sessions and interrupt a physician to present a case, when it is otherwise unnecessary, in order to get a signature on a referral. Some system must be set up to deal with referrals. If only physicians can be PCPs, it will ultimately fall on the practice manager to make sure that when there are physician-NP teams, the physicians are notified of what the NP is doing about referrals.
2. Physicians cannot have panels of unlimited size. At some point, to keep patients within a practice, there will have to be NP PCPs.

Arguments to Other NPs

Being deemed a PCP by an MCO may seem like a semantic issue rather than a substantive issue. Granted, the issue is more professional than clinical. An NP can provide primary care whether or not an NP is designated a PCP. For example, patient Smith may see NP Jones several times a year and may consider NP Jones to be her health care provider, whether or not an MCO has designated NP Jones as patient Smith's PCP. However, if NP Jones does not hold PCP status with patient Smith's MCO, the NP is invisible to the MCO. To the MCO, patient Smith's PCP is NP Jones's employer, Dr. Doe. In some clinics, patients have physicians whom they have never met named on their file as PCP. The clinic simply assigns some physician, any physician, to a patient who actually is cared for by an NP. Even though NP Jones evaluates patient Smith, orders diagnostic tests, makes referrals, and follows up to the MCO, this all is done by Dr. Doe.

The arrangement described above works well for patient Smith. As long as NP Jones does a good job, the MCO, patient, physician PCP, and clinic all will be happy with the arrangement. But to the "invisible provider," NP Jones, the arrangement means three things:

1. NP Jones is a ghost provider. His or her work is seen only through Dr. Doe's statistics and is indistinguishable from Dr. Doe's. The NP is a "helper."
2. Without data on NP Jones's work, the situation never will change. An MCO will never see how many patients NP Jones sees, never know the effectiveness of his or her diagnosis, treatment, preventive efforts, and teaching, and never know that NP Jones draws patients to the practice.
3. NP Jones always will be working for Dr. Doe or another physician. NP Jones cannot ever have his or her own practice, because he or she can never prove that he or she is an effective health care provider. NP Jones is forever tied to Dr. Doe.

The dynamics of human nature will begin to work as soon as Dr. Doe understands that NP Jones is forever tied to a physician, unable to care for MCO patients as a PCP. Dr. Doe will not give NP Jones as high a level of professional respect as if NP Jones were an equal PCP, able to take his or her patients and start his or her own practice down the block. A deficit in professional respect may reveal itself on a daily basis or only at contract negotiation time. At some point, however, it is sure to reveal itself.

The selfless NP who only wants to take good care of patients and has no interest in challenging the physician's role as captain of the health care ship should realize that the implications of this issue reach far beyond issues of pecking order. Patients will see their MCO's directory of providers and notice that NP Jones's name is not listed. Patients will notice that a physician's name, not NP Jones's name, appears on their referral forms and their medical card. Patients eventually will become aware that NP Jones is a "helper" rather than the PCP. The subtle message to patients is that NPs are second-class providers, not worthy of being relied on for advice about serious matters and not deserving of full attention when health care teaching is underway. The message may be completely erroneous, especially when an NP really is the patient's primary decision maker, diagnostician, teacher, gatekeeper, confidant, and advisor—in effect, the PCP.

How To Apply for Panel Admission

First, answer the following questions:

- Is the law in place?
- Does state law permit an NP to be a managed-care provider?
- Is your practice ready for scrutiny?

- Will it physically present well during a site visit? Are health maintenance efforts well documented? Are records orderly?
- Are policies written, recently reviewed, and organized?
- Are your relationships in place with a physician?
- If a written collaborative agreement is required by law, is it signed and approved by the appropriate board?
- Are your arguments ready? (See the arguments above.)

Give MCOs general information on NPs, such as educational requirements, malpractice actuarials, information on insurers that reimburse for NP services (e.g., Medicare, Medicaid, and Blue Cross), and scope of practice. Include articles on studies that demonstrate the cost-effectiveness and quality of NP practice. Also, give MCOs information on the specific practice, including credentials of each provider, description of the practice, location, and size.

What To Do if Rejected

If rejected, rework the arguments or address the counterarguments, wait six months, and try again. The climate may have changed, or the presentation may be better the second time.

Effective Negotiation of Managed-Care Contracts

Once an MCO agrees to admit an NP, it will offer a contract. This section provides basics on negotiating such contracts. The following basics about managed-care contracting should be understood:

- Under capitated-care contracts, everything the provider does is paid for in one lump sum, with exceptions.
- "Everything" means everything that is included in the contract and everything that is not excluded or excepted by the contract.
- Some MCOs pay providers on a fee-for-service basis.
- Some MCOs pay providers through a combination of fee-for-service and capitated fees.
- Currently, most MCOs and most physicians are using the fee-for-service model of care provision, superimposed on the capitated payment system.

Preparing To Negotiate

A practice owner should ask other providers, and possibly the state insurance commissioner's office, the following questions about an MCO with whom a practice is considering a contract:

- Have other providers been paid promptly?
- Are there specialists on the MCO's referral network of specialists with whom the provider is familiar?
- Does the MCO have a strong presence in the community?

- Is the MCO financially sound?
- Is there a history of complaints about the company with the Insurance Division?
- Does the company have decent quality data?

Use of Actuarial Data

Actuaries make predictions about risks, usually insurance risks. An actuary can predict such practice variables as how many visits patients will make a year and what the average payment per visit will be. If possible, an NP seeking a contract with an MCO should obtain actuarial data on the group of patients whom the contract would cover. Sometimes MCOs can provide actuarial data on their patients. If not, an NP could hire an actuary. If an actuary is unaffordable and the MCO cannot supply actuarial data, an NP who has data from the NP's own practice and/or access to charts can make some actuarial predictions on how many patient visits to expect per year and what the average payment per patient visit has been.

- Research the costs of the practice.
  1. Add up all salaries, rent, material costs, insurance costs, legal costs, cleaning costs, that is, all the costs of doing business. See Exhibit 11-1.
  2. Divide by the number of patients for which a practice can reasonably expect to get a year's capitation. The result will be the average yearly cap rate, per patient, needed to support the practice.
- Research the demographics of the practice.
  1. Age and gender will make a difference in the cap rate.
  2. Age and gender will make a difference in the time spent per patient.
- Decide upon the product line to be offered. Will the practice offer primary care service to all age groups? Will the practice offer full well-woman care? EKGs on site? Suturing? Sigmoidoscopies? Incision and drainage? Outpatient detoxification? Asthmatic nebulization? A practice that offers a wider range of services can expect to refer fewer patients to other providers and can argue for a large capitation rate when a capitation form of payment is being negotiated.
- Research the capitation and fee-for-service rates for that payer. Ask insurers for their capitation rates and fee-for-service schedules early on. If data on capitation rates offered other practices nearby are obtainable, obtain that information.

Negotiating

Here are some tips on negotiating a managed-care contract. They were suggested by physicians who signed whatever came their way in the first round and learned from their mistakes.

- Think of the unsigned contract as the presenter's opening offer. It is a biased offer. Understand that it is only a starting point in negotiations.

- Do not assume that any provision is nonnegotiable. It was written on a word processor and can be easily changed. Make counteroffers to strike unfavorable provisions and insert others that are favorable. Much will depend upon how much the MCO wants the practice.
- Read the whole contract carefully—even the fine print. Make a photocopy and write notes and questions on it. Have an attorney answer any questions in plain English. If the contract refers to manuals or "rules and regulations," review these before signing.
- Make certain the contract covers all important business. If something is not covered in the contract, the provision does not exist. Make sure oral promises are included in the written document.
  1. Ask: Is there a way out for the provider if the dealings with the MCO turn out to be unbearable?
  2. Watch the billing and payment provisions, details of quality and utilization reviews, restrictions on coverage arrangements, and limitations on referral and admission. Get it in writing that the MCO will pay "clean claims" within 30 days. Include a provision for regular utilization reports. Determine how the beginning and end of coverage for a client affects a provider's duty to give care. Determine the limitations on and procedures for referral and admission. Determine what the MCO expects as far as quality data.
- Pay attention to the definitions at the beginning of the document as definitions sometimes include substantive information, such as what is meant by "medically necessary services."
- Hold-harmless clauses usually work against an NP provider. They can be applied to a variety of situations: For example, a contract might state that "provider holds enrollee harmless for charges," even if the MCO becomes insolvent and does not pay the provider. Or it might state that "provider holds MCO harmless in regard to any lawsuit filed by a patient against provider." Do not agree to such a clause unless the practice's liability insurance carrier signs off on it.
- Indemnification clauses: *indemnification* means make whole or compensate for some loss or damage. Do not agree to indemnify the MCO for any loss by the MCO.
- *No-cause termination:* try to avoid a situation where an MCO could terminate the relationship at any time, without good cause. Instead, insert a due-process clause, which allows a hearing in front of peers to determine whether termination was being done with good cause.
- Do not negotiate jointly with anyone other than practice partners or other members of an integrated network. Practices differ greatly and need practice-specific contracts.
- Once the parties sign, the contract is binding.

For questions to ask the MCO, see "Managed-Care Organizations" in Chapter 9. Here are four questions to ask yourself, the provider:

1. Can I live with this MCO's rates?
2. Can I live with the other requirements?
3. Can I negotiate with the MCO on any of the issues important to me?
4. Can I alter the system of care from the traditional model to a more efficient and effective model?

Enlist the help of an experienced attorney in negotiating the terms of the contract. The practice's accountant should review the payment mechanisms. The practice's business manager should evaluate the mechanics of payment, the timing of reimbursement, and the requirements for approvals of referrals.

NOTES

1. Schuneman P. Master of the 'ABCs' of activity-based costing. Manag Care 1997; 6:43, 48, 53.
2. Borglum K. Practical tips to boost your efficiency and cut practice costs. Fam Pract Manag 1997; 4:86–92, 97–98.
3. Anderson AL, Gillis CL, Yoder L. Practice environment for nurse practitioners in California. Identifying barriers. West J Med 1996; 165:209–214.
4. Hospitals and Health Networks. Fraud . . . government fraud and abuse probes. June 5, 1997; 71:28.
5. National Committee on Quality Assurance. www.ncqa.org.
6. Salkever D, Skinner EA, Steinwachs DM, Katz H. Episode-based efficiency comparisons for physicians and nurse practitioners. Med Care 1982; 20:143–153.
7. Avorn J, Everitt DE, Baker W. The neglected medical history and therapeutic choices for abdominal pain: a nationwide study of 799 physicians and nurses. Arch Intern Med 1991; 151:694–698.
8. Hall JA, Palmer RH, Orav EJ, et al. Performance quality, gender and professional role: a study of physicians and nonphysicians in 16 ambulatory care practices. Med Care 1990; 28:489–501.
9. Mundinger MO, Kane RL, Lenz ER, et al. Primary care outcomes in patients treated by nurse practitioners or physicians: a randomized trial. JAMA 2000; 283:59–68.

APPENDIX 11-A

A Checklist for Setting Up a Practice

NPs who are contemplating going into private practice have few role model colleagues to consult with. Further, the NPs who run their own practices have little free time to consult with fledgling entrepreneurs.

This checklist gives NPs a description of things to do, think about, and decide before setting up a practice. Some of the things to do will vary from state to state, and some are common to NPs in all states.

ADMINISTRATION

A practice may have one owner or many. The three basic business forms are sole practitioner, partnership, and corporation. Each of these forms suggests administrative structure. If an NP is starting a business alone, there will be no confusion about who will make administrative decisions. Whenever more than one person is involved, decisions must be made about who will be making the many decisions necessary to run a practice and how the decision making will be done. Draw up an administrative chart as one of the first tasks in the planning process.

BILLING

Many practices have a billing clerk who does manual or electronic billing. Others hire outside companies to do the billing. An outside billing company may take a percentage of the income or charge a fee per bill.

BLUE CROSS/BLUE SHIELD AND OTHER PRIVATE INSURERS

Each insurance company has a procedure for enlisting providers. Develop a list of insurers' names, addresses, and telephone numbers. Call each company's Provider Relations office, and ask the following questions: What is the policy of the company regarding reimbursement for NP services? What is the process? How does an NP apply for a provider number? Ask for an application to become a provider, fill out and return the application, and deal with the responses one by one.

If a rejection comes in the mail, follow it up with telephone calls or letters to find out why. Some states have laws that require third-party payers to reimburse NPs for services performed. If there is such a law in your state, include a copy of it with your correspondence.

BUSINESS ASSOCIATES

As of April 14, 2004, the business associates of health care providers must be required by contract to protect the privacy of patient information, if a business associate has access to patient information. This is required by federal regulations (see Chapter 4, page 143), regarding patient privacy.

BUSINESS FORM

A sole proprietor is solely responsible for the business. Legal liability and liability for taxes lie with the sole proprietor. In a partnership, each partner shares the profits and liabilities. Each partner pays taxes on that partner's earnings. Each partner has personal liability for debts and judgments against the business.

There are several forms of corporations. A corporation is an entity apart from the individuals involved in the business. A corporation pays taxes on profits, the employees pay taxes on their income, and the shareholders pay taxes on their dividends. The corporation is liable for debts and judgments against the company. However, if corporate assets are insufficient to cover debts or other liabilities, corporate officers or directors may be personally liable. A corporation that provides medical services usually is required by state law to be a particular form of corporation: a professional corporation (PC) or professional association (PA).

A limited liability company (LLC) combines some aspects of the corporation and some aspects of partnership. In some states, an LLC may have the corporate purpose of delivering medical care. An LLC should be considered when there is more than one provider and the providers are considering partnership.

Consult an attorney about choosing a business form.

CALL

Set up a system for ensuring that patients have 24-hour access to providers. An answering service and beepers work well, coupled with a call schedule for providers and the answering service.

CHAPERONES

The need for a chaperone during a patient visit will rise and fall based on the nature of the visit and the gender of provider and patient. The provider often will not know the nature of the visit until the patient is in the room.

Consider the following patient-provider combinations:

- Male provider, female patient
- Same-sex provider and patient
- Female provider, male patient
- Unaccompanied minor patient of either sex with provider of either sex

The need for chaperones should be kept in mind when considering staffing.

Calling in chaperones for all patient visits may inhibit the back-and-forth between NP and patient. On the other hand, the practitioner who forgets to call in a chaperone may find him- or herself accused of improper behavior by a patient, and without a witness. The most reasonable policy regarding chaperones is to offer the patient the option of having a chaperone.

COMPUTER SYSTEM

Answer the following questions: What software will be used for billing? For medical records? For tracking quality data? How many terminals are needed? Will providers enter medical record data, and if so, will entry be done in the exam room with the patient present or later? What sort of networking is needed? Will Internet service be needed? E-mail? What are the provisions for patient confidentiality of data kept on a computer?

Point-of-care medical data entry is new and uncommon. It requires that practitioners be well versed in the data entry system or that a transcriptionist be hired. If research is a goal of the practice, a computerized medical records system is a must.

CONFIDENTIALITY

Answer the questions: How will patient confidentiality be maintained? Will patients have privacy when announcing their reason for the visit at the receptionist's desk? Will discarded notes and lab results be shredded? Is there an area where provider and assistants can talk about plans for patients without other patients' hearing the discussion? Are exam and conference rooms reasonably soundproof? Are rooms laid out such that a patient in a gown cannot be seen by waiting patients?

Concerning release of medical record information: Any provider, clinic, or hospital needs written permission from a patient to give out medical information on that patient, for any reason other than treatment, payment, or health care operations. When a patient's medical problem is substance abuse, federal law requires that certain language be used in the consent for release of information.

All employees should be aware of the need to protect patient confidentiality when responding to telephone inquiries from or about patients and the need for keeping progress notes, incoming lab tests, and mail about patients private.

COPY MACHINES, FAX

Some practice management consultants recommend that providers each have fax and copying machines within arm's reach. Every practice needs at least one of each.

CREDENTIALING

For each NP, the clinic manager should have:

1. A copy of the NP's current state license as an advanced practice nurse.
2. A copy of the NP's current certification by certifying organization.
3. A copy of two professional references, including name, address, telephone number, title, nature of professional association with employee, and recommendation as to clinical competence and ability to work with a team.
4. A statement signed by the NP declaring that the NP has never been convicted of a felony, is not under investigation for suspected commission of a felony, is not under investigation by the board of nursing for a licensing offense, and has not been suspended from Medicaid or Medicare provider status.
5. A statement of the NP's malpractice history. The National Practitioner Data Bank (NPDB) in Camarillo, California, keeps records of all damage awards for medical malpractice paid by a practitioner (MD, DDS, or NP). A practitioner can get his or her own report by requesting a form from the NPDB. Hospitals can subscribe to the service. Actions by state boards of nursing are not required to be reported by NPs, but reporting is required for MDs and DDSs.
6. The practice agreement under which the NP is practicing. In many states, each NP must have a written practice agreement with a physician specifying what the NP may do, what kind of oversight the physician will give, and the site of practice. The agreement must be signed by each party and approved by the board of nursing.
7. Prescribing authority. Providers need to obtain Drug Enforcement Administration (DEA) numbers (410-962-7580) and state Controlled Dangerous Substance (CDS) numbers. Contact the state health department and the DEA for an application.

DISABILITY

Patients with Disabilities

Each place of business should be wheelchair accessible so as to avoid unlawful discrimination against the patients with disabilities.

Screening Patients for Medicaid Eligibility

Clients may receive Medicaid because they are low income with children or because they, as adults, have disabilities. NPs may be asked to do disability evaluations. In the disability determination process, the client obtains a form from his or her local Department of Social Services (DSS) office, fills out the required information, and brings it to the clinic. The NP does a history and physical to determine (1) whether the client has a disability and is unable to work, and (2) how long the client will be disabled. The client's eligibility for services depends upon the projected length of disability. A clinic may obtain from the local DSS the financial criteria that qualify a family for welfare and refer to the DSS accordingly.

Screening Patients for Medicare Disability

As of the publication date of this book, NPs do not have the legal authority to determine disability under the Medicare program.

Employee Disability

An employee of the practice who injures him- or herself on the job will seek workers' compensation. Practices should carry insurance to cover such claims. Preventive measures—teaching employees to use proper body mechanics when lifting and the safe disposal of body fluids—of course are the best thing employers can do for their employees.

DOCTORS, MEDICAL

If a state requires physician collaboration, an NP may hire or contract with a physician to provide consultation services and develop and sign a written agreement as required by law. A physician's fee might be an annual or monthly retainer payment, a percentage of collections, a rate per hour of consultation time, or whatever arrangement is agreeable to the parties.

An NP may want to establish a partnership with a physician, contract with a physician for specific consulting services, or hire a physician as an employee. For an example of a contract between an NP and a physician for physician consultation services, see Appendix 11-D.

When an NP hires or contracts with a physician, the parties agree that the profits, as well as the liabilities, are the NP's. In a partnership, profits and liabilities are shared among the partners.

The owners of a new practice may find it most economical to engage a physician as an independent contractor rather than hire the physician as an employee. When taking on a physician consultant, specify in the contract that the physician is an independent contractor, specify an hourly rate of payment and terms of payment, and specify the duties and responsibilities of the physician and of the

NP. In addition to a practice agreement that fulfills the requirements of state law, the NP and physician should have an employment or professional services agreement. The former is the professional collaboration agreement; the latter is the business arrangement between the two individuals.

EMERGENCY PLAN

Establish a written emergency plan that answers the questions: How much emergency care will the NP give? What are the criteria for referral to the nearest emergency department? For calling 911? For ambulance transport? Each practice needs a plan for such emergencies as:

- Patient loss of consciousness or other life-threatening emergency.
- Fire on the premises.
- Threats to safety from intruders or unruly patients.
- Uncontained hazardous wastes.

EMPLOYEES

Anyone who hires another person legally must determine that the employee is an American citizen and that the employee is certified or licensed as necessary. An employer may be held liable for any injuries that an employee causes to a patient.

Employers are responsible for keeping records of employees' Social Security wages, Medicare wages, and income tax wages. Most employers pay at least a portion of employees' Social Security. All employers are required to withhold income tax from employee wages.

Employers should carry workers' compensation insurance, payroll insurance, and health insurance for employees in accordance with state laws.

FORMS

Forms should be developed for:

- Intake: (name, address, telephone, insurance company and numbers, birth date, etc.).
- History and physical.
- Tracking of health care maintenance and screening.
- Care plan/problem list.
- Progress note.
- Referral.
- Return to work.
- Appointment slips.
- Appointments (calendar).
- Encounter/billing.
- Release of medical information.

- General consent to treatment.
- Consent to procedure.
- Patient instructions.
- Lab report flowsheet.
- Vital sign flowsheet.
- Patient contact.
- Notice of patient privacy rights.

GUARDIANS

Any patient who has a legal guardian may not sign consents (or give consent) for care.

HEALTH MAINTENANCE ORGANIZATIONS

Some HMOs are contracting with NP practices for capitated care, and some are not. It is likely that changes will come about during the time it takes for this book to go through publication. When the practice address and telephone number are set, contact local HMOs about becoming a panel member.

HOURS OF PRACTICE OPERATION

Some managed-care organizations (MCOs) require by contract that a practice maintain certain hours. Barring that requirement, a practice is free to set its own hours.

HOUSEKEEPING

Housekeeping includes:

- *Cleaning:* Contract for a service, specifying how often cleaning is done and what is done. Three times a week is minimum.
- *Extermination:* Twice a month is reasonable.
- *Snow removal:* Businesses are usually responsible for removing snow or ice from the entranceway and parking lot.
- *Hazardous waste removal:* Separate red-bag trash cans need to be in each examination room. When those are filled, the bags are stored in a larger, marked box or can. Hazardous waste disposal companies pick up at a minimum rate of monthly.

INFORMATION SHEETS FOR PATIENTS

Collect effective patient handouts, videos, and tapes on an ongoing basis. Display them in waiting rooms, bathrooms, or offices.

INSURANCE

Practices will need premises, professional liability, payroll, workers' compensation, and employee health insurance.

JUSTIFYING NP EXISTENCE

Compile, on an ongoing basis, as many facts about the practice and clients as possible for use with insurers and other providers and for marketing purposes.

LABORATORY

Compliance

The laboratory for even a small practice that does only urine dipsticks and pregnancy tests must be approved by the state and federal governments. Obtain and fill out the necessary paperwork needed to comply with state (State Laboratory Administration) and federal (CLIA) requirements. This means applications, fees, and, most likely, a designated "laboratory director." In some states, the forms state that the laboratory director must be an MD, but on questioning, one may discover that a PhD in microbiology or biochemistry will be accepted as laboratory director.

Equipment

Buy a refrigerator with ice-making capabilities. Medications should be kept in a separate refrigerator from staff lunches and separate from specimens. Calibrate all equipment at least annually.

LAUNDRY

Linens can be rented and laundered by an outside company, or paper gowns and drapes can be used. Laundries often require a monthly minimum charge, which may not be cost-effective for a new clinic.

LIBRARY

Indispensable books are:

- Primary care handbook.
- Dermatology book with pictures.
- Lab test reference book.
- *Drug Facts and Comparisons* or *Physicians' Desk Reference.*
- *Sexually Transmitted Disease Guidelines* from the Centers for Disease Control and Prevention for current year.

- *Guide to Antimicrobial Therapy* from the Centers for Disease Control and Prevention for current year.
- A current algorithm for health care maintenance and screening.

MALPRACTICE INSURANCE

Several companies sell malpractice insurance to NPs. Promotions for these companies are found in any of the journals for NPs.

MARKETING

Consider generating newspaper articles about the opening of the practice, and ask for TV coverage if an NP practice is a novel idea in your area. See that the practice is listed in provider directories. Consider purchasing advertisements in local newspapers. Send direct mail flyers or have someone distribute flyers in local neighborhoods. Announce your practice to colleague NPs, in NP publications, and at NP meetings, and ask for referrals. Notify local physicians of your practice and ask for referrals. When you refer patients to MDs, dentists, podiatrists, or optometrists, send a letter with the patient so that the provider knows that the referral comes from you.

NURSES

For state-by-state education requirements of NPs, see Chapter 3, Appendix 3-B.

Family NPs are the most useful type of NP for a small clinic because they can see all age groups.

In terms of noneducational assets, experience in primary care, productivity, compatibility, resourcefulness, and flexibility are essential.

Depending upon patient needs, a practice may want to offer the services of addictions counselors and nurse psychotherapists.

RESEARCHERS

If there is a local nursing school, a connection for research expertise can be valuable.

RNs, LPNs

If payment for visits is not tied to NP or MD providers, a practice may find that visits to RNs or LPNs can be useful to patients.

ON-CALL SERVICE

Twenty-four hour on-call service is required by some insurers. Some practices use an answering machine that gives the beeper number of the person on call. Others use an answering service.

OSHA COMPLIANCE

The major requirements under the Occupational Safety and Health Act (OSHA) are for protective wear—gloves, gowns, masks, and goggles—when at risk for blood handling; collection of hazardous waste in separate, clearly marked trash cans; and proper disposal of hazardous waste.

In some states, the state administers the occupational health and safety program; other states have federal oversight. Inspectors generally concentrate on one of two areas: building safety or safe clinical practices.

PATIENTS

Think about sources for new patients and ways to keep established patients. Word of mouth about good experience of care is the best form of advertising. Also, see "Marketing."

PHARMACEUTICALS

Stock

State law may control the NP's authority to dispense medications and the conditions of dispensing. The practice may want to have a limited stock of commonly used pharmaceuticals. Or, if a pharmacy is nearby, the practice may not need to stock pharmaceuticals. As for stocking of controlled substances, a practice that does so increases the risk of robbery and drug-seeking behavior on the premises.

Samples

Drug representatives supply many practices with samples of the newest and most expensive pharmaceuticals. However, if patients do not have pharmacy insurance, it is unlikely that the patients will be able to afford to keep taking the medications dispensed as a starter dose.

Cost of Prescriptions

Some reference books give comparison cost information on medications. Pharmacists are good sources of such information. Some patients' insurance covers pharmaceuticals, and other insurers do not. Some patients are uninsured. Unless a patient has insurance that covers pharmaceuticals, patients will want to know the cost of prescriptions being written and the cost of alternative remedies. It is useful to establish a relationship with a pharmacy that can supply price lists for the prescribing NP.

Storage

Vaccines must be refrigerated, with a thermometer/thermostat keeping them at whatever temperature they require. Other, noncontrolled medications should be kept out of public display. Controlled substances should be behind double locks. Records of on-hand supply and the dispensing of each dose should be kept.

PHYSICAL PLANT

Consider need for the following types of space:

- Conference room
- Play area for children
- Exam rooms
- Waiting area
- Laboratory
- Utility room
- Offices
- Storage

PRESCRIBING

In some states, NPs need to obtain prescriptive authority separate from licensure. NPs who will be prescribing controlled substances need a DEA number and a state CDS number. There is a fee for DEA registration. There also may be a fee for the state registration.

State law may require that NPs follow specific procedures when prescribing or dispensing medications. The state board of nursing is a good starting point for information about prescribing requirements.

PURCHASING

Set up standing accounts with the following companies: medical supply company, pharmacy, medical waste disposal, answering service, telephone, utilities, medical equipment, equipment repair, printing, office supplies, and cleaning.

QUALITY ASSURANCE PLAN

Write a mission statement for the practice, and post it. Set up a method of evaluation for staff, and conduct periodic self-evaluations. Adopt a set of clinical practice guidelines and a set of health care maintenance and screening guidelines. Do periodic chart review to see that the practitioners are following the clinic's guidelines.

REFERRALS

Keep a referral directory, updated on a continuing basis, including names and phone numbers of referral sources for:

- Cardiac evaluation
- Chest X-rays
- Counseling regarding unwanted pregnancy
- Dentistry

- Dermatology evaluation
- Drug and alcohol counseling
- Genetic counseling
- Gastrointestinal/genitourinary evaluation
- Head, eyes, ears, nose, and throat evaluation
- HIV testing
- Mammograms
- Marriage/family counseling
- Neurologic evaluation
- Orthopedic evaluation
- Psychiatric care
- Sexually transmitted disease screening
- Social work
- Surgical evaluation
- Counseling
- Protective services

REGULATORY MATTERS

Every medical office lab needs either periodic inspection by CLIA or a letter of exception that states that an inspection is not required. For information, call the state department of health's laboratory division.

States do not necessarily require clinics to be licensed. However, the fire marshall will probably need to inspect and sign off on every public space.

REIMBURSEMENT

Develop a patient intake procedure by which the practice can ensure that insurance information is current. For example, check the patient's insurance card, copy the card, and verify current coverage through a telephone number on the card. If the patient has no insurance, obtain his or her credit card, or work out the payment process. Obtain copay. For more information on reimbursement, see Chapter 9.

Develop a fee schedule for visits and procedures, using appropriate CPT codes. Base the fee schedule on the income needs of the practice and the current reimbursements being paid by insurers.

SECURITY

Most clinics do not need a security guard, but it is something to contemplate. Consider drafting a policy about after-hours use of the clinic by staff members. Develop a policy on handling of cash collected during the day. Do not keep narcotics or large sums of cash in the clinic.

STANDARD OF CARE

Consult books, journals, and other providers, and attend at least one conference a year.

START-UP FUNDING

Write a business plan, or hire a consultant to write a business plan. Take the business plan to a bank and ask for a business loan. If turned down, contact the local Small Business Administration and request a loan.

SUPPLIES

Disposable Medical Supplies

No matter what a clinic starts with, additional supplies always will be needed. Any clinic needs a running account with a medical supply company and with a pharmacist, with a turnaround delivery time of no more than 48 hours.

Durable Equipment

Every state has durable medical equipment companies. Used medical equipment also is available through brokers or through newspaper advertisements.

Stationery

The practice will need letterhead and envelopes, business cards, appointment cards, prescription pads, promotional brochures, and patient education brochures.

Diagnostic Lab Supplies

Laboratories supply specimen collection materials. State health departments often provide supplies for infectious disease testing and sometimes offer free diagnostic testing, with specimens sent by mail. Commercial labs provide all of the materials and vessels necessary to transmit lab specimens.

SUPPORT STAFF

A receptionist is the most important employee, followed closely by the billing manager. Other staff to consider include: a lab technician, a marketing specialist, a handyman, and a housekeeper.

VOLUNTEERS

States differ on whether volunteers are liable for their own acts or whether a clinic is responsible for the acts of volunteers. Managers should follow the same credentialing process in taking on volunteers as they do with employees.

WASTE, HAZARDOUS

Red plastic containers specially made for sharp instruments and needles and clearly marked hazardous waste containers are required by law. Sharp instruments and needles are deposited in the red containers, which then go in boxes supplied by a waste disposal company, and the boxes are picked up monthly, at minimum. Diapers and bloody materials are deposited in red bags in trash cans. The red bags are tied and put into larger boxes. Personnel who pick up the hazardous waste must be certified in that area: that is, a staff person cannot cart it away. Therefore, clinics must hire waste disposal services.

WRITTEN AGREEMENT

In many states, each NP must have a written collaborative agreement with a physician specifying the scope of practice of the NP, what kind of oversight the physician will give, and the site of the practice. The agreement must be signed by each party and approved by the board of nursing.

YELLOW PAGES ADVERTISING

Advertising in the telephone book is expensive, yet for some practices it will be the major source of clients. It is a budgetary item to be considered and balanced among other necessary expenditures.

APPENDIX 11-B

Independent Contractor Agreement

Note: This is a sample contract for a situation where an NP is contracting for NP services with a business entity. It should not be used as a template because every arrangement is different and every arrangement needs its own contract. Consult an attorney for drafting of a contract to suit a particular arrangement.

THIS AGREEMENT made ______________, 2003, by and between Jane Doe, an individual, hereinafter referred to as "the Nurse Practitioner," and Heathrow School, a nonprofit educational institution in Maryland, hereinafter referred to as "the School."

Recitals

1. The School is an educational institution.
2. Jane Doe is an individual Nurse Practitioner certified to practice in Maryland.
3. The School has a health center that serves the needs of enrolled students when school is in session. The purposes of the health center is to (a) improve the health of children and adolescents by providing comprehensive physical and mental health services and (b) work with school faculty, parents, and students to create health-promoting environments.
4. The school year is September 5 to June 15, not including December 12 to January 4 and March 15 to 27.

NOW, THEREFORE, the parties agree as follows:

1. The School, through the Nurse Practitioner, will offer the following services: general primary health care; mental health, psychosocial, and family counseling; drug and alcohol abuse programs; treatment of minor injuries; sexuality education and counseling; gynecological exams and treatment of sexually transmitted diseases; AIDS education and counseling; nutrition education and weight reduction; health education; routine physical exams (including sports physicals); diagnosis and treatment of acute and chronic illnesses; referrals for illnesses and

injuries not suitable for treatment in the school clinic; pregnancy tests, early periodic screening and development testing; case management and support services for mainstreaming and preventing complications for children who have chronic health problems and special health care needs; and sick care for students with minor injuries and illnesses.

2. The School will have the following responsibilities for operations of the Center:

2.1. The School shall maintain physical plant, to consist of two rooms, including two telephone lines, copy machine, fax machine, desk, lamps, exam table, sink, file cabinets, all in safe working order.

2.2. The School shall arrange and pay for disposal of hazardous waste, compliance with state and federal requirements for health centers and laboratories, security, utilities, cleaning, and durable medical equipment and supplies.

2.3. The School will arrange and pay for physician consultation services, as required by Maryland law for nurse practitioner practice.

2.4. The School will maintain storage and confidentiality of medical records to the extent required by state law.

2.5. The School will bill for services provided by the Nurse Practitioner.

3. The Nurse Practitioner will have the following responsibilities:

3.1. Maintain her own certification, licensure, malpractice insurance, and continuing education.

3.2. Provide her own tools and examination instruments.

3.3. Pay her own taxes, Social Security, Medicare, workers' compensation, and unemployment contributions.

3.4. Set her own hours within the following parameters: she must be on premises five hours on school days, with a schedule prearranged and posted.

3.5. Provide on-call services for school hours when she is not on site.

3.6. Attend two school meetings per year.

3.7. Report to school authorities any student who is a danger to self or others, in accordance with the state laws regarding patient privacy.

3.8. Maintain patient confidentiality.

3.9. Maintain the accepted standard of care of school-aged patients.

3.10. Follow up outstanding diagnostic and treatment problems even if school has gone out of session.

4. Jointly, the parties will:

4.1. Establish procedures to adopt protocols and standards to evaluate quality and appropriateness of care provided at the health center.

4.2. Work cooperatively to generate reports and analyses required as a condition of grant or contract funding of the health center and submit to each other data and other information required by regulatory or funding agencies.

4.3. Work in concert to ensure compliance with all regulatory requirements relating to clinical services.

5. Term and termination.

5.1. This Agreement shall become effective September 1, 2003, and continue through June 15, 2004, and will be renewed annually, for a term beginning September 1. By agreement of the parties, this Agreement shall be amended to be effective for any subsequent school years in which the parties agree to continue the Agreement with compensation to be adjusted in such years in accordance with the procedure specified in clause 7.1.

5.2. Either party may terminate this Agreement upon the material default of the other party, provided that the party in default is given at least five (5) business days' notice of intention to terminate and fails to cure the default, or, if the default is such that it cannot be cured within five (5) business days, fails to undertake substantial efforts to begin cure and to continue such efforts until the default is cured. For this purpose, "business day" is defined as a day the School is open for regular business.

5.3. Either party may terminate this Agreement for any cause by giving the other party at least six (6) months' written notice.

5.4. If the parties agree that there are irreconcilable differences regarding the standard of care to be upheld at the health center, either party may give the other party thirty (30) days' notice of termination.

5.5. Either party may terminate this Agreement immediately if its performance becomes impossible, and is expected to remain impossible for an indefinite period of time, as a result of a cause described in clause 6.12.

6. Administrative and legal matters.

6.1. The School shall hold title to any equipment purchased by it. The Nurse Practitioner shall hold title to any equipment purchased by the Nurse Practitioner.

6.2. The parties shall comply with all federal, state, and local laws, ordinances, rules, and regulations that are applicable to the operation of the school health center.

6.3. Amendments to this Agreement must be stated in writing and executed by the authorized officials of the School and the Nurse Practitioner.

6.4. The relationship of the School and the Nurse Practitioner is that of independent contractor. Nothing in this Agreement shall be deemed to create or constitute a partnership, joint venture, employment, or agency relationship between the parties.

6.5. The parties agree that each is responsible for the actions and failures to act on the part of each party's own employees and agents in the performance of this Agreement and that each party shall have no responsibility for costs, judgments, or obligations resulting from or in any way connected with the actions and failures to act on the part of the other party's employees.

6.6. All notices, official correspondence, and requests for permission required by this Agreement to be sent from one party to the other shall be sent in writing by first-class mail, return receipt requested, or by any overnight courier or same-day delivery service that provides a receipt of delivery, to the address set forth in this paragraph or to such other address as a party may establish in the future by proper notice:

For the School:

Barbara Johnson
Headmistress
Heathrow School
Fulton, MD

For the Nurse Practitioner:

Jane Doe
11 Janeway Ct.
Fulton, MD

6.7. Each party represents that it has authority to execute and deliver this Agreement and to perform its obligations hereunder and that all necessary approvals for execution of this Agreement have been obtained.

6.8. This Agreement is not assignable, in whole or in part, by either party without the prior written consent of the other party.

6.9. This Agreement, the rights and obligations of the parties, and any claim or dispute arising from this Agreement shall be governed by and construed in accordance with the laws of Maryland.

6.10. If any part of any provision of this Agreement becomes invalid or unenforceable under applicable law, that provision shall be ineffective to the extent of the invalidity or unenforceability only, without in any way affecting the remaining provisions of this Agreement.

6.11. Any payment due the School that is rendered more than fourteen (14) calendar days after the date due shall accrue interest at the rate of ten percent (10%) per annum from the date due until the date paid.

6.12. Neither party shall have liability for breach of contract or delay in performance of its contractual responsibilities if the party is unable to perform required services under this Agreement as the result of performance becoming impossible due to governmental regulation, request or order, or due to circumstances beyond the reasonable control of the party, including, without limitation, acts of God, fire, flood, accident, labor strike, war or civil disobedience, inability to obtain supplies, or interruption of utility services, where such circumstances make it impossible to perform or to perform in a timely manner.

6.13. A party's waiver of any right under this Agreement, including without limitation the right to terminate for default, shall not be construed as an agreement to continue such waiver indefinitely or to grant a waiver in the event of a repetition of the action or omission in question.

7. Payment.

7.1 The School agrees to pay Nurse Practitioner $61,000 per year, payable in ten payments of $6,100, due on the first of the month starting September 1 and continuing through June 1.

7.2. The School agrees to mail payments to Nurse Practitioner at the address listed in clause 6.6.

IN WITNESS WHEREOF, the parties, by their undersigned representatives, have caused this Agreement to be executed.

____

Barbara Johnson
For Heathrow School

Date_______________________________________

____

Jane Doe, NP

Date_______________________________________

APPENDIX 11-C

Sample Business Plan

The following is an example of a simple business plan for a very simple NP practice. Any individual who is considering starting a business should research the income and expenses of the business to determine whether the business has potential for success. A business plan can be much more detailed than this example and should include a balance sheet. An NP should engage a business consultant to write or review a business plan, using research and projections supplied by the NP. An NP also should engage an accountant to compute a balance sheet and other computations based on the NP's research of income and expenses. The information below is what an NP should expect to supply to the business consultant and accountant.

ASSUMPTIONS

Assume that the business is a well-women clinic in a small town.

The business will be staffed by one NP, who will be assisted by a receptionist and a medical assistant.

The hours are noon to 4 PM, Monday to Friday, and 9 AM to 1 PM Saturdays.

The NP starting the practice has 15 years of experience as an OB-GYN NP but will not do obstetrics. She will refer pregnant patients to her collaborator.

Assume that the business is in a state where a written physician collaboration agreement is needed. The physician collaborator will be paid for reviewing and signing the written agreement and being available for consultation at the discretion of the NP.

The NP has elected not to bill insurance. The services will be provided on a fee-for-service, payment-at-time-of-service basis. The practice will accept credit cards. The fee for an exam is $60. Cultures (i.e., gonorrhea, chlamydia, and herpes) and HIV tests will be sent to the state public health lab, which will do the tests at no charge. The clinic will do urine pregnancy tests and wet mounts on site at a charge of $15 and $20, respectively. Pap smears will be read by a local laboratory, which has agreed to charge $20 each. If blood work is needed, the blood will be drawn by the NP and sent to a local laboratory. Bills for any blood work are sent from the laboratory directly to the patient.

Severna Park Well Women Care

111 Pinetree Lane
Severna Park, MD 20070
(410) 555-1212

Jane Jones, CRNP

July 30, 2003

1

Executive Summary 3
Mission Statement 4
Background Information on the Business 4
Objectives 4
Capital Requirements 5
Management Team 5
Product Strategy 5
Current Product/Service 5
Research and Development 6
Key Factors in Delivery of Service. 6
Definition of the Market 7
Analysis of the Market 7
Profile of Clients 7
Competition 7
Business Risks 8
Plan for Marketing the Practice 8
Marketing Strategy 9
Advertising and Promotion 9
Publicity Strategies 9
Financial Plan 10

Executive Summary

Severna Park Well Women Care (WomenCare) is a new business, to open January 2, 2004. The business will offer women who are essentially healthy routine annual gynecologic examinations, Pap smears, diagnosis and treatment of gynecologic infections, birth control, and pregnancy tests.

With the closing of Severna Park Planned Parenthood in June 2003 due to financial and management restructuring of that organization, there has been a lack of well-women services in Severna Park. Not only is the Glen Burnie office of Planned Parenthood inconvenient to the women of Severna Park, but also that office is not prepared to handle the volume of patients from Severna Park.

WomenCare will replace the services of the Severna Park Planned Parenthood office and will market itself differently so that women who would not go to Planned Parenthood will visit WomenCare. WomenCare will be located in a storefront location next to the town's main grocery store. WomenCare will offer basic gynecologic services, such as annual exams, breast exams, infection checks, prescription of birth control, and pregnancy tests. There will be no surgical services, no prenatal services, and no abortion services. Visits will be by appointment and on a walk-in basis.

Jane Jones, CRNP, is the owner and practitioner of WomenCare. Ms. Jones is an OB-GYN nurse practitioner, certified nationally and licensed in Maryland. Ms. Jones has 15 years of experience providing primary care to women at Planned Parenthood of Glen Burnie. John Evans, MD, an obstetrician-gynecologist in Glen Burnie, will provide consultation and sign the written agreement as is required by Maryland law for nurse practitioner practice. Patients who need surgery, or further consultation, or who are pregnant, will be referred to Dr. Evans or another obstetrician-gynecologist of the patient's choice.

The business strategy of WomenCare is to offer low-cost, high-quality primary care women's health services in a convenient storefront setting. WomenCare will operate on a cash or credit card payment basis, with fee paid at time of service. WomenCare will not bill insurance companies. The strategy underlying this payment system is that avoiding the clerical work necessary to establish provider status and bill multiple insurers will allow WomenCare to offer services at a rate below that of other local providers. Furthermore, WomenCare's services will be performed by a nurse practitioner, whose services can be offered at less cost than a gynecologist's services.

The charge for a routine annual examination from a private physician in Severna Park is $120. WomenCare will offer the exam for $60 and therefore will be attractive to uninsured women. Forty percent of the women in

3

Severna Park do not have health insurance ("Uninsured Lack Care in Area," *Baltimore Sun*, January 2, 2002, p. 2). Women who are insured may visit WomenCare, pay the bill, and attempt to obtain reimbursement from their insurer.

Start-up funding is needed in the amount of $30,000.

Mission Statement

To provide convenient, high-quality, affordable primary women's health care services to generally healthy women aged 13 and over.

Background Information on the Business

During her 15 years of practice in Severna Park, Jane Jones has established a following of patients. She is now working at the Glen Burnie Planned Parenthood but will leave that position on December 30 to open WomenCare. The location for WomenCare has been secured. An agreement has been reached with the consulting physician. Opening publicity has been planned.

Hours will be noon to 4 PM Monday to Friday and 9 AM to 1 PM Saturdays, 50 weeks of the year. Patients will be scheduled for half-hour appointments. Therefore, the volume will be 48 visits per week, or 2,400 visits per year. The charge will be $60 per visit, $15 for a pregnancy test, and $20 for a wet mount.

Objectives

1. Secure start-up funding by October 15, 2003.
2. Sign lease on December 1, 2003.
3. Purchase equipment for delivery on December 15, 2003.
4. Outfit office from December 15 to 30, 2003.
5. Hire two employees to start December 26, 2003.
6. Open WomenCare on January 2, 2004.
7. Repay start-up loan by December 31, 2007.

Capital Requirements

Start-up funding of $30,000 is needed to cover initial rent, furnishings, equipment, legal fees, initial salaries, cleaning, and other business expenses. It is not anticipated that further business loans will be needed unless expansion is needed.

4

Management Team

Jane Jones is the provider/manager. Because there is no billing of insurers, there is little need for a professional office manager. Ms. Jones will be assisted during office hours by a part-time medical assistant. A receptionist will cover the front desk during office hours.

Attorney Carolyn Buppert will provide legal services, including contracts between Ms. Jones and Dr. Evans, review of the lease, and laboratory contracts, filing of the CLIA application, and employment contracts for the staff.

Accountant James Edwards will provide accounting services. Payroll will be handled by PayCheck, a local payroll service.

Product Strategy

Every woman needs a gynecologic exam every year. The strategy of WomenCare is to provide that service at a convenient neighborhood location at a reasonable cost through a provider already well known to many neighborhood residents. Women will be reminded of WomenCare's services every time they visit the grocery store, which is located in the same strip shopping center as WomenCare.

Current Product/Service

There is no current service by WomenCare. The services to be offered by WomenCare are offered at a higher cost by three local obstetrician-gynecologists, who are located in a less convenient location in the Severna Park Medical Park. Similar services to WomenCare are offered currently through Planned Parenthood of Glen Burnie, which is 20 miles away from the proposed WomenCare location.

Research and Development

Ms. Jones surveyed the patients who visited Planned Parenthood of Severna Park in the final three months of that clinic's operation. Two hundred patients responded. Patients responded that they did not have an alternative provider in mind at the time of the survey, that they were interested in continued service from Ms. Jones, and that they were primarily in need of the following services:

- Annual gynecologic exam, once a year (100 percent of patients)
- Infection checks, approximately once a year (25 percent of patients)
- Exam for menstrual pain or dysfunctional menses, approximately once every three years (10 percent of patients)
- Renewal of birth control pills every six months (20 percent of patients)
- Pregnancy test approximately once every six months (10 percent of patients)

Planned Parenthood of Severna Park had 800 patients at the time the center closed.

A survey conducted at the local YWCA in April 2002 of 200 women attending a seminar for unemployed women revealed that 50 percent of the women would visit a women's health office every year if the cost were $60 or less. Seventy-five percent of surveyed women stated that they would prefer a woman provider. Ninety-eight percent of women surveyed were amenable to having their primary care services provided by a nurse practitioner. Two percent preferred a physician.

Of the five internists in Severna Park, only three do gynecologic examinations. Two internists refer their patients to gynecologists for annual examinations. Ms. Jones met with the two internists who do not do gynecologic exams and asked whether they would consider referring to WomenCare. Both internists agreed to refer "some" of their patients to WomenCare.

Key Factors in Delivery of Service

Key factors distinguishing WomenCare and contributing to its success are:

- Convenience.
- Service by one well-known nurse practitioner.
- Reasonable cost.

Definition of the Market

The market for WomenCare is all females aged 13 and over living in Severna Park, Maryland, or within a 15-mile radius of WomenCare.

Analysis of the Market

Fourteen thousand people live in Severna Park. Approximately 35 percent of Severna Park's residents are females aged 13 and over. The potential market in Severna Park, therefore, is 4,900 people. If WomenCare acquired one-half of the potential market, WomenCare would have 2,450 patients, each visiting at least once per year.

Arnold and Pasadena are neighboring communities with 10,000 and 15,000 residents, respectively. If 35 percent of Arnold and Pasadena residents are women over 13 years of age, and 10 percent of the eligible population visited WomenCare, then WomenCare will have an additional 875 patients who will visit at least once a year.

Profile of Clients

There are three subsets of "average patients" who will patronize WomenCare.

One subset of clients will be sexually active females of childbearing age who are employed but without health benefits or are unemployed. Such clients will be seeking birth control services for some portion of their childbearing years and will be seeking diagnosis of symptoms that they will suspect are sexually transmitted.

A second set of average patients will be menopausal women who will need attention to menopause-related symptoms and hormone replacement therapy or alternative therapies.

A third subset of patients will be teenagers who are seeking care for complaints that they would prefer not to discuss with their parents. These patients are considered emancipated under Maryland law for issues of birth control and sexually transmitted disease screening, and parental consent is not required.

Competition

There are three obstetrician-gynecologists in Severna Park. Two are male, and each has been in practice for approximately 20 years. The third is female and has been in practice approximately five years. Approximately 50 percent of the practice of each physician is obstetric care. The two male physicians have approximately 3,000 patients each. The female physician has 2,000 patients. The physicians draw patients from Annapolis, Arnold, Pasadena, and Glen Burnie.

WomenCare could be expected to draw approximately 500 patients from the physicians. These patients would be those who are uninsured and do not want to pay $120 per visit.

Planned Parenthood of Glen Burnie offers the same services proposed by WomenCare and therefore is a competitor. However, because Ms. Jones practiced in Severna Park with Planned Parenthood until June 2003 and now practices at the Planned Parenthood in Glen Burnie, it is reasonable to expect that Ms. Jones has former patients in Severna Park and that a portion of the Glen Burnie patients will visit WomenCare.

Business Risks

The biggest risk is insufficient patient visits, primarily because of inability of patients to afford the $60 fee plus lab fees when necessary. Another risk is the withdrawal of Dr. Evans as collaborator. This risk is minimized for the first year, because Dr. Evans has agreed to sign a yearlong contract.

Plan for Marketing the Practice

A direct-mail announcement will be sent to all of Ms. Jones's former patients at Severna Park Planned Parenthood. Flyer-type advertisements will be posted at the grocery stores and on the high school and community college bulletin boards.

Because of WomenCare's storefront location next to the grocery store, WomenCare will be seen by almost everyone in the neighborhood. An "Opening Soon—WomenCare" sign will appear on December 1, 2003, at the location.

Dr. Evans has agreed to refer patients to WomenCare when they are uninsured and cannot afford the $120 he charges.

Marketing Strategy

The strategy for marketing WomenCare is to get a core number—approximately 250 patients—through direct mail to former patients of Ms. Jones at the now-defunct Planned Parenthood of Severna Park, through the flyers at the store and schools, and through the "Opening Soon" sign at the business location. It is anticipated that each of the core 250 patients will tell one other potential patient of WomenCare in the first three months of operation and that one-half of the word-of-mouth contacts will visit. Therefore,

8

by month 4, WomenCare will have seen approximately 375 women. Each quarter, it is estimated that a patient will tell at least one friend, neighbor, or family member about WomenCare and that a significant portion of those contacts will visit within the year.

Advertising and Promotion

No advertising will be purchased. However, the WomenCare sign at the location in the strip shopping center will advertise the business.

Ms. Jones and her staff will attempt to make every patient a permanent patient through close attention to personal service and attention to individual needs.

One Saturday a month will be "Teen Day," when female teenagers will be encouraged, through an announcement posted on the door of the business location, to come and ask any question of Ms. Jones, free of charge. Through this promotion, teenaged girls will begin to establish a relationship with Ms. Jones so that when they are in need of services, they will think of WomenCare.

Publicity Strategies

Each visitor to WomenCare will receive a business card that includes the services provided and their prices, along with the usual business card information.

Ms. Jones will do one presentation per year at the high school on a topic of interest to female high school students and one presentation per year at the local college on a topic of interest to female college students.

Financial Plan

Projected Operating Expenses, Year 1	
Rent	$18,000
Utilities	$6,000
Supplies	$2,500
Continuing Education	$1,000
Cleaning	$6,000
Insurance	$1,000
Hazardous waste disposal	$600
MD consultant	$10,000
Total nonsalary expenses	$45,100
Salaries, annual	
NP, 0.6 FTE	$40,000
Medical assistant, 0.6 FTE	$14,000
Receptionist, 0.6 FTE	$14,000
Social Security/Medicare, 1.8 FTEs	$5,202
Total salary expenses	$73,202
Total operating expenses	$118,302
Expenses of start-up (equipment, attorney, licenses, etc.)	$18,300

Table A11-C-1 Projected Expenses, Month by Month, Year 1 ($)

	Jan	*Feb*	*Mar*	*Apr*	*May*	*June*	*July*	*Aug*	*Sept*	*Oct*	*Nov*	*Dec*
Operating Expenses												
Rent	1,500	1,500	1,500	1,500	1,500	1,500	1,500	1,500	1,500	1,500	1,500	1,500
Utilities	500	500	500	500	500	500	500	500	500	500	500	500
Salary	6,100	6,100	6,100	6,100	6,100	6,100	6,100	6,100	6,100	6,100	6,100	6,100
Supplies	1,500					500			500			
Cont. ed.					1,000							
Insurance	1,000											
Cleaning	500	500	500	500	500	500	500	500	500	500	500	500
MD consult	1,000	1,000	1,000	1,000	1,000	1,000	1,000	1,000	1,000	1,000		
Haz. Waste	50	50	50	50	50	50	50	50	50	50	50	50
Expenses/mo	12,150	9,650	9,650	9,650	10,650	10,150	9,650	9,650	10,150	9,650	8,650	8,650
YTD expenses	12,150	21,800	31,450	41,100	51,750	61,900	71,550	81,200	91,350	101,000	109,650	118,300
Loan Payments	500	500	500	500	500	500	500	500	500	500	500	500

11

Table A11-C-2 Projected Income, Month by Month, Year 1 ($)

	Jan	Feb	Mar	Apr	May	June	July	Aug	Sept	Oct	Nov	Dec
Visits	60	80	100	110	120	120	120	100	140	160	180	192
Test, preg.	8	10	10	15	20	20	20	25	30	40	60	72
Tests, wet mount	15	20	25	26	30	30	30	25	35	40	44	48
Income	4,020	5,350	6,650	7,345	8,100	8,100	8,100	6,875	9,550	11,000	12,580	13,560
Projected total income, year 1				101,230								
Projected operating expenses, year 1				118,300								
Year 1 operating loss				(17,070)								
Loan payments, year 1				(6,000)								
Year 1 loss				(23,070)								

Table A11-C-3 Projected Income, Month by Month, Year 2 ($)

	Jan	Feb	Mar	Apr	May	June	July	Aug	Sept	Oct	Nov	Dec
Visits	200	200	180	205	195	205	190	180	205	200	190	190
Test, preg.	80	80	70	50	40	50	50	50	50	45	40	40
Tests, wet mount	50	50	60	50	45	45	45	35	50	45	45	45
Income	14,200	14,200	13,050	14,050	13,200	13,950	13,050	12,250	14,050	13,575	12,900	12,900
Projected total income, year 2				161,375								
Projected operating expenses, year 2*				124,215								
Loan payments, year 2				12,000								
Total expenses, year 2				136,215								
Profit, year 2				25,160								

*It is projected that operating expenses will increase at 5 percent per year.

Table A11-C-4 Projected Income, Month by Month, Year 3 ($)

	Jan	*Feb*	*Mar*	*Apr*	*May*	*June*	*July*	*Aug*	*Sept*	*Oct*	*Nov*	*Dec*
Visits	200	200	180	205	195	205	190	180	205	200	190	190
Test, preg.	80	80	70	50	40	50	50	50	50	45	40	40
Tests, wet mount	50	50	60	50	45	45	45	35	50	45	45	45
Income	14,200	14,200	13,050	14,050	13,200	13,950	13,050	12,250	14,050	13,575	12,900	12,900
Projected total income, year 3				161,375								
Projected operating expenses, year 3				130,425								
Loan payments, year 3				12,000								
Total expenses, year 3				142,425								
Profit, year 3				18,950								

Payback Plan

Loan of $30,000 on October 1, 2003.
Repay nothing until January 1, 2004, at which time payments will be made as follows:

January 1 to December 31, 2004: $500/month

January 1 to December 31, 2005: $1,000/month

January 1 to December 31, 2006: $1,000/month

January 1 to December 31, 2007: $550/month

Total repaid: $36,000

Professional Services Agreement

Note: This is a sample contract between an NP and a physician collaborator. It is not meant to be a template. Each agreement between two parties is different, and participants should consult an attorney to determine the best contract to suit the particular agreement.

THIS AGREEMENT ("Agreement"), effective ____________, 20__, is between C.B. Bosco, CRNP, PC, a Maryland professional corporation (the "Nurse Practitioner") and George Oaks, MD, PC, a Maryland professional corporation (the "Physician").

RECITALS
WHEREAS, the Physician is engaged in the practice of medicine in Maryland;
WHEREAS, the Nurse Practitioner is engaged in practice of a nurse practitioner in Maryland;
WHEREAS, the Nurse Practitioner is required by law to have a collaborative association with a physician;
WHEREAS, the Physician wishes to collaborate with the Nurse Practitioner;
NOW, THEREFORE, for good and valuable consideration, the receipt and sufficiency of which is acknowledged, the parties agree as follows:

1. Definitions

1.1. "Contract Year" shall mean the twelve-month period following the effective date of this Agreement. Thereafter, each additional twelve-month period during the term or any successive term shall constitute a Contract Year.

1.2. "Nurse Practitioner" shall mean C.B. Bosco, located at 102 Goldleaf Ave., Suite 2, Jasonville, MD.

1.3. "Physician" shall mean George Oaks, located at 102 Goldleaf Ave., Suite 3, Jasonville, MD.

1.4. "Term" shall mean the period from ____________, 20__, through __________________, 20__, unless sooner terminated or extended as provided herein.

2. Representations and warranties
   - 2.1. The Nurse Practitioner represents:
     - 2.1.1. That she holds a current license from the State of Maryland as an Adult Nurse Practitioner;
     - 2.1.2. That her license or certificate to practice as a registered nurse or nurse practitioner in Maryland has never been revoked, suspended, restricted, or subject to possible disciplinary action;
     - 2.1.3. That her privileges to practice as a nurse practitioner at a hospital or other health care facility have never been revoked, suspended, restricted, or subject to possible disciplinary action;
     - 2.1.4. That there has never been entered against the Nurse Practitioner a final judgment in a malpractice action, and that there has never been an allegation of malpractice by the Nurse Practitioner that has been settled by payment to the plaintiff;
     - 2.1.5. That the Nurse Practitioner has never had malpractice liability insurance canceled, restricted, or not renewed;
     - 2.1.6. That the Nurse Practitioner has never been found guilty of a crime of any nature;
     - 2.1.7. That the Nurse Practitioner has never been reported to any state or federal health care program for alleged violations of state or federal health laws or regulations or been found by such program to be in violation of such laws or regulations.
   - 2.2. The Physician represents: .
     - 2.2.1. That the Physician holds a current license from the State of Maryland as a physician;
     - 2.2.2. That the Physician's license to practice as a physician in Maryland has never been revoked, suspended, restricted, or subject to possible disciplinary action;
     - 2.2.3. That the Physician's privileges to practice as a physician at a hospital or other health care facility have never been revoked, suspended, restricted, or subject to possible disciplinary action;
     - 2.2.4. That the Physician has never been found guilty of a crime of any nature;
     - 2.2.5. That the Physician has never been reported to any state or federal health care program for alleged violations of state or federal health laws or regulations or been found by such program to be in violation of such laws or regulations.

3. Duties of the Nurse Practitioner

The Nurse Practitioner shall:

3.1. Practice the profession of a nurse practitioner in accordance with the laws and regulations governing the practice of a nurse practitioner in Maryland.

3.2. Provide all medical services within reasonable and accepted medical standards and in conformance with all requirements that may be imposed from time to time by the applicable health licensing boards.

3.3. Maintain neat, timely, and legible medical records for all patients evaluated and treated by the Nurse Practitioner.

3.4. Maintain Nurse Practitioner's own malpractice insurance; maintain a license to practice as a nurse practitioner in Maryland in good standing during the term of this Agreement or any renewal thereof; maintain nurse practitioner board certification; and maintain nurse practitioner continuing education credits according to the prevailing standard, which is a minimum of seventy-five (75) credits every five (5) years.

3.5. Maintain her own schedule of patients.

3.6. Pay the Physician a sum of $5,000 per contract year, with one payment made on the date this Agreement is signed and one payment made six months after the signing of this Agreement, plus $200 per hour for consultation time initiated by the Nurse Practitioner.

- 3.6.1. Consultation time includes telephone consultations, in-person, face-to-face consultations, and review of charts.
- 3.6.2. The minimum segment billed for a consultation is ten minutes.
- 3.6.3. Nurse practitioner will pay consultation fees monthly, within thirty (30) days of receiving a bill from the Physician.
- 3.6.4. When patients are admitted to a hospital, Nurse Practitioner shall pay Physician for consultation time until such time as the patient is admitted. After hospital admission, Physician may bill patient or patient's insurance company for services provided the patient in the hospital until such time as the patient is discharged.

4. Duties of the Physician

The Physician shall:

4.1. Respond to a telephone call from Nurse Practitioner within two (2) hours, unless Nurse Practitioner characterizes the call as an emergency, in which case the Physician will respond to a call within fifteen (15) minutes.

4.2. Keep a record of consultations and bill the Nurse Practitioner once a month.

4.3. Sign the Nurse Practitioner's written agreement as required by Maryland law.

4.4. Meet with the Nurse Practitioner once a month, for one-half hour, for discussion of clinical guidelines and management of difficult patients.

- 4.4.1. Agree that the meeting shall take place at a mutually agreed-upon location, which may vary from time to time.
- 4.4.2. Agree that payment for monthly meeting time is included in the $5,000 per contract year that Nurse Practitioner pays Physician.

4.5. Agree to conform, in Physician's consultations, to the standard of care of a reasonably prudent Physician practicing as an internist in suburban Maryland.

4.6. Assist Nurse Practitioner, to the best of Physician's ability, in any other requirements for physician collaboration that may arise and that are necessary to conform to the laws and regulations governing the practice of a nurse practitioner in Maryland.

4.7. Agree not to bill a patient's insurance company directly for any consultative services Physician provides a nonhospitalized patient of the Nurse Practitioner unless the Nurse Practitioner and Physician agree that the Physician, and not the Nurse Practitioner, will bill the services.

4.8. Bill a patient of the Nurse Practitioner or the patient's insurance company for visits to such patient while the patient is hospitalized.

4.9. Return the care of hospitalized patients of the Nurse Practitioner to the Nurse Practitioner after discharge from the hospital.

4.10. Cosign charts where the Nurse Practitioner and Physician are comanaging patients.

4.11. Maintain Physician's own malpractice insurance; maintain a license to practice as a physician in Maryland in good standing during the term of this Agreement or any renewal thereof; maintain physician board certification; and maintain physician continuing education credits according to the prevailing standard.

4.12. Maintain hospital admitting privileges at at least one hospital within a 20-mile radius of the Nurse Practitioner's office.

4.13. Physician agrees that this is not an employment relationship.

4.13.1. Physician agrees that Physician is responsible for federal and state income taxes on any amount paid to Physician by Nurse Practitioner; for Physician's own health insurance, workers' compensation, and unemployment insurance; and for Physician's own expenses of practice.

5. Term

5.1. The Term of this Agreement shall be from ________________, 20__, and shall automatically renew for successive one-year terms unless terminated earlier as provided herein.

5.2. In the event that either party intends not to renew, such party shall give the other party ninety (90) days' notice of its intent not to renew, and the term or renewal term shall end upon the completion of the applicable contract year.

6. Termination

6.1. The Agreement shall be terminated immediately upon the happening of any of the following events:

6.1.1. The death of Nurse Practitioner or Physician;

6.1.2. Nurse Practitioner is legally disqualified or restricted in Nurse Practitioner's ability to render professional medical services in the State of Maryland as a nurse practitioner, or disciplinary action is taken against Nurse Practitioner's license in any other jurisdiction. For purposes of this section, the lapse of license for nonpayment of applicable licensing fees in a jurisdiction other than Maryland shall, by itself, not be considered disciplinary action;

6.1.3. Physician is legally disqualified or restricted in his ability to render professional medical services in the State of Maryland as a physician, or disciplinary action is taken against Physician's license in any other jurisdiction. For purposes of this section, the lapse of license for nonpayment of applicable licensing fees in a jurisdiction other than Maryland shall, by itself, not be considered disciplinary action;

6.1.4. Physician's loss or restriction of staff membership or professional privileges at any hospital or health care facility at which Physician has privileges, unless such loss or restriction was due to the occasional violation of the facility's record-keeping requirements or Physician shall have previously notified Nurse Practitioner that such loss or restriction will not terminate this Agreement;

6.1.5. Physician's disability as defined by federal or state law, or to the extent that the Physician cannot reasonably or competently perform the Physician's duties;

6.1.6. Nurse Practitioner's disability as defined by federal or state law, or to the extent that Nurse Practitioner cannot reasonably or competently continue to practice;

6.1.7. Ninety (90) days after Nurse Practitioner or Physician gives written notice to the other of termination without cause;

6.1.8. At any time by mutual agreement of the parties;

6.1.9. Nurse Practitioner's material breach of this Agreement, provided, however, that if Nurse Practitioner's breach of this Agreement is of a type and nature that may be cured, Nurse Practitioner shall have the opportunity immediately to cure breaches to the reasonable satisfaction of the Physician;

6.1.10. Physician's material breach of this Agreement, provided, however, that if Physician's breach of this Agreement is of a type and nature that may be cured, Physician shall have the opportunity immediately to cure breaches to the reasonable satisfaction of the Nurse Practitioner;

6.1.11. Upon Physician's conviction of a crime;

6.1.12. Upon Nurse Practitioner's conviction of a crime;

6.1.13. Upon adjudication that Nurse Practitioner is insane or determined to be legally incompetent;

6.1.14. Upon adjudication that Physician is insane or determined to be legally incompetent;

6.1.15. In the event that professional malpractice insurance for Nurse Practitioner is denied or lost or is limited by restriction or endorsement;

6.1.16. In the event that professional malpractice insurance for Physician is denied or lost or is limited by restriction or endorsement;

6.2. Upon termination of this agreement, the original records of patients followed by Nurse Practitioner or in Nurse Practitioner's office are understood by the parties to be the property of Nurse Practitioner.

7. Notices

All notices provided in this Agreement shall be directed to the parties in writing, by registered or certified mail, return receipt requested or by hand delivery at the following addresses:

If to Nurse Practitioner:
C.B. Bosko, NP
102 Goldleaf Ave. Suite 2
Jasonville, MD
If to Physician:
George Oaks, MD
102 Goldleaf Ave. Suite 3
Jasonville, MD

8. General terms

8.1. Applicable law. This Agreement shall be construed and enforced under Maryland law.

8.2. Nonassignment.

8.2.1. The Physician shall not be entitled to assign any of the benefits or burdens imposed on the Physician hereunder.

8.2.2. The Nurse Practitioner shall not be entitled to assign any of the benefits or burdens imposed on the Nurse Practitioner hereunder.

8.3. Binding effect. This Agreement shall be for the benefit of and be binding upon the parties hereto, their respective representatives, heirs, assigns, and successors-in-interest.

8.4. Execution. This Agreement shall be executed in duplicate, and each executed copy shall constitute an original, but the two copies shall be deemed one and the same instrument, and this Agreement shall not be modified or changed, except in writing, signed and acknowledged by the parties hereto.

8.5. Entire agreement. This Agreement contains the entire understanding between the parties hereto and supersedes any prior written or oral agreement between the parties. There are no representations, agreements, or understandings, oral or written, between or among the parties hereto relating to the subject matter of this Agreement that are not fully expressed herein.

WITNESS the following signature and seals;

Nurse Practitioner: ______________________

Date: ________________________________

Physician: ____________________________

Date: ________________________________

CHAPTER 12

Lawmaking and Health Policy

Health care is regulated for the public good, to ensure quality to a public that is powerless to assert quality control as individuals. That is the theory at least. In the real world, health care is regulated for quality reasons and because professional groups lobby for regulations that support their profession and businesses lobby for regulations that help their businesses. Regulation is imposed through statutes, regulations, and policies, and, when a statute or regulation is challenged in court, through the judicial system.

THE LEGAL PROCESS

Statutes

A statute is a law enacted by a state legislature or Congress. Laws are found in state and federal codes. For example, Maryland statutes are found in the Maryland Code Annotated, and federal statutes are found in the US Code Annotated (U.S.C.A.).

Citizens have input into the enactment of statutes by electing representatives who they think will vote as they would wish and by lobbying those representatives for passage of bills about specific issues.

For example, in many states, NPs' prescriptive authority is found in a statute. In those states, the legislatures have considered the issue of NP prescribing and have approved.

Regulations

A regulation is law written by a state or federal agency in accordance with a statute. Agencies are a part of the executive branch of government. A regulation cannot directly contradict a statute but may expand upon a statute, supplying details not included in the statute. The divided responsibility—between the legislature to enact statutes and the executive branch agencies to write regulations—is part of the balance of power constructed by the US Constitution.

Citizens have input into regulations in that regulations, prior to being adopted, usually are published for public review, with an opportunity for public comment. Agencies may or may not accept the comments. Further, citizens who are unhappy with a current regulation could enlist their legislators to enact laws that would require agencies to change the regulations. For example, if state regulations addressing nursing homes do not address NP practice in nursing homes, a state NP organization will want to: (1) ask the director of the appropriate state agency for a change of regulation to include NPs as providers in nursing homes; (2) ask legislators to request a regulation change, and, if necessary; (3) ask legislators for a statute that would require the agency head to change regulations to allow NPs to practice in nursing homes.

Policies

Policies are rules, made by companies or government agencies, that do not have the force of law but that dictate day-to-day decisions. Citizens have input on policies only insofar as they can convince whoever has authority for the policy to change it. Or citizens may lobby legislators for a law that requires companies or government agencies to change policy. For example, a hospital may have a policy to give admitting privileges to physicians only. Local NPs who want admitting privileges will want to persuade the appropriate hospital decision maker, through facts, figures, and a presentation of projected benefits to the hospital, of the need to change policy and allow NPs to admit patients.

THE JUDICIAL SYSTEM

A state court may hold that a state law is unconstitutional, and a federal court may hold that a federal law is unconstitutional. Courts may interpret laws and determine whether laws have been applied as the legislature, or Congress, meant the law to be applied. A citizen who believes that a law has been misapplied and who has suffered damage as a result may bring suit for a court decision in an effort to force correct application of a law. For example, in 1983, the Medical Board in Missouri brought legal action against two NPs practicing in a women's services clinic on the basis that the NPs were practicing medicine without medical licenses. The lower court found that the NPs were practicing medicine without a license, but the NPs took the case to the highest court in Missouri, and after reviewing historical documents, the state's highest court held that the intent of the legislature in expanding the nurse practice act had been to expand the scope of practice to include the activities performed by the NPs.

HEALTH POLICY

Policy is defined by the *New Merriam-Webster Pocket Dictionary* as "a definite course or method of action selected to guide and determine present and future decisions."[1] Presidents and governors have policies on health care. Executive branch policies may influence the activities of federal and state agencies. However, unless policy becomes law, policy is like nursing theory: it may or may not have any effect on the way people do things.

An example of the influence of policy on the health care industry is President Clinton's 1994 effort at health care reform. The president had a definite course of action, a move toward a one-payer system: that is, government run health care. The president's plan was not enacted; in fact, it was criticized so soundly that it never was introduced as a bill in Congress. However, the threat implied by the Clinton health care reform policies—that if the health care industry did not change itself, the government would impose changes—encouraged the private sector to reform itself. Health care in 2003 is quite different from health care in 1993. For one thing, managed care is now a household word.

LAWS AND RULES THAT AFFECT NPs

NPs are affected by laws, regulations, policies, and court decisions that address:

1. Scope of NP practice.
2. Reimbursement for health services.
3. Qualifications for NP licensure and renewal.
4. Delegation of authority by physicians.
5. Quality of care.
6. Requirements for collaboration.

NPs have found laws, regulations, and policies to be barriers to the practice for which they were educated. A 1995 survey of 2,741 California NPs reported that perceived barriers to practice included lack of prescriptive authority, lack of support from physicians, reimbursement difficulties, and lack of public awareness.[2] Two of these four barriers are legal. How can NPs change these legal barriers?

CHANGING LAWS

NPs who seek to change laws generally do so because they find that a statute, regulation, or a policy keeps them from doing something necessary for practice. For example, NPs who were enrolled as Medicaid providers found that once Medicaid patients began enrolling in managed-care health plans, the NPs could no longer be the primary providers for the patients because the policies or the managed-care organizations (MCOs) precluded NPs from being admitted to primary care provider (PCP) panels.

In some states, the quest to change MCO policy has turned into an effort to enact new statutes. That is because MCOs, when asked to admit NPs to provider panels, said that state law was unclear. So NPs are seeking to clarify state law such that NPs are specifically designated by statute as PCPs.

UNDERSTANDING THE BIG PICTURE

Currently, as managed care goes, so goes health care. Managed care is the aspect of the big picture that will most affect NP practice in the next decade at least.

What Is Going on in Managed Care?

Simply put, managed care is a system where the insurer is not only the payer, but also the provider of health care. Prior to managed care, insurance companies paid bills submitted by providers. The insurer had no control over the quality or quantity of care being given. The insurer had no responsibility to the patient other than to pay the bills. Under managed care, the insurer is responsible for the care given. The insurer keeps close tabs on the services provided. The insurer monitors how the health care services are utilized and sometimes denies, in advance or retrospectively, payment for services. Under fully developed managed care, insurers agree with purchasers to give care—whatever care is needed—for a fixed monthly or yearly fee, and clinicians agree with insurers to give whatever care is needed for a fixed monthly fee. The clinician shares with the insurer the financial risk that a patient will need more care than a payment covers.

Insurers are not only concerned with cost. They now monitor the quality of care given by providers and practices.

The health care industry has recently come under scrutiny regarding quality of care from the people who purchase the most services—employers who buy health care for employees—and from consumer-oriented groups such as the National Committee for Quality Assurance (NCQA), which accredits health plans and monitors and reports on quality of care. Employers are beginning to base decisions about which health plan services to offer employees upon quality data gathered and reported by NCQA. Employers monitor the NCQA data, NCQA monitors health plans, health plans monitor practices, and practices monitor individual providers.

State and national legislators, wanting to ensure that citizens' best interests are not overshadowed by the goals of employers and insurers to make money, are introducing bills to improve quality and to make sure that citizens get the care they want or need. For example, some state legislatures have passed bills requiring that health plans allow postpartum mothers to stay overnight in the hospital for 24 hours after delivery. Health plans had been requiring mothers to go home after delivery. Citizen groups felt that good care required that postpartum mothers have at least a one-night hospital stay. Thus, legislatures have been delving into health care decisions formerly made only by clinicians, and lately made by insurers and clinicians.

Stages of Managed Care

NPs' place in the managed-care landscape will depend upon the stage of managed care in the region. In the early stages of managed care, most patients are covered by traditional insurers, and MCOs try to encourage employers who purchase health plans to enroll employees by offering premiums that cost less than those of traditional insurers. In the middle stages of development of managed care, more patients are enrolled, and MCOs try to control costs by decreasing hospital visits, length of stay in hospitals, and emergency department visits and by bargaining with medical practices for reduced rates on visits. In the advanced states of managed care, most patients are enrolled in managed care, and medical practices have agreed to share the risks. In other words, medical practices agree to take care of patients for a fixed amount of money per year. If care costs more than the set fee, providers will lose money. If care costs less than fees, providers will make a profit. In the later stages of development, much attention is paid to providing care that will prevent hospitalization and other high costs in the future, and to providing the nuts and bolts of care most cost-effectively. It is at these later stages that NPs are most likely to fulfill the needs of MCOs.

Where Do NPs Appear in the Managed-Care Landscape?

The position of NPs is well described by a favorite quote of the late Congressman Sonny Bono: "We have good soap to sell, but we have to go out and sell it." NPs are likely candidates for the position of PCPs, responsible for their own panels of patients. Consider the endorsement of NP practices given by Dr. Stephanie Seremetis, director of the Women's Health Program at Mount Sinai Medical Center: "Probably in the future the best use will be nurse practitioners in independent practice, using a physician as a backup for complex conditions and for system analysis."[3] Or consider the endorsement by Joseph A. Califano, Jr.:

> We should develop a three-tiered medical system: non-physician practitioners, primary care physicians, and physician specialists. The first tier—the front line of delivery—should be the non-physician practitioners: physician assistants, nurse practitioners, and certified nurse midwives. These professionals are capable, reliable and cost-efficient. . . . They should be licensed to diagnose ailments, treat common diseases, prescribe drugs, admit patients to hospitals, and release them. . . . The second tier should be composed of primary care physicians: the family doctors, pediatricians, and general internists, including geriatric practitioners. These physicians should handle the more complex cases that do not require specialist care and be available to consult, guide, and, where appropriate, supervise the non-physician practitioners. . . . The third tier should be specialists.[4]

The views expressed by Dr. Seremetis and Mr. Califano concern the general welfare. What about the welfare of the NP? Consider the view of Joseph Tommasino, a physician assistant writing about both physician assistants and NPs:

> Our professional growth . . . is essentially stunted by the simple fact that we have nowhere to go. We all grapple with, but seldom talk about, our lack of vertical mobility. . . . Want to change jobs? Submit your curriculum vitae and join the throng of PAs or NPs that apply for the job. True, your experience should ultimately speak for itself, but even if it does, will you get the salary you deserve? I doubt it, especially given the propensity of administrators to fill slots with the least expensive PAs or NPs. . . . One thing is certain: NPs and PAs must be proactive in designing their own career tracks.[5]

Salary aside, NPs who are practice owners have the opportunity to design a flow of care that makes sense from the point of view of the NP owner. It is not cast in stone that care must be given through the office visit. The office visit mode of health care delivery came about because of a physician-driven effort to tie reimbursement to physician services. Under capitated managed care, any model of care delivery that keeps patients satisfied and meets quality standards is a good model. That could mean increased use of community health nurses, home visits, and school-based health care. Groups of NPs with open and creative minds could design effective models that get out of the box established by fee-for-service medicine. Currently, however, NPs are giving primary care but are doing so under the auspices of a physician. NPs are not generally PCPs at this time. The present situation is a function of: (1) past history; (2) the present law; and (3) public perceptions of physicians as givers of medical care.

Past History

Physicians "professionalized" their practice before nurses or other health care practitioners did and before NPs existed. Physicians convinced lawmakers to draw the legal lines such that only physicians could diagnose and treat and only physicians could order and perform tests, procedures, and medication. For many years, nurses went along with physician dominance.

NPs are now trying to climb a hill where physicians work at the top, and the entrances are barricaded and are being shored up on all sides by physicians, who want to maintain their status as "king of the hill." Many state laws governing the practice of medicine and health care contain protectionism for physicians, while other health care providers have had to fight for the right to provide the services they have been educated to provide.

The successes of NPs in getting protective language for their practice have been limited to the state and federal laws governing Medicaid and the underserved populations. Generally, state laws regarding who can be a PCP for the commercially insured population either are nonexistent or do not specifically name NPs. Laws governing Medicaid, however, often do permit NPs to be PCPs.

Present Law

Reimbursement goes to PCPs and specialists. Therefore, if NPs want to have their own practices, they need to be legally designated PCPs.

In many states, physician collaboration is a matter of law, not of clinical judgment. Collaboration should be a matter of clinical and professional judgment for NPs, not something mandated by law. The majority of states require physician collaboration for NP practice, especially if prescription writing is involved. Most states allow NPs to prescribe if they have a collaborative agreement with a physician.

Public Perceptions

While research indicates that patients are highly satisfied with the experience of care given by NPs, and while some patients specifically request NPs as their providers, it is unclear whether there is a general awareness that NPs could be PCPs in their own right without physician oversight or collaboration.

Television shows have impressed the image of the kindly family physician on the minds of the public. There is no nurse counterpart to Marcus Welby, MD. The American Medical Association and the American Academy of Family Physicians have active public relations campaigns that seek to maintain the public perception of the physician as primary care provider.

HMO policies initially called for physician PCPs, even though NPs were delivering much of the care of patients enrolled in HMOs. Some HMOs are changing their policies, however.

What Must Happen for NPs To Be PCPs?

For NPs to achieve PCP status, three things must happen. Laws have to permit NPs to be PCPs, the public must accept and be comfortable with the concept of the NP as PCP, and MCOs must agree to designate NPs as PCPs. States that do not define a PCP as an NP will need to be convinced to add this legal permission. Public relations efforts should be aimed at convincing the public that they are safe with NPs. Simultaneously, MCOs need to be convinced of the advantages of having NPs as PCPs. For more information about marketing NPs to the public, see Chapter 13.

Laws can prohibit NPs from practicing, permit NPs to practice, and protect NP practice. An example of a prohibitive law is: "Expanded role . . . means a process of diffusion and implies multidirectional change . . . but does not permit medical diagnosis or medical prescription of therapeutic or corrective measures" (S.C. CODE ANN. REGS. § 91-3).

Examples of permissive laws are: "APRNs perform medical acts, independently, within a collaborative practice with a licensed physician" (VT. CODE R. 04 052001-44) and:

The nurse practitioner provides holistic health care to individuals, families, and groups across the life span in a variety of settings, including hospitals, long term care facilities and community-based settings.

Within his or her specialty, the nurse practitioner is responsible for managing health problems encountered by the client and is accountable for health outcomes. This process includes:

- Assessment
- Diagnosis
- Development of a plan
- Intervention
- Evaluation

The nurse practitioner is independently responsible and accountable for the continuous and comprehensive management of a broad range of health care, which may include:

- Promotion and maintenance of health
- Prevention of illness and disability
- Assessment of clients, synthesis and analysis of data and application of nursing principles and therapeutic modalities
- Admission of his/her clients to hospitals and long term care facilities and management of client care in these facilities
- Counseling
- Consultation and/or collaboration with other care providers and community resources
- Referral to other health care providers and community resources
- Management and coordination of care
- Use of research skills
- Diagnosis of health/illness status
- Prescription and/or administration of therapeutic devices and measures, including legend drugs and controlled substances, . . . consistent with the definition of the practitioner's specialty category and scope of practice

The nurse practitioner is responsible for recognizing limits of knowledge and experience, and for resolving situations beyond his/her nurse practitioner expertise by consulting with or referring clients to other health care providers.

Citation: OR. ADMIN. R. 851-050-0005.

Examples of protective laws (protective of physicians) are:

A hospital may not refuse to act upon an application for staff membership or professional privileges, or deny privileges for a physician, podiatrist, optometrist or dentist, without stating the reasons therefor, or if the reasons stated are unrelated to standards of patient care, patient welfare, the objectives of the institution or the character or competency of the applicant.

Citation: N.Y. PUB. HEALTH LAW § 2801-b.1.

and "If a hospital does not follow proper procedure, above, the physician, podiatrist, etc. may file a complaint with the public health council, which will make a prompt investigation and may recommend that the hospital review its actions" (N.Y. PUB. HEALTH LAW §§ 2801-b.2. & 3).

NPs need to work to erase the laws that are prohibitive. NPs need more laws that are permissive and protective. An example of a law protective of NPs would be:

> A managed care organization may not refuse to act upon an application for staff membership or professional privileges, or deny privileges for a nurse practitioner, without stating the reasons therefor, or if the reasons stated are unrelated to standards of patient care, patient welfare, the objectives of the institution or the character or competency of the applicant.

This is a slight alteration of New York's law quoted above, that protects physicians, dentists, podiatrists, and optometrists from being denied hospital privileges without fair reason.

The first step for state and national NP organizations is to have an attorney analyze the law to identify the barriers. Sometimes, when arguing about a professional issue, competitors will cite as barring NP participation laws that NPs were not even aware of.

The top priority areas where laws need to be changed to reflect NP training and practice are:

- Authorization of PCP status.
- Reimbursement.
- Hospital privileges.
- Loosening of legal requirements for physician collaboration.

NPs who are not familiar with the law and with government agencies may be surprised that an MCO cannot grant PCP panel membership to whatever form of provider the MCO chooses to admit. However, there are laws created prior to the emergence in the 1960s of NPs, laws that give physicians authority to care for patients. Insurance commissioners, for example, do not want to exceed their authority by allowing MCOs to admit NPs when the law does not specifically name NPs.

Once prohibitions are erased from the law, and once permission is certain, NPs will want to work toward legal protection. Other professions, notably physicians, have remarkable legal protection of the profession. The legal protection of physicians has been so great that the public associated "health care provider" with "physician" until recently, when other providers began to be assertive about their roles.

The stage is set for more permission and protection of professions other than physicians. For example, Medicaid law requires an insurer to offer a variety of choices to enrollees. Some state laws require insurers to pay NPs for services.

THE PROCESS OF CHANGING THE LAW

Law change involves certain steps, including:

- Developing a set of goals and legislative strategies for achieving the goals
- Analyzing present state law for barriers to NP practice
- Monitoring of law changes proposed by other groups
- Responding to proposed law that affects NPs adversely
- Following up to see how bills that have been introduced have progressed
- Arranging testimony when bills come up for a hearing
- Arranging for communication with legislators
- Drafting and arranging support for legislation that supports the NP agenda
- Following through until the bill is written into regulations
- Debriefing to see how the process can be done better next time

Developing Goals and Strategies

Clinicians know what gets in their way. NPs who have considered starting practices or who have done so know what stopped them from getting paid, know how difficult it can be to get a good physician collaborator, and know whether they need hospital privileges. NP organizations should poll their members to develop a list of goals for the organization. Then, keeping in mind that law must be in place, public perception must be favorable, and payer policies must be permissive, organizations can develop strategies for overcoming barriers. Strategies might include hiring a lobbyist, drafting a bill, hiring a public relations firm, brainstorming about ideas for news articles on NPs, meeting with researchers about data collection on NP practices, or meeting with MCO executives to tell them the benefits to their business of having NPs as providers.

Analyzing Law for Barriers to NP Practice

An attorney familiar with the NP role should analyze the law of each state for each state organization. First, the attorney will analyze the law that names NPs to determine whether any prohibitions exist or whether permission or protection is needed. The attorney will look for laws that do not name NPs but that regulate health care in a way that affects NPs. For example, the attorney will analyze state insurance law even if it does not name NPs as reimbursable providers. The attorney can locate the clause that should name NPs as reimbursable providers. The attorney should analyze state law that addresses health care quality. If a law says a physician must oversee all care of patients in MCOs, the attorney will locate the clause that neglects NPs and suggest language changes that will remedy the barrier for NPs.

Monitoring Law Changes Proposed by Other Groups

NPs will not be the only group looking to change the law. NP organizations will need to have someone monitoring proposed statutes and regulations to see how incoming law might affect NPs. Physicians will be going for protective language, as will physical therapists, physician assistants, chiropractors, and other professionals. It is frustrating enough that NPs must change laws that were enacted before NPs existed. It is doubly frustrating when NPs are caught off guard and new law is made that excludes NPs.

Responding to Proposed Law That Affects NPs Adversely

Sometimes a law is proposed that adversely affects NPs but is not a result of professional competition. Instead, the proposed law is aimed at solving some unrelated problem. For example, the agency that administers Medicare, the Center for Medicare and Medicaid Services (CMS), sets rates of payment for visits by Medicare patients. Physicians, NPs, physical therapists, chiropractors, and many other groups all may be working toward the same end: increasing those rates. In such situations, NPs may find allies in other professional groups. Again, to participate, NPs must be aware of the proposed law changes.

Following up on Bills in Progress

A bill may be changed many times between introduction and passage. The job of the lobbyist includes checking on bill status nearly every day to determine when the hearings are, what amendments have been proposed, when the votes will be held, who is in favor and who is opposed, and what bills have been introduced that may counteract any given bill. Sometimes an NP organization, to get the legislative support to get its bill passed, will need to agree to support another group's bill. In that case, a lobbyist must know who backs which bills, who will give what support in return for support, and what the NP organization's parameters are in terms of what can be supported and what cannot.

Arranging Testimony

Bills come up for hearings before legislative committees before a vote is taken to pass the bill out of committee and to the full legislative body, house or senate. At hearings, citizens are permitted to address the committee or legislative body about the effect a bill will have on a citizen or a group. Committee members may question those who testify. Often there are many people wanting to testify on a particular bill. There may be several hearings in a day. Keeping in mind that legislators can only digest so much information, testifying parties are advised to keep testimony short and to the point. Three minutes is often all an individual has to make the point.

Legislators will be more affected by testimony that a bill will affect many people or will affect some people greatly. For example, a legislator is going to be more swayed by testimony that a particular bill will open health care to 17,000 uninsured citizens than by testimony that a bill will give reimbursement to five self-employed NPs. On the other hand, if an NP can show legislators how the number of self-employed NPs could, with release of barriers, soon grow to 2,500 self-employed NPs who can participate in a state program for the uninsured by offering reduced rate services, legislators' interest will be stimulated. Legislators, like the population in general, are moved by issues that affect mothers and children, the elderly, public safety, and public expenditures. Testimony that shows how a bill touches on these issues can be very effective.

Lobbyists often help NP organizations develop testimony and testifiers. If a bill affecting NPs also affects patients, it is often helpful to have patients testify on behalf of a bill.

Arranging for Communication with Legislative Representatives

Citizens can communicate their opinions to legislators through telephone calls and visits as well as in hearings. Legislators make themselves available to citizens at such gatherings as "nurses' night at the legislature" and other receptions. All legislators have aides who can hear citizen concerns and pass those concerns along to the legislator. NPs wanting to communicate with legislators about professional issues might arrange for a personal visit with their individual legislators in their districts, telephone the legislator or aide, ask patients to contact their legislators about an NP issue of interest to the patient, and/or hire a lobbyist to communicate with the legislators.

It is a fact of life that legislators need money to conduct reelection campaigns. Legislators do, in fact, take the time to listen to contributors. Legislators do remember the individuals and groups who contribute to their campaigns. Many NP organizations have political action committee funds that they use to support legislative campaigns. This is an important use of association funds.

Drafting and Arranging Support for Legislation That Supports the NP Agenda

The drafting of legislative language is an art. Lobbyists, legislators, and attorneys do it. Citizens and associations do not do it, or rather, do not do it well. A bill has to take into account the existing law, the form that state law takes, possible unintended consequences of particular language, the state defined meaning of particular words, the possible reaction to opponents and competitors to specific language, and the need for conciseness and clarity of expression.

NP associations usually begin a bill-drafting process by discussing with a lobbyist the problem NPs are trying to solve. The lobbyist then locates the section of law that needs to be changed and proceeds to draft language changes that will solve the problem. Lobbyists, when drafting bills for NPs, often will get opinions from selected legislators and other professional groups about possible language in an attempt to pretest reactions to specific language. Often, between the time a bill is conceptualized and the time it is introduced, the bill's language has been changed and rearranged many times. And after the bill is introduced, the language may be changed several times through amendments.

After there is a draft of language for a proposed bill, or during the drafting process, a lobbyist seeks sponsors. A bill's sponsor introduces the bill and shepherds the bill through the legislature. There can be companion bills in both houses of the legislature, in which case there should be a sponsoring senator and a sponsoring representative. The selection of a sponsor is crucial because the personality, committee position, affiliations, and popularity of a sponsor will have an effect on how the bill progresses. For example, a well-positioned sponsor may decline because the legislator is trying to curry favor from an opposing group. Therefore, it is not uncommon to shop for sponsors.

After a lobbyist gets a bill sponsor, the search is on for cosponsors. A bill with many cosponsors is a bill likely to get passed. No legislator likes his or her name on a bill that fails. So, cosponsors can be expected not only to support the bills they cosponsor, but to work for passage of those bills.

After obtaining sponsors and cosponsors, a lobbyist's next task is to line up testimony for committee hearings. Then, after a hearing, a lobbyist turns attention to getting votes locked in. Lobbyists ask legislators directly whether they intend to vote for or against a bill. If the vote is no, a lobbyist can ask why. If something about the bill can be changed to change a "no" vote to a "yes," a lobbyist can draft an amendment and seek the approval of sponsors, cosponsors, and other favorable voters on the amended language.

Finally, a bill comes to a vote. A bill must pass each house of the legislature. A bill that passes both houses then goes to the governor for approval. The final hurdle is escaping a gubernatorial veto. Lobbying is done even at this final stage to convince the governor and his or her staff of the worth of the bill.

After a bill becomes a law, the bill is codified: that is, written into the state's code of laws. Many bills are further expanded upon in regulations written by state agencies that carry out the laws. Regulations may include detail not specified in the law, but regulations cannot directly contradict a statute.

NPs who are working toward legal change will want to work closely with their lobbyist all the way through regulation writing. After it is over, debrief to see how things could be done better next time.

Hiring Lobbyists and Attorneys

Lobbyists and attorneys often serve many clients and may or may not know the issues of most importance to NPs. An NP association that is fortunate to have a lobbyist and attorney well versed in NP issues and already familiar with the law regarding NPs has a head start.

When interviewing an attorney, or lobbyist, ask:

1. What is your experience with NP issues?
2. Have you personally experienced the care of an NP?
3. Who are your other clients whose issues might conflict with NP issues?
4. Do you have any opinions about NPs?
5. What does an NP do?

One would think a lobbyist or attorney who has scheduled an interview with an NP organization would have done enough research to answer Question 5. But surprisingly, this is not always the case. A prospective lobbyist or attorney who cannot answer Question 5 should not be hired.

Do-It-Yourself Lobbying

Some NPs are very good at testifying. Usually the best testifiers are those who have had the most practice. When called to testify, ask who the committee members are and whether any are health care providers. Ask about a time limit. Ask who else will be testifying, and coordinate the testimony if possible. The best testimony has an introduction, a middle, and a conclusion, just like a speech. Polish is not a necessity, but preparation is essential.

Should NPs Join with the State Nurses' Association for Lobbying?

In some states, the NP association is a separate organization from the state nurses' association. In other states, NPs are an interest group within the state nurses' association. Ideally, from the point of view of an outsider, the state nurses' association would be taking care of legislative issues for all nurses. However, NPs sometimes find that their issues get a lower priority with the state's nurses' association than NPs would like. So NPs have formed their own organizations and hired their own lobbyists.

It is worth noting that in Oregon, where state law is quite favorable to NPs, lobbying has always been done by a strong state nurses' association, of which NPs are an interest group. Officers of NP associations should attempt to work with the state nurses' association on legislative issues. If, after attempts to work with the state nurses' association, NPs find they cannot get what they need from the state nurses' association, then NPs can hire their own lobbyist.

Dealing with Government Agencies

Many people who work for government agencies lack understanding of health care and specifically the role of NPs. Though an NP might expect that a state or federal agency might research an issue when knowledge is lacking, many state agencies rely on citizens and their representatives to bring problems to light and to do the legal research to support the proponent's position. When NPs or their hired representatives become familiar with the personnel of state and federal agencies and seek person-to-person communication about an NP issue, questions and problems can often be taken care of efficiently at the agency level without resorting to legislative action. Further, NPs will be included in government policy making when NPs sit on the advisory panels and commissions making the policies. It is part of a lobbyist's job to know the influential policy-making commissions in a state and attempt to get NPs appointed to the commissions and boards.

The Competition

Change would be easy were there no competition. There is competition, however, and it is useful to know where it comes from and what competitors' interests are.

Physician Competition

Physicians have fought for their position in health care and now fight to maintain it. The fight is by no means limited to NPs. Physicians fought hard against other providers such as homeopathic physicians and optometrists, and now they fight hard against MCOs, which physicians perceive as threatening physician autonomy.

Through capturing the mechanisms of reimbursement, physicians were able to secure and maintain a dominant position among health care providers. They are not going to give up their position now.

Although NPs made significant strides in the 1970s because of a physician shortage in certain areas, and although NPs made some progress in the 1990s because of a funds shortage, there are still many legal and policy barriers to NPs, many of which were established through physician influence and are maintained through physician influence.

Whereas the climate in the early 1970s was conducive to the proliferation of "physician extenders" due to the physician shortage, in recent years the NP has been increasingly viewed by some physicians as a competitor rather than simply an extender of physician services. Now, a more abundant supply of physicians is anticipated, which results in a different and more competitive atmosphere in the medical community.

For a sense of the effort that physicians are putting into fighting NP independence, consider the following policy statements from the American Academy of Family Physicians: "The nurse practitioner should not function as an independent health practitioner" and "The AAFP believes . . . that interests of patients are best served when their care is provided by a physician or through an integrated practice supervised directly by a physician."[6]

Physician groups are big spenders when it comes to lobbying. The American Medical Association spent $8.7 million in 1997 on lobbying; the American College of Emergency Physicians spent $1.6 million; the American Society of Internal Medicine spent $860,000; and the American Academy of Family Physicians spent $550,000.[7] While physician competition will not go away, neither will NPs.

Competition is something NPs always will need to budget for in terms of time, energy, and money.

Competition from Physician Assistants

Physician assistants (PAs) have many of the same goals as NPs: professional recognition and respect, the ability to make a good living, and the ability to control one's work product. PAs will have to fight their own battles, as their profession was set up differently from its inception. By nature of their name and mission, PAs are not meant to be independent providers. While individual NPs may compete with individual PAs for specific jobs, it is not fruitful for NP professional organizations to engage PA organizations in competition in the public arena.

Competition from Other Nurses

Some NP associations find that when they go for inclusion in the law as PCPs, other nurses, particularly clinical nurse specialists (CNSs), want to be included as well. At that point, there is a possibility that the legislature will be hearing competitive arguments from NP and CNS groups about the relative merits of each group. As with PAs, NPs and CNSs have many of the same goals. It will not serve either group well to fight, and public fighting will definitely cause harm. Peaceful coexistence is the key. If NPs only put forth efforts to further their profession and decline from efforts to hold back other professions, not only will time and expenses be saved, but public relations will be better.

How Can Individual NPs Make a Difference?

Individuals can influence lawmakers and lawmaking in the following ways:

- Ask candidates in local elections their position on NPs, and vote accordingly. Support good candidates with campaign contributions, noting on the check that you are an NP.
- When a bill concerns NPs or health issues of concern to NPs, call or write legislators, noting that you are an NP.
- When regulations are proposed that affect NPs, write and send comments on how the proposed regulations will affect NPs.
- Join an NP association.
- Write letters to the editor of the local newspaper about news events affecting NPs or affecting your patients.

CONCLUSION

The process for making law conform to NP goals for the profession is:

1. Analyze the current law for prohibitions, lack of permission, and lack of protection where it matters. Have an attorney work with the NP organization to do the analysis.

2. Draft a bill that erases prohibition, gives permission, or affords protection for NP practice. Have an attorney, lobbyist, or legislator work with the organization to do this.
3. Gather support for the bill among lawmakers and the public. Enlist the participation of association members in each legislative district.
4. Introduce the bill, and follow its progress, testifying when necessary, educating lawmakers when necessary, and arranging give-and-take with other groups when necessary. At this stage, professional lobbyists should be running the show.
5. Follow the bill through to the regulation-writing stage, monitoring the language of proposed regulations and commenting on the proposed regulations through letters. Have an attorney do this.
6. Refine the approach, based on what was learned with previous law changes. Association officers, attorneys, and lobbyists should do this.

NOTES

1. *New Merriam-Webster Pocket Dictionary.* New York, NY: Pocket Books; 1971:83.

2. Anderson AL, Gillis CL, and Yoder L. Practice environment for nurse practitioners in California: identifying barriers. *West J Med* 1996; 165:209–214.

3. The Future Wears White: Nurses Treading on Doctors' Turf. *New York Times* Week in Review section, November 2, 1997. Available at www.nytimes.com. Accessed August 2003.

4. Califano JA Jr. *Radical Surgery: What's Next for America's Health Care.* New York, NY: New York Times Books, 1994; 218.

5. Tommasino J. The dilemma of the one-rung ladder. *Clinician Reviews* 1998; 8:31.

6. American Academy of Family Physicians, Policy Statement (1997). Available on the Web at http://www.aafp.org. Accessed July 2003.

7. Weissenstein E. Lobbying on rise. Budget plan leads healthcare groups to use checkbooks. *Mod Health* 1997; 27:50.

CHAPTER 13

Promoting the Profession to the Public

According to studies of patient satisfaction, patients who have seen NPs like NPs. But not everyone has seen an NP. People who are healthy and rarely visit any health care provider may not have experienced care given by an NP. Those who have had a long relationship with a physician may not have experienced the care of an NP.

NPs have had little if any exposure on television or in movies. There are no NPs on prime-time television. There are no equivalents of Marcus Welby, Dr. Quinn, or ER doctors for the NP profession. These TV characters, doing their work on the air week after week, have given the general public a sense that they know what physicians do.

There are no well-known figures in literature or in the popular culture who are NPs. Children do not grow up reading books about NPs. There is no Nancy Drew, NP. There are no NP dolls. No movies have been done about NPs or having NPs as central characters. There are no NP senators or congressional representatives. Fortunately, no NPs have become prominent for their misdeeds.

No advertising campaign keeps NPs in the public eye in the way that advertising keeps Coca-Cola in the public eye. The American Medical Association (AMA), on the other hand, budgeted $2.5 million in 1997 for a major public relations (PR) effort with the goal of making the AMA a symbol of "all that is good in medicine and patient care" and establishing the AMA as an "American icon" on par with McDonald's and IBM.[1] The campaign was initiated even though the association had shortfalls in dues projections in the previous year and did not have the money to spend.

NP organizations are just beginning to realize that organized PR campaigns are needed for NPs. NPs who want to see the passage of legislation favorable to NPs' practice and NPs who have their own practices and want to see them thrive will want the public to have an opinion about NPs, and will want that opinion to be favorable. NPs have made great progress on a one-on-one basis. Perhaps the main way the public will understand what an NP does is by experiencing the care. Those who have not experienced the care of an NP can be encouraged, through PR efforts, to seek the care of an NP.

PUBLIC RELATIONS STEPS

There are systematic ways of raising public awareness about NPs. Marketing, public relations, and sales all have the same process: (1) develop a message; (2) determine whom the message should reach; (3) determine the best way to disseminate the message; (4) disseminate the message; and (5) evaluate the success of the effort and fine-tune the process.

The steps in a PR strategy for NPs are:

1. Set a goal.
2. Develop a plan.
3. Develop a budget.
4. Work the plan.

SETTING THE GOAL

A likely PR goal for NPs is to establish NPs as experts on primary care. The ultimate goal might be getting primary care provider (PCP) status for NPs. An alternative goal for an individual NP with a private practice may be getting patients to come in the door.

DEVELOPING THE PLAN

Either way, the plan will revolve around establishing NPs, or the NP, as a high-quality professional who gives primary care. The most effective forms of publicity will be those that show the expertise of NPs in a way the public can understand. NPs can convey expertise in a number of ways:

- Providing high-quality care to each patient, one-on-one.
- Suggesting word of mouth when a friend or family member had a good experience of care.
- Including testimonials from patients in brochures, promotional videos, or paid advertising.
- Arranging for articles by NPs on health topics in local newspapers.
- Arranging for radio or television talk show appearances by NPs.
- Arranging for advice from NPs to be included in newspaper or magazine articles on health topics.
- Speaking on health care topics at community forums.
- Serving on health care advisory boards in the area.
- Endorsing as an association particular sets of preventive care guidelines and standards.

A simple PR plan that focuses on a series of news releases is described in Appendix 13-A.

DEVELOPING THE BUDGET

PR can be done on a champagne budget or a beer budget. Either way, there must be a budget, or nothing will happen. The majority of a PR budget will go toward services. The researching and writing of news releases, the searching for names and addresses of editors, and the follow-up with telephone calls will consume the most monetary resources.

Even a small NP organization should count on spending $15,000 to $18,000 a year on PR. Where will the money come from, other than dues? From other business ventures. One job of a PR professional could be to promote an NP educational conference that would have a registration fee and would presumably turn a profit. Another job of a PR professional would be to develop written materials—brochures and fact sheets on NPs—that could be sold to individual NPs and practices and distributed to patients.

WORKING THE PLAN

Proactive PR

In a proactive PR plan, an NP organization would seek to generate articles or television pieces about NPs or to showcase the expertise of NPs, not in response to some attack on NPs, but as a regular, systematic promotion of NPs. For example, an NP organization might arrange for an article to appear in the local newspaper giving an NP's advice for staying well in flu season. The article serves three purposes: It keeps NPs in the news in a positive light, demonstrates the information an NP can offer, and gives people useful information. The article satisfies the needs of NPs, the needs of readers, and the needs of newspaper editors to run informative articles.

A message about NP expertise in primary care could be disseminated on television, in newspapers and magazines, at health fairs, by word of mouth, and through advertising. It is generally agreed that television stories and newspaper articles are an effective way of getting a message to a large segment of the population with little expenditure.

When developing a PR plan, NPs need to keep in mind that newspapers and television station owners need readers (or viewers) and advertisers. An NP may not be able to offer a newspaper advertisers but can offer readers if the NP is providing information on a topic of interest to many people. Health, and particularly primary care, is interesting to many people.

To generate one article in a newspaper, the following things have to happen:

1. Generate an idea for an article.
2. Generate the information to be conveyed.
3. Write the news release.
4. Identify the appropriate vehicle for the article.

5. Identify the decision maker (editor) who can ensure that the article will get into the paper.
6. Give the editor the name of a contact if the editor wants more information.
7. After the release is sent to the editor, follow up by telephone call.
8. Arrange for more information to be given to the editor, or arrange for accompanying photograph or art.

A statewide media campaign would involve something like sending a news release to every newspaper in the state once a month. When the process described above is done 12 times a year and multiplied by 50 or 100 newspapers, it is close to a full-time job.

Each NP organization and each private practice needs a person designated to handle PR. PR services may be purchased or performed by a volunteer NP. Obviously, a volunteer is less expensive, will know more about NPs than a PR professional, and will be motivated. However, a volunteer probably will have a job as an NP, and the volunteer PR efforts may not get the regular attention that is needed. Further, when NPs organize into associations and there is a treasury, it makes sense for all NPs to share in contributing to PR efforts, and that is best done by purchasing PR services rather than imposing on one NP to do the work.

Reactive PR

Public relations is reactive when it is in response to a particular event or criticism. For example, if a physicians' group came out with a statement that only physicians should be PCPs, the rebuttal of an NP organization would be reactive.

The keys to effective reactive PR are speed and a consistent and logical message. Therefore, NP organizations should have a set of "talking points" ready for use in the event that a speedy reaction is needed. Talking points are a PR method for ensuring that a spokesperson for a group has something to say and that the message is consistent with the group's goals. For examples of talking points for NP organizations, see Appendix 13-B.

THE SUBSTANCE OF THE MESSAGE

When NPs are asked how NPs differ from physicians and why NPs should be incorporated into payment systems, NPs must be ready with hard facts and data that answer the questions.

Compare the following two statements: "Nurse practitioners are good listeners and are safe and effective providers of health care" and "A health services research team studying 799 episodes of otitis media and sore throat in a Columbia, Maryland HMO found that NPs were more effective at resolving the problem. And NPs' care was 20% less expensive than MDs'." Which statement will more effectively persuade business people and lawmakers that NPs are value-added providers? The second statement is what an NP will want to tell an insurance executive, an employer, or a congressperson. NPs know that the first statement is true, but everyone else wants hard facts and numbers.

SUPPORTING DATA

Three recent studies and one not-so-recent study that is nevertheless powerful compared NP and MD practice and found NPs to be as good as or better than MDs as PCPs. These four studies, done by non-nurse researchers, should be on the tip of the tongue of anyone trying to "sell" the concept of the NP as the preferred health care provider.[2]

Study 1: NPs Match MDs on Primary Care Tasks

Hall set up audit criteria, with input from the practitioners being studied, and then audited charts of 426 MDs and NPs in 16 ambulatory care practices.[3] The researcher looked at eight tasks: (1) follow-up of a low hematocrit to detect patients with anemia caused by colorectal cancer or other serious gastrointestinal disease; (2) screening for cancer using breast examination and Pap smears in women; (3) follow-up of a high serum glucose to detect and treat diabetes; (4) monitoring of patients on digoxin to detect drug toxicity or symptomatic relapse; (5) follow-up of a positive urine culture to treat persistent bacteriuria; (6) compliance with the American Academy of Pediatrics standards for screening and immunization of infants; (7) assessment of the risk of dehydration in children at the start of an episode of gastroenteritis; and (8) monitoring and follow-up of children with otitis media to detect and treat failure to resolve the middle-ear effusion.

The findings: NPs' performance was comparable or superior on seven of the eight tasks. Female MDs were better at cancer screening for women, but male MDs were worse at this than NPs. The sample of male "nonphysicians" was too small to make any generalizations about and was therefore excluded from the results.

Study 2: NPs Are Cost-Effective

Salkever et al. compared NPs and MDs on cost and effectiveness.[4] To study costs, Salkever paid observers to time NP and MD visits with patients. The research team then analyzed costs of office space, costs of follow-up visits, and costs of ancillary services and drugs ordered by the providers. To study effectiveness, the researchers randomly surveyed patients regarding problem severity and changes in problem status after treatment. The researchers then computed the cost per episode of care for two conditions, sore throat and otitis media.

The findings: NPs were 20 percent less costly in their care.[5] NPs were at least as effective as MDs at resolving the problem.[4 p152]

Study 3: NPs Get to the Root of the Problem

Avorn et al. asked 799 MDs and NPs to consider the following case vignette and answer two questions:[6]

Case vignette: A man you have never seen before comes to your office seeking help for intermittent sharp epigastric pains that are relieved by meals but are worse on an empty stomach. The patient has just moved from out of state and brings along a report of an endoscopy performed a month ago showing diffuse gastritis of moderate severity but no ulcer. Is there a particular therapy you would choose at this point, or would you need additional information?

Questions: What more do you want to know? What would you do?

The findings: Nurses were far more likely to collect more historical information about the patient before deciding upon therapy. The NPs asked an average of 2.6 questions about the patient as opposed to 1.6 for physicians. A third of physicians (and 19 percent of NPs) chose to initiate therapy without any additional information. Nurses were far more likely to ask about the patient's diet and psychosocial information (but less likely to ask about alcohol intake). NPs were more likely to suggest nonprescription approaches to therapy, such as a change in diet or counseling to help the patient deal with stress. NPs were far less likely than physicians (20 percent versus 63 percent) to recommend a prescription drug.[7] NPs were much less likely to state that a prescription drug would be the single most effective therapeutic intervention for this patient (12 percent versus 46 percent).[8]

No analysis of cost of therapy was done. However, when the cost of MDs' treatment plan—prescription medication, but no counseling about unhealthy lifestyle—is compared with NPs' treatment plan—no prescription, but counseling regarding aggravating factors—the NPs' treatment plan certainly shows itself to be the more economical approach to care.

Study 4: Patients Are Satisfied with NPs

Medical Economics, a magazine written for physicians, conducted a survey of patient satisfaction with NPs and MDs.[9] Patients were as satisfied with NPs as with physicians.

Study 5: Patients Are Satisfied with NPs

Harrocks et al. systematically reviewed randomized controlled trials and prospective observational studies and found that patients were more satisfied with care by a nurse practitioner, that there were no differences in the health status of patients treated by nurse practitioners versus medical doctors, and the quality of care was in some ways better for nurse practitioner consultations.[10]

Study 6: NPs More Successful at Getting Patients Blood Pressure Down

Mundinger et al. conducted a randomized trial comparing outcome measures for care provided by nurse practitioners and medical doctors. Among other things, Mundinger found a statistically significant difference in the diastolic value of patients treated for hypertension by nurse practitioners. Nurse practitioners' patients had a lower diastolic blood pressure after treatment than physicians' patients.[11]

Further Data on the Value of NP Practice

A survey study (N = 3,257) comparing OB-GYN practices that used nonphysician providers with physician-only practices found that patients preferred the "collaborative" practices.[12] Of the nonphysician providers, 45 percent were NPs, 19 percent were midwives, 16 percent were PAs, and 9 percent were CNSs. Reasons for preferring practices with nonphysician providers were:

- The patient got an appointment faster.
- More time was spent with the provider.
- More health information was given.
- More diet information was given.

Patients felt that nonphysicians were less rushed in their care. However, patients believed that physicians provided more complete information.

For a quick reference to substantive arguments supporting NP practice and citations for the arguments, see Exhibit 13-1.

COLLECTING IMPRESSIVE FACTS

Not all hard facts and data come from research studies. When a practice gets a contract as a provider with an HMO, the practice receives quarterly performance reports from the HMO.

Exhibit 13-1 Effective Arguments for NPs

Argument 1: Effective care requires a proper match between provider and patient problem. NPs are the appropriate first-line provider.
Data: Hall, Salkever, and Avorn studies (see notes 3, 4, and 6 of this chapter)
Argument 2: Patients are highly satisfied with NPs.
Data: Perry and Harrocks studies (notes 9 and 10)
Argument 3: NPs have been proven cost-effective in their evaluations/treatments.
Data: Avorn and Salkever studies (notes 4 and 6)
Argument 4: NPs give high-quality primary care.
Data: Hall, Salkever, Avorn, and Mundinger studies (notes 3, 4, 7, and 11)
Argument 5: NPs emphasize disease prevention and health care maintenance.
Data: Hall and Avorn studies (notes 3 and 6)

Source: Adapted with permission from Buppert C. Reimbursement for nurse practitioner services. *The Nurse Practitioner* 1998; 23: 67, 70–74, 76. Springhouse Corporation.

The reports compare the practice to the aggregate (average practice) on such qualities as: (1) number of emergency department visits by covered patients; (2) number of admissions; (3) length of stay of admitted patients; and (4) monthly cost of care per patient.

NP practices are getting contracts with MCOs. One NP practice that has contracted with an MCO as a primary care provider performed significantly better than the aggregate. The NP practice, Abbottsford Community Health Center, had 48 fewer admits than the aggregate per 1,000 patients, the average stay of admitted patients was 1 1/2 days shorter, and the facility cost per admission was more than $1,000 less for the NP practice (D. Torresi, personal communication, July 1994).

NPs who do not have their own practices but who work as employees of MDs or HMOs may find that practice managers are collecting data to compare NPs' performance with that of local MDs. NPs who collect such data and pool it with other NPs will have substantive answers to such questions from businesspeople and legislators as "Why should we want NPs?"

PRESENT BARRIERS TO FACT COLLECTION

Though data from the NP-only practice is impressive, NP practices are rare. Far more common are MD/NP practices. However, when HMOs or state agencies want to study NP participation in the practice, efforts are stymied. This is because the easiest way for agencies to collect data on practice is the CMS 1500 form, the standard billing form that the practice transmits to Medicare, Medicaid, and most private insurers.[13] If billing clerks in doctors' offices designate the physician as the "provider," rather than an NP who actually sees a patient, then the NP's practice patterns will be invisible to researchers.

A billing clerk may be in the habit of billing for visits with an NP under a physician's provider number because the physician owns the practice. Or the billing clerk may put the physician's number in the box because, until recently, NPs have not been able to get UPIN numbers. A claim with a blank box is likely to be rejected. Or the NP may be working under an "incident to" arrangement with a physician, and the practice may be billing at 100 percent of Medicare rates. (See Chapter 9 for a definition of "incident to.") NPs should inquire of billing clerks whether the NP's or the MD's provider number is used for billing. If there is no compelling reason for using an MD's number, then an NP's number should be used on the CMS 1500 when an NP is the provider of care.

NOT-SO-IMPRESSIVE FACTS ABOUT NPs

While some of NPs' problems with acceptance are brought on by physicians who are guarding their professional territory or by the response of the public to physicians' successful and persistent PR, some of NPs' problems are self-inflicted. The argument put forth by physician organizations that the education required for entry into NP practice is less than the education required for physician entry into practice is true. Likewise, the argument that the continuing education requirements of NPs are less than physician requirements is true. The *Washington Post* gave this advice to NPs in an editorial:

> If nurses' role is to go on changing as quickly as it has, it will be up to nursing schools to look closely at that training—as some clearly have done—and make sure it corresponds to reality. It remains true that nurses receive far less medical training than doctors (typically two years or less) and a far lower proportion have been to college.[14]

DEALING WITH THE DOWNSIDE

NPs need to be able to respond positively to comparisons between NP and MD education. NPs need a standard minimum entry into practice. NPs need a standard continuing-education requirement similar to that of family physicians.

NPs can deal with the PR problem in two ways. They can upgrade the entry-into-practice requirement to a master's degree. Thirty states already have done this. They can upgrade the continuing education requirements. The present continuing education requirements of NPs differ depending on the certifying organization. A wise move on the part of NPs would be to match continuing education requirements to those of family physicians.

NPs need to be able to respond that all NPs are required to have master's degrees.[15] The American Association of Colleges of Nursing is working toward that goal.[16] NPs need to urge their credentialing body to increase the continuing-education requirements to parallel the requirements for family physicians. At least one pharmacology course needs to be on every nursing graduate school's list of required courses. Nursing graduate schools would do well to add physicians to their faculty, specifically for the illness management portion of the program. Medical schools also would benefit from adding NPs to their faculty teaching primary care. Finally, nursing schools should offer a clinical doctorate in primary care. The curriculum logically might include pharmacology, physiology, clinical psychology, and advanced medical management.

Even if NPs place the requirement for entry into practice at a master's degree, the education of NPs will be shorter than physician education. One counterargument to physicians who argue that their education is longer is that there are no data to support the necessity of four years of medical school and three years of residency to perform primary care. Physicians set those educational requirements with no research to support that level of education. The data that show that NPs are excellent primary care providers support an argument that master's-level preparation is appropriate education for PCPs.

A second not-so-impressive fact about NPs is that there is too much humility among NPs. Humility does not serve nurses well in day-to-day work situations, when nurses defer to physician dominance.[17] It does not serve researchers well when they fail to approach journalists with their findings.[18] It does not serve NP spokespeople or testifiers well when reacting to jabs from physician organizations. It is time for NPs to state, publicly and consistently, that "NPs are experts in primary care," not that "NPs do primary care in a collaborative relationship with a physician."

Every NP organization, whether state or national in focus, should devote at least 25 percent of its budget toward PR services. Recent college graduates make a yearly salary in the low $20,000s. Experienced PR professionals earn $125 an hour. If an organization purchases ten hours per month from an experienced PR professional, the yearly bill will be $15,000. Compare this with the expenditure on PR of a 160-provider medical group (including 15 physician assistants and NPs) in Ames, Iowa: $608,207 in 1997, of which $79,922 went for a PR specialist and an assistant.[19]

Among the projects for a PR professional hired by an NP organization would be to generate publicity, particularly through news releases that establish NPs as experts in primary care. Another likely project would be to generate a fact sheet or brochure on NPs to give out to anyone who expresses interest in and has questions about NPs. See Appendix 13-C for an example of the information that could be included in a fact sheet on NPs.

An NP organization can evaluate the success of PR services through an additional expenditure, a "clipping service." Clipping services extract all published articles about any subject a client specifies. An NP organization can see just where its news releases are printed and can then judge the effect of its PR professional. Clipping services start at about $150 per month and $1.50 per article.

Finally, each NP organization should designate an NP in the organization who will be the spokesperson when a reactive comment is called for. This NP should be familiar with the organization's talking points and should be unafraid of talking with the news media.

NOTES

1. News at deadline: AMA spends big to burnish its image. Hosp Health Net 1997; January 5: 55. Available at: http://www.hhnmag.com. Accessed August 2003.
2. The Salkever study was done by two public health PhDs, an MSW, and an MD. The Hall study was done by four PhDs, an MB, and an MA, from departments of psychology, health policy, biostatistics, and information technology. The Avorn study was done by MDs.
3. Hall J, Palmer RH, Orav EJ, et al. Performance quality, gender and professional role: A study of physicians and nonphysicians in 16 ambulatory care practices. *Med Care* 1990; 28:489–501.
4. Salkever DS, Skinner EA, Steinwachs DM, Katz H. Episode-based efficiency comparisons for physicians and nurse practitioners. *Med Care* 1982; 20:143–153.
5. For otitis media, NP cost per episode was $14.98; MD cost was $18.22. For sore throat, NP cost per episode was $11.80; MD cost was $15.64.
6. Avorn J, Everitt DE, Baker MW. The neglected medical history and therapeutic choices for abdominal pain: a nationwide study of 799 physicians and nurses. *Arch Intern Med* 1991; 151:694–698.

7. A month's supply of both Ranitidine and Tagamet costs close to $100.
8. There was no relationship between nurses having prescription authority in their state and their reliance upon prescription versus nonprescription therapy.

9. Perry K. Patient survey: physician extenders. Why patients love physician extenders. *Med Econ* 1995; 72:58, 63, 67.
10. Harrocks S, Anderson E, Salisbury C. Systematic review of whether nurse practitioners working in primary care can provide equivalent care to doctors. *Brit Med J* 2002; 324:819–823.
11. Mundinger M, et al. Primary care outcomes in patients treated by nurse pracitioners or physicians: A randomized trial. *JAMA* 2000; 283:59–68.
12. Hankins GD, Shaw SB, Cruess DF, et al. Patient satisfaction with collaborative practice. *Obstet Gynecol* 1996, 88:1011–1015.
13. Maryland's Health Care Cost and Access Commission, mandated by the Maryland legislature to study health care cost and access and come up with payment systems, ran into this problem. As a result, they have postponed data collection on NP practice until after MD data collection is done.
14. Doctors vs. nurses? Editorial. *Washington Post*, December 13, 1993, A20. Available at: http://washingtonpost.com, archive. Accessed August 2003.
15. Medical education was a mishmash of courses and apprenticeships until standardized at its present form in the early 1900s by the American Medical Association. See Starr P. *The Social Transformation of American Medicine*. New York, NY: Basic Books, Inc.; 1982:116–123.
16. The AACN position as of November 18, 1994, is: (1) all advanced practice nursing certification must meet a recognized and uniform national certification standard, integral to which is a requirement for a graduate degree in nursing, and (2) use uniform national standards when certifying nurses for advanced practice. Currently, more than 30 organizations offer advanced practice certification via at least 56 procedures for attaining the desired certification. Fickeissen JL. 56 ways to get certified. *Am J Nurs* 1990;90: 50–57.
17. Buresh B, Gordon S. Subtle self-sabotage. *Am J Nurs* 1996; 96:22–23
18. Buresh B, Gordon S. Publicizing nursing research. *Am J Nurs* 1996; 96:62, 64.
19. Chesanow N. How one group builds market leadership. *Med Econ* 1998; 75:84–86, 92–94, 98–100.

APPENDIX 13-A

A Simple PR Plan for a State NP Organization

This plan will work for a state organization or for an individual NP. It is a simple plan, using newspapers only. Much more elaborate plans could be made with the aid of a good PR expert. More elaborate plans might look into television news coverage, television features, prime-time shows featuring NPs, public TV pieces on NPs, national magazine pieces, radio talk show appearances, speaking engagements, and/or advertising.

For each topic below, four things need to happen:

1. Develop the substance of the news release. Two or more NPs could do this in less than 30 minutes.
2. Write the news release in the form that news editors are used to seeing. Have a PR professional do this.
3. Place the release. Decide which newspapers and whom at the newspapers to send it to, and send it. A PR professional should do this.
4. Arrange for follow-up. Have a contact name on the release. The contact should place a follow-up telephone call if there is no response in two weeks. The contact should deal with any responses that come in by helping to arrange interviews and photos and answering questions.

JANUARY

It is the new year. Place an article on NP advice on annual health maintenance. Suggestions include time to schedule mammogram, Pap smear, yearly cholesterol check.

FEBRUARY

It is flu season. Place an article on NP advice on the "Five Best Ways To Avoid Passing the Flu."

MARCH

It is spring break time. Place an article on NP advice to avoid ruining spring break, such as: wear seat belts, consume alcohol only in moderation, don't ski alone.

APRIL

It is pollen season. Place an article on NPs' advice to allergy sufferers.

MAY

It is prom season. Place an article on NP advice on avoiding the consequences of unprotected sex. Recycle the information from March because it applies to prom season and can never be said too many times.

JUNE

It is sunbathing season. Place an article on NP advice for maintaining healthy skin.

JULY

It is poison ivy season. Place an article on NP advice for treating and avoiding poison ivy.

AUGUST

It is hot. Place an article on NP advice for avoiding dehydration and overheating, especially for individuals with other medical problems.

SEPTEMBER

It is back-to-school time. Place an article on NP advice on up-to-date immunizations.

OCTOBER

It is Halloween. Place an article on NP advice to mothers about how to oversee safe trick or treating.

NOVEMBER

It is holiday season. Place an article on NP advice on the benefits of moderate diet and exercise.

DECEMBER

It is Christmas. Place an article on NP advice on how to recognize depression and discuss current treatments.

APPENDIX 13-B

Some Talking Points for NPs

1. Every study of NP cost-effectiveness has shown that NPs are cost-effective primary care providers.
2. Every study of NP quality of care has shown that NPs are effective and safe.
3. Every study of patient satisfaction done about NPs has shown that patients are very satisfied with NPs.
4. Research has been corroborated, no matter whether the researchers were nurses or physicians.
5. New York [or your state, if applicable] law does not preclude NPs' being on HMO provider panels. In the case of Medicaid and the Child Health Insurance Plan, NY law specifically names NPs as PCPs.
6. Federal law does not preclude NPs as PCPs. In fact, CMS policy for Medicaid patients mandates that managed-care organizations offer NP services.
7. MDs are fighting NP admission to provider panels because of the pressures of economic competition.
8. The American Medical Association surveyed physicians who employ NPs and found that the physicians think NPs operate with a high level of autonomy. In practice, physicians who hire NPs do not supervise NPs but provide consultation when the NP requests it. It is only when it is suggested that the flow of money go straight to the NP that physicians begin to protest.
9. Experts agree that NPs are the way to go. See Chapter 12 for some endorsements of NPs by experts.
10. Unless NPs are admitted to provider panels, there will be no realworld data on NP costs, effectiveness, attention to preventive measures, outcomes, or utilization. That research cannot be done unless NPs have a panel of patients and their practice patterns are tracked, as is done with physicians.
11. Patients deserve to have a choice of NP as provider. Let the customers decide what kind of health care provider they want.
12. Take the reins for controlling NPs out of the hands of physicians. Physicians have an economic conflict of interest.

13. Put the reins for controlling quality of the NP profession in the same hands that control quality over other health care providers:
    a) Licensing boards
    b) Consumer-oriented groups (such as the National Committee for Quality Assurance, Foundation for Accountability, and Joint Commission on Accreditation of Healthcare Organizations)
    c) The MCO credentialing process
    d) MCO audits
    e) Health Employer Data and Information Set (HEDIS) report cards
14. NPs provide a perfect fit of provider and patient need.
15. There is still a shortage of PCPs in the Northeast [or your region].
16. The position of NPs is: NPs do primary care. If physicians want to do it too, fine. But don't try to impede NPs from practicing their profession.
17. When the American Medical Association surveyed its physicians who work with NPs, the majority saw NPs as functioning at a medium or high level of autonomy. All physicians surveyed "endorsed the NPs' judgment, cited their high degree of acceptance by patients [and] praised their contributions" (American Medical Association Council on Medical Service Report 15-I-94).

COUNTERARGUMENTS TO MEDICAL SOCIETY TALKING POINTS

Here are some arguments that physician organizations will make in attempting to erect barriers:

Admitting Privileges

Argument: NPs don't have admitting privileges. How will they care for hospitalized patients?

Answer: Some NPs have admitting privileges. Some physicians don't have admitting privileges but still get on provider panels by arranging with other physicians to take care of admitted patients. Some family practice physicians assert that they do a better job by concentrating on office visits and turning over admitted patients to "hospitalists." NPs without admitting privileges arrange with a provider who does cover hospitalized patients.

Credentialing

Argument: We don't know how to credential NPs.

Answer: The following is the credentialing information most often asked of NPs:

- Geographic area of practice
- Types of patients cared for (i.e., adults, pediatric, OB-GYN)
- Procedures done
- Partners practicing with
- MD collaborator

- States where licensed as NP, license number
- DEA number
- Degrees, year of graduation, and schools attended
- Certification (year, type, and granting agency)
- Specialty training, year, agency giving training
- Three references
- Work history
- Are there any suits against you that have resulted in damages? Are you listed with the National Practitioner Data Bank? Are you currently being sued for malpractice?
- Malpractice insurance policy number, carrier, limits, claims made, or occurrence

Malpractice Insurance

Argument: If we allow NPs to be PCPs, then their employer physician will be more likely to be sued.

Answer: Ask your insurer about that. Our experience is that insurers have the policy that an NP is responsible for the NP's actions and a physician is responsible for the physician's actions. If an NP is the PCP, it makes common sense that the NP, not the employer physician, is likely to be found liable. The physician employing an NP PCP is actually safer than if the NP is caring for the physician's patients, the NP makes a mistake, and the physician is the official PCP.

APPENDIX 13-C

Sample Fact Sheets on NPs

FACT SHEET ON NURSE PRACTITIONERS

About Nurse Practitioners

Nurse Practitioners are registered nurses with advanced preparation who provide primary health care services. Nurse Practitioners provide medical and educational services such as:

- **Complete physical examinations**
- **Health assessments and screenings**
  Examples include monitoring blood pressure, monitoring blood sugar levels for diabetic patients, giving routine gynecologic exams, and screening for high cholesterol levels.
- **Treatment of common acute illnesses**
  Examples include bronchitis, skin infections, urinary tract infections, and gynecologic infections.
- **Treatment of chronic stable medical conditions**
  Examples include diabetes, high blood pressure, asthma, ulcers, and high cholesterol levels.
- **Health counseling services**
  Examples include smoking cessation, weight reduction, diet and exercise, medications and their side effects, effects of heavy drinking, and effects of high blood pressure on long-term health.

Education Requirements

Nurse Practitioners must complete a two-year master's degree program in addition to obtaining a college degree. All Nurse Practitioners have advanced training beyond their license as a registered nurse, but some may not have received the master's degree because this is a relatively new requirement.

Source: Courtesy of Better Life Health Care Systems, Inc., Annapolis, MD.

FACT SHEET ON NURSE PRACTITIONERS

MARYLAND LAWS REGULATING ACTIVITIES FOR NURSE PRACTITIONERS

Licensure

Nurse Practitioners have licenses as registered nurses for which they must pass a national board examination. They must then pass an additional national board examination to become certified as a Nurse Practitioner.

Diagnosis and Treatment

Nurse Practitioners may diagnose and treat patients under the Nurse Practitioner's own license. Maryland requires that Nurse Practitioners have a written agreement with a physician, who agrees to consult with the Nurse Practitioner as needed. The written agreement stipulates the types of evaluations and treatments that will be performed by the Nurse Practitioner. These agreements are approved by, and filed with, the state board of nursing.

A physician is not required to be on site during treatment of patients. The Nurse Practitioner determines when consultation with a physician or other health professional is necessary. The Nurse Practitioner may choose to consult with the physician listed in the written agreement, or with other health providers. Consultation may be in person, by telephone, or by fax.

Scope of Practice

The Practice Act is written so that Nurse Practitioners may practice within the scope of an approved written agreement. There are no proscribed evaluations or treatments.

All primary care evaluations, procedures, and treatments are within the scope of practice for Nurse Practitioners. In addition, Nurse Practitioners may assist with surgery, do sigmoidoscopies, oversee exercise stress testing, excise skin lesions, and suture. Nurse Practitioners may write for both controlled and noncontrolled medications without the cosignature of a physician.

As of October 1, 1995, HMOs may not reject a provider who applies for admission to an HMO panel on the basis of class of license so long as the provider is certified under Maryland law to provide the type of care for which the provider is applying.

FACT SHEET ON NURSE PRACTITIONERS

The Opportunity: A Practical Alternative for Primary Care Services

In today's health care market squeezed by tightening profitability margins, Nurse Practitioners provide a primary care service already recognized by physicians who regularly employ them to provide such care for their patients. Typically, physicians will bill for Nurse Practitioner services at their regular, higher rate and then pocket the marginal cost difference. This cost is then passed on to the paying patient or third-party insurer.

The favorable regulatory environment in Maryland provides Nurse Practitioners with the opportunity for opening up their own private practices that directly compete with services provided by neighboring primary care physician practices. Although this competitive development has not been favorably received by some physicians, several entrepreneurial ventures have been launched and have been in successful operation for many years. This pattern and the results of such practices are well documented by other states.

The Results: Quality Care for Patients at Less Cost

- **Excellent quality of care.** Many published studies prepared by physicians report that the care given by Nurse Practitioners is as good as or better than the care given by physicians in similar settings.
- **High patient satisfaction.** Patient satisfaction level with Nurse Practitioner treatment is extremely high, often because Nurse Practitioners are perceived as accessible and because they focus on education and the lifestyle needs of the patient.
- **Greater cost efficiency.** Cost of primary care by Nurse Practitioners in private practice is roughly 20 percent less than cost of care provided by primary care physicians. Many patients opt for care by a Nurse Practitioner when they perceive better value for their health care dollar.

FACT SHEET ON NURSE PRACTITIONERS

Malpractice Actuarials

Lawsuits against Nurse Practitioners are rare. The rate of lawsuits per 1,000 Nurse Practitioners is 0.6, compared with a rate for physicians of 38.

Nurse Practitioners may be sued for malpractice, and the physician affiliated through the written agreement may be named as codefendant. However, the physician is not automatically considered to be liable for a colleague Nurse Practitioner's negligence. In fact, the Maryland insurer of physicians does not charge physicians an extra premium for having a written agreement with a Nurse Practitioner. The physician is liable for the physician's acts, and the Nurse Practitioner is liable for the Nurse Practitioner's acts.

Reimbursement

Medical Assistance (Medicaid) reimburses Nurse Practitioners directly. So do Blue Cross and other Maryland insurers. Although out-of-state third-party payers are not required by law to reimburse Nurse Practitioners, many do so.

Medicare reimburses Nurse Practitioners directly only in rural areas. In urban or suburban areas, Nurse Practitioners may treat patients, but "incident to physician services" rules apply, and the payments must go to a physician practice or clinic, rather than directly to the Nurse Practitioner.

Employer Familiarity with Nurse Practitioner Services

A recent informal survey of employers revealed that:

- Company presidents are familiar with Nurse Practitioners because they are seeing Nurse Practitioners when they themselves "visit the doctor."
- Company presidents have reported satisfaction with the care that they received from Nurse Practitioners.
- Employers are hungry for quality health care plans that offer savings on premiums.

CHAPTER 14

Standards of Care for Nurse Practitioner Practice

The standard of care for NPs is changing under the influence of managed care. Even the definition is changing.

DEFINITIONS OF STANDARD OF CARE

The traditional definition of standard of care was, "such reasonable, ordinary care, skill, and diligence as used by practitioners in good standing in the same general type of practice, in similar cases." Today, NPs and other clinicians are judged not so much by what other clinicians would do, but by what is best for the patient. Today, the standard of care addresses the questions:

- Did the clinician do the right thing at the right time?
- Was effective care provided to the patient?
- Was care provided safely and in an appropriate time frame?
- Was the outcome as good as expected, given the patient's condition and personal characteristics and the current state of medical science?

WHO IS MONITORING STANDARD OF CARE?

In the past, compliance with standard of care was voluntary, performance was not measured, performance was not reported to the public, and often, the standard of care for a particular set of circumstances became clear only after a mistake was made, a lawsuit was filed, expert witnesses were hired, dual versions of the "standard of care" were argued by both sides of a malpractice case, and a jury accepted one or the other side's version. Today, while the standard of care for NPs still may be scrutinized in a court of law, there is a recognition that a minimum acceptable level of care may be determined outside the judicial system by consensus, with participation by consumers, providers, and agencies. The standards that are being developed will be continually reassessed and reset on the basis of results of outcomes research, analysis of costs and benefits, and results of patient satisfaction measures.

The 1990s brought increased attention to quality standards for health care from people outside the medical profession, namely consumers and government agencies. Corporate and government purchasers of health services have joined medical and nursing professional organizations, licensing boards, and the judicial system in setting standards for health care providers. Standards of care are being monitored, publicized, and changed by several national consumer-oriented groups, with only minimal input from clinician groups. Traditionally, standards of medical and nursing care were developed by clinicians and monitored by:

- Professional societies.
- Licensing boards.
- The Joint Commission on Hospitals.
- The judicial system.
- Employers.

Standards of care are now being set, modified, monitored, and publicized by certain self-appointed consumer-oriented agencies as well as a government agency. Those groups include:

- National Committee for Quality Assurance (NCQA)
- Joint Commission on Accreditation of Healthcare Organizations (Joint Commission)
- Foundation for Accountability (FAcct)
- Agency for Health Care Research and Policy (AHRP)

Professional Societies

The American Academy of Nurse Practitioners (AANP) has written the following standards for the process of care:*

Assessment of Health Status
The nurse practitioner assesses health status by:
- Obtaining a relevant health and medical history.
- Performing a physical examination based on age and history.
- Performing or ordering preventive and diagnostic procedures based on the patient's age and history.
- Identifying health and medical risk factors.

Diagnosis
The nurse practitioner makes a diagnosis by:
- Utilizing critical thinking in the diagnostic process.
- Synthesizing and analyzing the collected data.
- Formulating a differential diagnosis based on history, physical examination, and diagnostic test results.

*Courtesy of American Academy of Nurse Practitioners.

- Establishing priorities to meet the health and medical needs of the individual, family, or community.

Development of a Treatment Plan

The nurse practitioner, together with the patient and family, establishes a mutually acceptable cost-awareness plan of care that maximizes health potential. Formulation of the treatment plan includes:

- Ordering additional diagnostic tests
- Prescribing/ordering appropriate pharmacologic and non-pharmacologic interventions
- Developing a patient education plan
- Appropriate consultation/referral

Implementation of the Plan

Interventions are based upon established priorities. Actions by the nurse practitioner are:

- Individualized.
- Consistent with the appropriate plan of care.
- Based on scientific principles, theoretical knowledge, and clinical expertise.
- Consistent with teaching and learning opportunities.

Actions include:

- Accurately conducting and interpreting diagnostic tests.
- Prescribing pharmacologic agents and nonpharmacologic therapies.
- Providing relevant patient education.
- Making appropriate referrals to other health professionals and community agencies.

Follow-up and Evaluation of the Clients' Status

The nurse practitioner maintains a process for systematic follow-up by:

- Determining the effectiveness of the treatment plan with documentation of patient care outcomes.
- Reassessing and modifying the plan as necessary to achieve medical and health goals.

Care Priorities

The nurse practitioner's practice model emphasizes:

A. Patient and Family Education

The nurse practitioner provides health education and utilizes community resource opportunities for the individual and/or family.

B. Facilitation of Patient Participation in Self-Care

The nurse practitioner facilitates patient participation in medical and health care by providing information needed to make decisions and choices about the:

- Promotion, maintenance, and restoration of health
- Consultation with other appropriate health care personnel
- Appropriate utilization of health care resources

C. Promotion of optimal health
D. Provider of continually competent care
E. Facilitation of entry into the health care system
F. The promotion of a safe environment

Interdisciplinary/Collaborative Responsibilities
The nurse practitioner participates as a team member in the provision of health and medical care, interacting with professional colleagues to provide comprehensive care.

Accurate Documentation of Patient Status and Care
The nurse practitioner maintains accurate, legible, and confidential records.

Responsibility as Patient Advocate
Ethical and legal standards provide the basis of patient advocacy. As an advocate, the nurse practitioner participates in health policy activities at the local, state, national, and international levels.

Quality Assurance and Continued Competence
Nurse practitioners recognize the importance of continued learning through:

- Participation in quality assurance review, including systematic review of records and treatment plans on a periodic basis.
- Maintenance of current knowledge by attending educational programs.
- Maintenance of certification in compliance with current state law.
- Applying standardized care guidelines in clinical practice.

Adjunct Roles of Nurse Practitioner
Nurse practitioners combine the roles of provider, mentor, educator, researcher, manager, and consultant. The nurse practitioner interprets the role of the nurse practitioner to individuals, families, and other professionals.

Research as Basis for Practice
Nurse practitioners support research by developing clinical research questions, conducting or participating in studies, and disseminating and incorporating findings into practice.

Some states have adopted the AANP's standards or those of other nursing professional organizations as their standards for NP practice.

Regarding accountability, the AANP says:

> The autonomous nature of the nurse practitioner's advanced clinical practice requires accountability for health care outcomes. Ensuring the

> highest quality of care requires certification, periodic peer review, clinical outcome evaluations, a code for ethical practice, evidence of continuing professional development and maintenance of clinical skills. Nurse practitioners are committed to seeking and sharing knowledge that promotes quality health care and improves clinical outcomes. This is accomplished by leading and participating in both professional and lay health care forums, conducting research, and applying research findings to clinical practice.[1]

Adherence to the AANP standards is voluntary.

State Legislatures and State Agencies

Some states address NP standards of care in their law.

In Montana, the board of nursing must approve the method of an advanced practice nurse's (APN) quality assurance prior to issuance of prescriptive authority. Montana law mandates that the quality assurance method include the following:

- Thirty charts, or 5% of all charts handled by the APN, must be reviewed quarterly (by peer and by physician).
- Reviewers must use standards which apply to APN area of practice.
- Reviewers must use preestablished criteria.
- Reviewers must write an evaluation of the review with steps for corrective action if indicated and follow-up.

Citation: MONT. ADMIN. R. 8.32.1508.

Indiana law sets the following standards for each NP:

1. Assess clients by using advanced knowledge and skills to:
   a. Identify abnormal conditions
   b. Diagnose health problems
   c. Develop and implement nursing treatment plans
   d. Evaluate patient outcomes
   e. Collaborate with or refer to a practitioner as defined in IC 25-23-1-19.4 in managing the plan of care
2. Use advanced knowledge and skill in teaching and guiding clients and other health team members.
3. Use appropriate critical thinking skills to make independent decisions, commensurate with the autonomy and responsibilities of an NP.
4. Function within the legal boundaries of their advanced practice area and have and utilize knowledge or the statutes and rules governing their advanced practice area, including the following:
   a. State and federal drug laws and regulations
   b. State and federal confidentiality laws and regulations
   c. State and federal medical record access laws

5. Consult with and collaborate with other team members.
6. Recognize the limits of individual knowledge and refer as appropriate.
7. Retain professional accountability for any delegated intervention, and delegate only as authorized by IC 25-23-1 of this title.
8. Maintain current knowledge and skills in the NP area.
9. Conduct assessment of clients and families which may include health history, family history, physical examination, and evaluation of risk factors.
10. Assess normal and abnormal findings obtained from the history, physical examination, and laboratory results.
11. Evaluate clients and families regarding development, coping ability, and emotions and social well-being.
12. Plan, implement, and evaluate care.
13. Develop individualized teaching plans with each client based on health needs.
14. Counsel individuals, families, and groups about health and illness and promote attention to wellness.
15. Participate in periodic joint evaluation of services rendered, including but not limited to chart review, client evaluations, [and] outcomes statistics.
16. Conduct and apply research findings appropriate to each area of practice.
17. Participate when appropriate, in the joint review of the plan of care.

Citation: IND. ADMIN. CODE tit. 848, r. 4-2-1.

Licensing Boards

Licensing boards carry out the statutes of the state and write and administer rules and regulations for nursing practice, based on statute.

Licensing boards enforce standards by:

- Ensuring that qualifications are up to date by authorizing licensing.
- Responding to complaints from consumers, employers, colleagues, or patients.
- Following up on malpractice awards monitored through the National Practitioner Data Bank to determine whether a nurse was grossly negligent in providing care.

Boards of nursing do not test NPs or do audits of NP practice. An NP who is sued for malpractice will not necessarily be investigated by the state board of nursing. If, however, a judge, attorney, or plaintiff reports a nurse for suspected gross negligence, the board of nursing will investigate.

Accreditation Commissions

The Joint Commission on Accreditation of Health Care Organizations, formerly called the Joint Commission on Accreditation of Hospitals, has accredited and monitored hospital practice and now evaluates health plans, clinics, and medical groups through an accreditation program. The accreditation program is voluntary; however, hospital accreditation became synonymous with staying in business. Health plan accreditation is becoming a business necessity. Clinics and medical practices are not routinely accredited, but it is reasonable to expect that accreditation may become a standard in the future.

Through accreditation, committees set standards and conduct site visits to ensure that the standards are met. Providers of health care want to publicize the fact that they are accredited, so they make sure they meet the current standards.

The Judicial System

The judicial system becomes involved in NP practice only when a patient is injured and files suit. Whether a health care provider is negligent is decided by a judge or a jury on the basis of the law and facts of the case. In a court case, each side may present, through expert witnesses, the "standard of care." The plaintiff will argue that the standard of care has been violated. The defendant is likely to argue that there has been no violation of standard of care.

When a judge or a jury accepts one side's version of the standard of care, that version is affirmed for future cases, and for health care providers, because previous case decisions (precedent) affect future decisions.

Although one organization may publish one standard of care and an expert may testify to an alternate version of the standard of care, the judicial system is a final arbiter of standards.

Employers

Some employers develop performance standards for NPs. The following is an example of an employer-generated performance standard for NPs, addressing patient education:

> *Criterion for evaluation:* Provides health education to patients about ways to improve, promote, and maintain their health status, including but not limited to providing educational information on disease/disease processes, self-care practices, and positive lifestyle choices.
>
> *Performance standards:*
> 1. Assesses learning capabilities and readiness of population or individuals, and tailors education to meet age, developmental, and educational needs.
> 2. Prioritizes learning needs and documents them accordingly.

3. Ensures that time frame and subject matter are appropriate for target audience/individual.
4. Utilizes appropriate teaching materials.
5. Initiates, designs, and completes educational programs for patients, families, and targeted audiences.

(Exceeds) Demonstrates a high degree of effectiveness in fulfilling standard as observed by supervising physician.[2]

The National Committee for Quality Assurance

NCQA is a consumer-oriented group directed by representatives from major employers, insurers, and government. NCQA accredits MCOs and health plans. It has developed a set of clinical performance measures and patient satisfaction surveys that the group believes represents the consumer's interests. Those performance measures are being applied to health plans around the country, and the results of the measures are being reported in the news media. Health plans voluntarily collect the performance data, hoping to rate high, receive accreditation, receive media attention, and attract more enrollees.

Health plans and MCOs turn to medical groups and physician practices for much of the performance data. The most prominent of the performance measures is the Health Plan Employer Data and Information Set (HEDIS®). NCQA is now the premier organization that monitors the quality of managed care, and the core set of performance criteria it endorses—HEDIS—is being widely publicized and accepted. The NCQA changes HEDIS measures from time to time, so one most order their materials or check their Web site to ascertain the current measures. Some examples of HEDIS are*:

1. Immunizations of children
   Measure: By the second year of life, children should have received four shots of diphtheria-tetanus-pertussis, three polio vaccines, one dose of measles-mumps-rubella vaccine, a minimum of three *Hemophilus* influenza type B vaccines, and three hepatitis B vaccines.
2. Immunizations of adolescents
   Measure: By age 13, children should have received the second dose of measles-mumps-rubella, hepatitis B vaccine, tetanus-diphtheria booster, and chicken pox immunization.
3. Smoking cessation
   Measure: Adult patients who smoke or have recently quit report in Member Satisfaction Survey that they received advice to quit smoking from a health professional in the plan.

---

*Source: http://www.ncqa.org. Accessed July 2003.

4. Flu shots for older adults
   Measure: Patients over 65 received influenza vaccine prior to the past year's flu season.
5. Breast cancer screening
   Measure: Female patients aged 52 to 69 had at least one mammogram in the past two years.
6. Cervical cancer screening
   Measure: Women aged 21 to 64 had at least one Pap smear during the past three years.
7. Prenatal care in the first trimester
   Measure: Pregnant women began prenatal care during the first 13 weeks of pregnancy.
8. Checkups after delivery
   Measure: Women who had live births had a postpartum visit within six weeks after delivery.
9. Beta blocker treatment after a heart attack
   Measure: Patients discharged from a hospital after a heart attack (without allergies to or contraindications to beta blockers) were dispensed a prescription for beta blockers.
10. Eye exams for people with diabetes
    Measure: Diabetic patients received an eye exam in the past year.
11. Health of seniors
    Measure: Seniors rate, on a survey, whether their ability to function has improved or worsened over time.
12. Follow-up after hospitalization for selected mental illnesses
    Measure: Patients aged six and over who were hospitalized for selected mental disorders (including manic depression, paranoia, schizophrenia) were seen on an outpatient basis by a mental health provider within 30 days after discharge.[3]

For more on HEDIS measures, visit www.ncqa.org.

The Agency for Health Care Research and Policy

AHRP is a government agency that studies what works in health care. AHRP has convened panels of experts that developed standards on certain illnesses, including:

- Acute Pain Management (February 1992)
- Urinary Incontinence in Adults (March 1992)
- Prevention of Pressure Ulcers (May 1992)
- Cataract in Adults (February 1993)
- Depression in Primary Care (April 1993)
- Sickle Cell Disease in Infants (April 1993)
- Early HIV Infection (January 1994)

- Benign Prostatic Hyperplasia (February 1994)
- Management of Cancer Pain (March 1994)
- Unstable Angina (March 1994)
- Heart Failure (June 1994)
- Otitis Media with Effusion in Children (July 1994)
- Quality Determinants of Mammography (October 1994)
- Acute Low Back Problems in Adults (December 1994)
- Treatment of Pressure Ulcers (December 1994)
- Post-Stroke Rehabilitation (May 1995)
- Cardiac Rehabilitation (October 1995)
- Smoking Cessation (October 1996)
- Recognition and Initial Assessment of Alzheimer's and Related Diseases (October 1996)

Some of these standards have been changed or retired, as new evidence has become known. For access to current guidelines, visit www.ahcpr.gov.

AHRP, while encouraging clinicians to use the guidelines, states that the recommendations may not be appropriate for use in all circumstances and that decisions to adopt any particular recommendation must be made in light of available resources and circumstances presented by individual patients.

HOW SHOULD NPs KEEP CURRENT ON STANDARD OF CARE?

NPs should use the traditional methods of keeping current, including:

- Books
- Continuing education seminars
- Journals
- Other practitioners

In addition, and in light of the emerging standards, NPs should consult:

- Audit tools used by managed-care organizations
- Accreditation guidelines supplied by accrediting organizations
- NCQA standards
- AHRP standards or guidelines
- State law, if standards are mandated by law
- Established, credible Web sites, such as Medscape.com

CREDENTIALING

Another standard being developed under managed care is credentialing. Although there are no published standards on what combinations of credentials are acceptable, some MCOs will accept only board-certified physicians and will ask NPs whether their board certification is equivalent to physician board certification. Some MCOs will not accept a clinician who has a malpractice history.

Given the quantity and detail of questions being asked on applications for admission to provider panels, it is reasonable to expect that a set of standards based on credentials will emerge. For a listing of questions frequently asked of NPs and physicians seeking admission to managed-care provider panels, see Appendix 9-A.

Utilization

Under managed care, not all standards for clinicians are related to the quality of patient care. Some standards look at quantity of care delivered. For example, NPs can expect that health plans will be looking at NP utilization of emergency room visits, hospitalization, specialist visits, and diagnostic testing.

Patient Satisfaction

There are emerging standards regarding patient satisfaction. For example, some health plans want practices to answer a telephone call within five rings, want patients to be able to get appointments within 72 hours, and do not want patients to have to wait more than 20 minutes after arrival for an appointment. These standards have evolved from research showing that patients are annoyed with unanswered telephones, long waits for appointments, and long waits in waiting rooms. Because health plans compete for patients, and because medical practices compete for admission to provider panels, it is reasonable to expect that certain customer service standards that now are informal will be more forthrightly stated in the future.

NOTES

1. American Academy of Nurse Practitioners. Standards of Care 2002. Available at http://www.aanp.com. Accessed August 2003.

2. Smith MA. Job description for primary care nurse practitioners. *Nurse Pract* 1996; 21:160, 162–163.

3. National Committee for Quality Assurance. *HEDIS 3.0: Narrative*, vol. 11. Annapolis Junction, MD. 1997; 35–51. Available at http://www.ncqa.org. Accessed August 2003.

CHAPTER 15

Measuring Nurse Practitioner Performance

Standards of care and measures of performance are interrelated. Measures of performance are used to determine the extent to which standards of care are met. Measuring performance without standards is like playing a game without rules. Setting standards without measuring performance is like making laws when there are no police to enforce the laws.

MEASURING QUALITY

In general, quality of clinical care is assessed by asking the following questions:

- Did the clinician do the right thing?
- Was the care effective?
- Was care given in an appropriate time frame?
- Was the outcome as good as could be expected, given each patient's condition and personal characteristics and the current state of medical science?

A standard of care for a particular episode of illness would answer the questions:

- What was the correct treatment?
- What was the correct timing of treatment?
- What was the correct teaching?

Measures would include:

- Did the clinician follow the standard?
- Did the patient's problem resolve?
- Did the problem resolve within the expected time frame?
- Were the resources used to solve the problem in line with what would be expected for that problem?

MULTIPLE MEASURES, MULTIPLE MEASURERS

NP performance is evaluated on several levels: productivity, utilization, and patient satisfaction, as well as clinical decision making. An NP's performance is going to be judged by employers, patients, health plan auditors, peers, and possibly researchers.

If an NP's performance is employer defined, then the NP will need to ascertain the values of the employer. To one employer, good performance might be high billings, which could, by nature of time constraints, preclude much time and attention given each patient. For another employer, good performance might be high scores on surveys of patient satisfaction. An NP who satisfies patients might not be a high biller. To yet another employer, good performance might be close communication with the physician consultant. To another, it might be independent functioning without need for communication with a physician.

If performance is defined by the health plan, then a good performer is one who uses expensive resources—hospitals and emergency rooms—relatively infrequently.

If an NP's performance is defined by present performance measures developed by consumer-oriented groups, such as NCQA, an NP who sees that all children are properly immunized, who gets patients to quit smoking, and who raises the functional status of elderly patients will be a good performer.

If an NP's performance is defined by peers, a good performer will be one who is an expert diagnostician and who shares knowledge willingly with other NPs.

If performance is defined by researchers, a good performer is one who meets the particular testing criteria studied by the researcher.

If performance is defined by patients, a good performer is one who did not make the patient wait more than 20 minutes in the waiting room before being seen, who is patient and polite, and who hires friendly receptionists.

There is no single, widely accepted set of measures of an NP's worth or performance. In this chapter, several measures of performance are summarized.

PRODUCTIVITY

A definition of productivity may depend upon the setting and the method of payment to the practice.

In a practice that gets reimbursed according to fee-for-service, a productive NP will be one who sees many patients, at a 99213 level or above, and who bills often for additional services that bring revenue, such as suturing, incision and drainage, and endometrial biopsy.

In a practice that receives mostly capitated payments, then an NP who efficiently handles a large panel of patients with little use of the practice's resources—staff, materials, time—will be a good performer.

If an NP is employed by a nursing home, productivity may mean keeping elderly patients out of the hospital, while imparting to their families the feeling that their loved one is being closely monitored and well cared for.

In a fee-for-service practice, a simple way of measuring performance would be to set the number of visits conforming to the evaluation and management Current Procedural Terminology (CPT) codes. For example, good performance could be set at 20 visits at levels 99211 to 99215 per day. One would not want to set a specific code as a performance measure because it is the patient's need for evaluation and management services that determines the CPT code billed, and a provider cannot predict what level of visit will be needed.

In a capitated practice, good performance could be set at maintenance of an 1,800-member panel of patients, with patient satisfaction, as measured by a particular tool, at 80 percent or above.

In a nursing home practice, good performance could be measured by decreasing, over a previous year, the number of hospital visits among the nursing home's residents.

HOUSEKEEPING PERFORMANCE MEASURES

NPs may have more experience with "housekeeping" forms of performance measurement than with substantive forms like HEDIS measures. For example, many NPs' charts are audited for such things as clear labeling of allergies, laboratory results initialed and dated, name of patient on every page, and problem list filled in. What may be an emphasis on the less important aspects of performance may be simply a sign that managed care is in its initial phases.

In the initial stages of managed care, when a minority of patients are enrolled in managed care, health plans pay attention to high-cost areas of primary care: admissions, length of stay, and emergency room visits. Health plans may or may not give feedback to practices on whether a practice's numbers were consistent with the aggregate or high or low.

Also in the initial stages, health plans are interested in auditing housekeeping matters, possibly because audits can be conducted by less highly trained staff than are required for auditing HEDIS measures. In the future, however, NPs should expect that audits will follow the HEDIS measures developed by NCQA.[1]

NCQA MEASURES OF CLINICAL PERFORMANCE

Nonclinicians have begun to get involved in measurement of clinical performance. After putting out a call for performance measures, NCQA received 800 suggestions and developed HEDIS and a set of clinical performance measures aimed largely at primary care providers. Presumably HEDIS is some indication of what employer purchasers, consumers, and health plan executives think is important for health care providers to accomplish.

The HEDIS measures are still being refined. In some cases, NCQA gives a measure but no guidance on what is good performance.

Among the evaluation measures set by HEDIS for primary care providers are:

- Ninety percent of children received four shots of diphtheria-tetanus-pertussis, three polio vaccines, one dose of measles-mumps-rubella vaccine, a minimum of two *Hemophilus* influenza type B vaccines, three hepatitis B vaccines by their second birthday, and one dose of VZV (chicken pox).
- Ninety percent of 13-year-olds received the second dose of measles-mumps-rubella, had received three doses of hepatitis B vaccine, and had been immunized against chicken pox.
- At least 70 percent of female patients aged 52 to 69 had at least one mammogram in the past two years.
- Ninety percent of women aged 21 to 64 had at least one Pap smear during the past three years.
- Ninety percent of pregnant women began prenatal care during the first trimester of pregnancy.

Some of these data are collected from Center for Medicare and Medicaid Services (CMS) 1500 (billing) forms. Other data are collected by auditors who review charts.

HEDIS also looks at:

- Whether women who have live births have a postpartum visit on or between 21 and 56 days after delivery.
- Whether patients who are hospitalized for depression, schizophrenia, attention deficit disorder, and personality disorders are seen on an outpatient basis by a mental health provider within 30 days after discharge.
- Whether patients who are discharged from the hospital after a heart attack are dispensed a prescription for beta blockers upon discharge.
- Whether diabetic patients received an eye exam in the past year.

HEDIS measures change from time to time. For the current measures, visit www.ncqa.org.

OTHER MEASURES

HEDIS is not the only set of performance measures, and NCQA is not the only organization looking after consumer interests and rating health plans and providers. Among the other organizations publishing performance measures are the Foundation for Accountability (FAcct), the Joint Commission on Accreditation of Healthcare Organizations (Joint Commission), certain managed care plans, certain state health departments, and AHRP. The performance measures advocated by these organizations overlap to some extent.

FORMAL RESEARCH

Researchers who have studied NP performance and compared it with physicians' performance have looked at the following measures:

- Whether NPs took thorough history and gave appropriate treatment to a patient with a particular set of symptoms and history.[2]
- Whether NPs performed or followed up on a set of primary care tasks, such as follow-up of a low hematocrit and obtaining appropriate cancer-screening tests.[3]
- Whether patients reported, on a survey, that their experience of care was satisfactory.[4]
- Whether NPs' care was cost-effective when all of the costs of care were tallied.[5]
- Whether level of care in nursing homes was improved by NP participation.[6]
- Whether NPs controlled the blood pressure of patients diagnosed with hypertension to below 140/90.[7]

The performance of NPs was found to be at least as good as physicians' on these measures.

PATIENT RATINGS

Many difficulties and intervening factors become apparent when one attempts to get patients to rate NP performance. For example, patients come with their own set of beliefs about health and illness, which may affect their interpretation of the quality of care given them. Patients may focus on nonclinical aspects of care that affect their experience of care. Patients may feel compelled to give a provider a good rating, fearing a turn in the relationship if the patient is critical. And surveys may reach a patient at a date much later than the care was given, when a patient has forgotten the bad or the good aspects of the care.

Nevertheless, patient-rated measures of performance are to be striven for. Whether or not a NP believes a patient's rating to be valid, much information can be gleaned from patient survey results. If a patient's experience of care was influenced negatively by a grouchy receptionist, then attitude adjustment on the part of the receptionist is a relatively easy alteration for a practice to make.

NCQA will be seeking data from health plans on patient satisfaction. Health plans can be expected to conduct surveys, and NPs would be wise to get copies of various patient satisfaction surveys and survey results and to conduct visits and make corrections in problem areas accordingly.

PEER REVIEW

Some accrediting organizations require that medical offices conduct regular peer review. There are many peer review tools in the NP literature.

UTILIZATION

Because hospitals, emergency rooms, and specialists are high cost centers for health plans, health plans want providers to keep admissions and referrals to the emergency room and specialists at a minimum. Whether an NP works for a physician or is in independent practice, the NP can expect that in the world of managed care, someone will be looking at the numbers of admissions and referrals.

An NP who wants to shine on performance evaluations will determine who in a work setting is interested in what measures and will adapt his or her practice accordingly. If there are no adopted performance measures, the NP may want to adopt the self-evaluation routine given in Appendix 15-A.

HOW TO GET AN "A" ON PERFORMANCE REPORT CARDS

The number of hoops through which NPs must jump continue to rise. Many more tasks are coming under scrutiny than ever before.

NPs with 15 minutes in which to take care of a patient's episodic problem know the frustration of leafing through a patient record to check on details. Whether a patient has been a smoker, whether a patient has been advised to quit, or whether a patient is up to date on health care maintenance—mammograms, immunizations, and Pap smears—often takes longer than 15 minutes to ascertain, even when the patient is sitting in the adjacent chair.

Documentation of health maintenance checks was a problem long before the terms *HEDIS, NCQA,* and even *primary care provider* came into common usage. Every primary care provider is familiar with the feeling of uneasiness that comes from scanning a chart for an established patient that contains no record—all in one place—of routine screening efforts and results. Occasionally, some thoughtful physician assistant, NP, or physician will have summarized a patient's chart in a progress note. The trick then becomes finding that progress note.

Some practices keep flowcharts to document health care maintenance. Practices that do this are far ahead of those that do not keep such information in a central place. But even practices that keep the flowcharts need to know what NCQA has decided to "grade" in the next few years.

ENSURING COMPLIANCE

Several simple tools, kept in the front of a chart or in a special section called "Performance Measures" or some similar title, prompt busy providers to ask the pertinent questions, arrange the pertinent screens, tests, medications, classes, or counseling, and note the date when the work was done. One format for a tool is given in Appendix 15-B.

Health care maintenance flowcharts, which have been around for years but are updated here to include the HEDIS measures, save time for providers and make it very difficult for an auditor or chart reviewer to miss.

NPs who are employees can be motivated to keep these checklists and flowcharts up to date by: (1) tying compliance to bonuses; (2) conducting internal quality assurance audits and giving feedback to providers on their performance; and (3) including this activity in job descriptions and evaluation tools.

Self-employed NPs will find their own rewards in keeping up with outside measures of performance. Finding a health care provider is no longer a matter of word of mouth. Patients usually go to providers who will be reimbursed by the patient's health plan. Retention on provider panels is likely to be contingent on satisfaction of performance measures. Those providers who meet the standards now being set by consumer-driven groups will end up with thriving practices, which, after all, is the most traditional measure of performance.

The organizations doing the measuring, grading, and reporting have the mission of helping consumers. How logistically difficult it is for health plans and providers to comply with these measures is not the concern of these organizations.

The hoops are not limited to clinical performance measures. HEDIS includes measures of access and availability of care, patients' satisfaction with their care experience, health plan stability, utilization of selected services, cost of care, and such services as new member orientation and translation services.

HEDIS details are not particularly accessible to consumers, health plans, or providers. Anyone can purchase HEDIS reports and explanations from NCQA, but they are expensive.

Strategies for complying with the performance criteria set by NCQA include increasing clinicians' and administrators' knowledge of specific performance measures, delegating responsibility for continuous quality improvement, implementing systems for tracking compliance, attending to patient satisfaction, addressing the functional level of elderly patients, and rewarding clinicians and practice managers for compliance and high scores.

NOTES

1. National Committee for Quality Assurance. The Health Plan Employer Data and Information Set (HEDIS®). Available at: http://www.ncqa.org. Accessed August 2003.

2. Avorn J, Everitt DE, Baker MW. The neglected medical history and therapeutic choices for abdominal pain: a nationwide study of 799 physicians and nurses. *Arch Intern Med* 1991; 151:694–698.

3. Hall JA, Palmer RH, Orav EJ. Performance quality, gender and professional role. A study of physicians and nonphysicians in 16 ambulatory care practices. *Med Care* 1990; 28:489–501.

4. Perry K. Patient survey: physician extenders. Why patients love physician extenders. *Med Econ* 1995; 72:58, 63, 67.

5. Salkever DS, Skinner EA, Steinwachs DM, Katz H. Episode-based efficiency comparisons for physicians and nurse practitioners. *Med Care* 1982; 20:143–153.

6. Mahoney DF. The appropriateness of geriatric prescribing decisions made by nurse practitioners and physicians. *Image* 1994; 26:41–46.

7. Mindinger MO, Kane RL, Lenz ER, et al. Primary care outcomes in patients treated by nurse practitioners or physicians: a randomized trial. *JAMA* 2000; 283:59–68.

APPENDIX 15-A

NPs' Self-Evaluation

To ensure that an NP will fare well on clinical performance evaluations, an NP should set up a routine for self-evaluation. For example:

1. For each visit, have I asked the patient:
   - Are you smoking? If so, advise patient to quit.
   - Did you get an appointment promptly?
   - How long did you spend in the waiting room? Too long?
   - Has this visit satisfied your expectations?
2. On each visit, have I consulted the chart for:
   - Up-to-date immunizations, for patients under 18?
   - Up-to-date cancer screening: Pap, mammogram, colonoscopy?
   - Eye exam in the past year for diabetic patients?
   - Follow-up visit within six weeks of giving birth for postpartum patients?
3. If a patient has been hospitalized:
   - If for myocardial infarction, is the patient on beta blockers?
   - If for mental illness, was the patient seen by a mental health clinician within 30 days after discharge?

To do utilization self-monitoring, for each quarter, keep a notebook noting:

- Patient admissions to hospitals
- Referrals to emergency department
- Referrals to specialists
- Number of patients seen per day

APPENDIX 15-B

Health Maintenance Flowchart

Name: ______________________ Date of Birth: ______________________

Patient number: ______________________

Female Cancer Screening	Date	Result	Date	Result	Date	Result	Date	Result
Pap (21–64)								
Mammo (52–69)								

Adult Immunizations	Date	Date	Date	Date	Date	Date	Date	Date	Date	Date	Date
Tetanus (all patients, q 10 yrs)											
Flu (q yr. > 65 y.o.)											
Pneumococcal (only for individuals > 65 y.o.)											

Childhood Immunizations	Date	Date	Date	Date
Diphtheria-tetanus-pertussis				
Polio				
MMR				
HIB				
Hep B				
Chicken Pox				

CHAPTER 16

Resolving Ethical Dilemmas

There are a multitude of ethical questions that come up in daily practice, including:

- Whether or not to disclose to a patient that the nurse practitioner or someone else at the practice made a mistake regarding the patient's care.
- Whether the availability or lack of reimbursement should determine whether or not a service is provided.
- Whether participation in a research study is the best thing for a patient.
- Whether a promise to a patient or family member not to disclose information to a family member or patient best serves the patient or family.
- Whether and when curative treatments should be stopped.
- When and how to terminate a relationship with a patient.
- Whether or not to accept a gift or meal from a vendor or pharmaceutical representative.
- Whether to discuss the deficiencies of a patient's insurance coverage with the patient.
- Whether and how to tell a patient you are moving to another practice.
- Whether and how to inform a patient that you believe the surgeon he or she has chosen is not competent.

EXAMPLES

Consider these four situations:

Situation 1:

While standing in line at the grocery store, you hear "Help! This lady is having a seizure!" Behind you, a woman is on the floor, jerking around in a way you know is characteristic of a grand mal seizure. Several people are standing over her, calling out for help. You feel compelled to help, but worry that you will a) get sued, if something goes wrong, and b) be accused of practicing medicine without a physician collaborator.

Situation 2:

You get a letter from a pharmaceutical company inviting you to participate in a round table discussion hosted by the company. There will be 15 attendees, all nurse practitioners who provide women's health care. The topic will be treatment of hypercholesterolemia in the older woman. The company has a prescription product for reducing cholesterol. The letter offers you $500 plus a gourmet dinner. The writer wants to send you a consulting contract.

Situation 3:

You are arranging the annual conference for NPs in your state. You have heard from past conference chairs that some pharmaceutical manufacturers will do any and all of the following sponsorship activities:

1) Purchase booth space in the exhibit hall.
2) Provide unrestricted grants for general conference overhead in return for a listing as sponsor on the program.
3) Fund specific speakers, including speaking fee, travel, slides and handouts.
4) Purchase books as gifts for attendees.
5) Fund the travel expenses of some high volume prescribers.

You have the names and telephone numbers of several drug reps in your area. You aren't sure what to ask for or what is appropriate under the new Federal compliance program guidance for pharmaceutical manufacturers.

Situation 4:

A patient of yours wants to quit smoking. His health plan will pay for Wellbutrin (buproprion) for depression but not Zyban (buproprion) for smoking cessation. You wonder whether it is "insurance fraud" to save a patient money by treating smoking cessation with a prescription for Wellbutrin, given the medication and dosing is the same as Zyban.

ANALYZING THE ETHICAL CHOICES INHERENT IN THESE SITUATIONS

Situation 1: Providing Care on the Street

When faced with Situation 1, a nurse practitioner who ignores the patient having a seizure is doing nothing illegal. There is no legal requirement that a health care provider pay attention to patients, even when a patient is sitting in front of the provider in a clinic. However, most health care providers feel an ethical as well as business responsibility to provide care for patients who come to the office. As for the individual who falls down in the street, has a seizure in public or has had an automobile accident, the individual clinician may make his or her own decision whether to become involved. The decision will be based on the clinician's analysis of whether he or she is ethically obligated to respond and whether other considerations outweigh any ethical dictates. Any two nurse practitioners may come to opposite conclusions.

Four forces encourage clinicians to provide care:

1. Fear of a lawsuit for malpractice, if he or she neglects to treat an illness;
2. Fear of a charge of patient abandonment, if one does not give care;
3. The need for compensation; and
4. The clinician's own values, which include the clinician's sense of ethical responsibility.

Malpractice

For a successful lawsuit for malpractice, four elements have to be satisfied. First, there must be a duty of care owed the patient by the clinician. Second, the clinician has to have breached the standard of care. Third, there must be an injury to the patient. Fourth, the patient's injury must be causally related to the clinician's breach of the standard of care.

A clinician who provides care or advice for a person on the street establishes a duty of care. A clinician who walks by without offering advice or service does not establish a duty of care. Thus, the clinician who chooses not to become engaged is shielded from a lawsuit for malpractice, because there is no duty of care.

Patient Abandonment

In the case of the woman seizing in the grocery store, a clinician cannot be charged with patient abandonment if the clinician never becomes engaged in the woman's care. Patient abandonment is defined slightly differently in different states, and often is addressed on the Web sites for the Board of Nursing. For example, the Colorado Board of Nursing states that for patient abandonment to occur, the registered nurse has to have accepted the assignment and severed the relationship without giving reasonable notice to the appropriate person (such as supervisor or patient) so that arrangements can be made for care by others. It is not patient abandonment, therefore, to refuse to accept an assignment or a patient-nurse relationship. Therefore, a nurse who walks by a person in distress on the street could not be accused of patient abandonment.

Reimbursement

In a roadside assistance situation, reimbursement is not an issue, as there is no system under which a clinician can submit a bill for such care. The reimbursable settings of care are office, hospital, nursing home, patient's home, and domiciliary facility, and there are no procedure codes for the setting "sidewalk" and "grocery store."

Ethics

The clinician faced with a decision to ignore or become involved with an individual in distress will weigh his assessment of right and wrong, and attempt to come to a decision in which his behavior conforms to a standard of right behavior. Some considerations might be:

- Are there other people already helping the individual?
- Are my skills any more helpful than what is already being done for the individual? The NP can help shield the patient's head from hard or sharp surfaces, but so can the non-clinician bystander. If the nurse practitioner has no education or experience in emergency medicine, the nurse practitioner may not be any more qualified to help than another bystander.
- What, exactly, can I do for the patient? For example, the treatment for seizures is IV Valium. The NP on the street has no Valium to offer the patient. On the other hand, if the situation is that an individual has fallen to the ground, apparently unconscious, and a nurse practitioner knows cardiopulmonary resuscitation, then there is something the nurse practitioner can offer.
- Do I have the legal authority to diagnose and treat in this situation? In most states, a NP needs a collaborative agreement with a physician to diagnose and treat, and those agreements do not usually extend to on-the-street encounters.
- Will I feel that I did not meet my own expectations of myself if I pass by without offering help?
- If I were the patient, and a nurse practitioner walked by and saw me, would I want the nurse practitioner to offer to help?

Nurse practitioners make situation-by-situation decisions on whether to become involved with clinical care on off hours. There is no legal mandate to offer services. A clinician may choose to become involved or not, depending upon the situation and the clinician's analysis of what is the humane and reasonable thing to do.

Situation 2

When a pharmaceutical company offers a clinician substantial remuneration for not much work, one has to wonder whether the company is looking to create a situation where a clinician feels obligated to prescribe the company's medication.

Both the pharmaceutical industry and the federal government recently have adopted guidelines addressing the relationships between clinicians and pharmaceutical companies. The guidelines attempt to provide pharmaceutical companies with a yardstick by which to judge whether a gift or payment from a pharmaceutical company is a kickback to a clinician or a payment at fair market value for personal services rendered.

The questions which separate a kickback from a business arrangement for services are:

- Is the clinician in a position to generate health care business for the manufacturer directly or indirectly?
- Is any one purpose of the remuneration to induce or reward the referral or recommendation of business payable in whole or in part by a federal health care program.[1p14]
- Does the arrangement have a potential to interfere with, or skew clinical decision-making?
- Does the arrangement or practice have a potential to increase costs of the federal health care programs, beneficiaries, or enrollees?
- Does the arrangement or practice have a potential to increase the risk of over-utilization or inappropriate utilization?
- Does the arrangement or practice raise patient safety or quality of care concerns?[1p15]

The pharmaceutical industry's own "Code on Interactions with Health Care Professionals" provides the following guidance:

> It is appropriate for consultants who provide services to be offered reasonable compensation for those services and to be offered reimbursement for reasonable travel, lodging, and meal expense incurred as part of providing those services. Compensation and reimbursement that would be inappropriate in other contexts can be acceptable for bona fide consultants in connection with their consulting arrangements. Token consulting or advisory arrangements should not be used to justify compensating health care professionals for their time or their travel, lodging, and other out-of-pocket expense. The following factors support the existence of a bona fide consulting arrangement . . . :

- A written contract specifies the nature of the services to be provided and the basis for payment of those services;
- A legitimate need for the services has been clearly identified in advance of requesting the services and entering into arrangements with the prospective consultants;
- The criteria for selecting consultants are directly related to the identified purpose and the persons responsible for selecting the consultants have the expertise necessary to evaluate whether the particular health care professionals meet those criteria;
- The number of health care professionals retained is not greater than the number reasonably necessary to achieve the identified purpose;

- The retaining company maintains records concerning and makes appropriate use of the services provided by consultants;
- The venue and circumstances of any meeting with consultants are conducive to the consulting services;
- Activities related to the services are the primary focus of the meeting; and
- Any social or entertainment events are clearly subordinate in terms of time and emphasis.[2p3,4]

The Office of Inspector General (OIG) "Federal Register Notice on the Compliance Program Guidance for Pharmaceutical Manufacturers" dated April 2003 states: "In general, fair market value payments to small numbers of physician for *bona fide* consulting or advisory services are unlikely to raise any significant concern. Compensating physicians as 'consultants' when they are expected to attend meetings or conferences primarily in a passive capacity is suspect."[1p32] The OIG guidance applies to health care professionals other than physicians.[1p28]

While the Pharmaceutical Research and Manufacturers of America (PhRMA) Code and the OIG Guidance are targeted to the pharmaceutical industry, clinicians can get a sense of what is considered right and wrong on their part.

Hence, a clinician faced with Situation 2 should apply the tests now accepted as standard in the industry, before accepting the invitation. Specifically, will the nurse practitioner, having accepted the $500 and a fine dinner, be more likely to prescribe the company's medication, even though it will cost the patient or the patient's insurer much more than a generic product, than if the nurse practitioner did not accept the money and dinner? And, if the answer is "no," is the nurse practitioner being ethical accepting the money and dinner? Will the nurse practitioner provide $500 worth of consultative services to the pharmaceutical company at the dinner?

Situation 3

The PhRMA Code has these caveats about pharmaceutical company involvement in third-party educational or professional meetings:

- Financial support should be given to the conference's sponsor rather than to an individual participant.
- Responsibility for and control over the selection of content, faculty, educational methods, materials, and venue should remain with the conference organizers.
- Financial support for meals or receptions may be provided to the CME sponsors who can provide meals for all attendees, or a company may provide meals or receptions directly if it complies with the organization's guidelines.
- Meals or receptions should be modest.
- Meals and receptions should be conducive to discussion among faculty and attendees.

- The amount of time at meals or receptions should be clearly subordinate to the amount of time spent at the educational activities of the meetings.
- The main incentive for bringing attendees together should be the educational presentation.

For arrangements between physicians and other persons in a position to make or influence referrals, orders, or prescriptions which do not fit a safe harbor from the anti-kickback rule, the analysis that the OIG recommends is:

- What degree of influence does the physician have, directly or indirectly, on the generation of business for the manufacturer?
- Does the remuneration take into account, directly or indirectly, the volume or value of business generated?
- Is the remuneration more than trivial in value?
- Do fees-for-services exceed the fair market value of any legitimate, reasonable, and necessary services rendered by the physician to the manufacturer?
- Does the remuneration have the potential to affect costs to any of the federal health care programs or their beneficiaries or to lead to over utilization or inappropriate utilization?
- Would acceptance of the remuneration diminish, or appear to diminish the objectivity of professional judgment?
- Are there patient safety or quality of care concerns?
- If the remuneration relates to the dissemination of information, is the information complete, accurate and not misleading?

A safe harbor from violation of the anti-kickback is described as follows:

> Personal services and management contracts. As used in section 1128B of the Act, "remuneration" does not include any payment made by a principal to an agent as compensation for the services of the agent, as long as all of the following seven standards are met:
>
> (1) The agency agreement is set out in writing and signed by the parties.
>
> (2) The agency agreement covers all of the services the agent provides to the principal for the term of the agreement and specifies the services to be provided by the agent.
>
> (3) If the agency agreement is intended to provide for the services of the agent on a periodic, sporadic or part-time basis, rather than on a full-time basis for the term of the agreement, the agreement specifies exactly the schedule of such intervals, their precise length, and the exact charge for such intervals.
>
> (4) The term of the agreement is for not less than one year.
>
> (5) The aggregate compensation paid to the agent over the term of the agreement is set in advance, is consistent with fair market value in arms-length transactions and is not determined in a manner that takes

into account the volume or value of any referrals or business otherwise generated between the parties for which payment may be made in whole or in part under Medicare, Medicaid, or other Federal health care programs.

(6) The services performed under the agreement do not involve the counseling or promotion of a business arrangement or other activity that violates any State or Federal law.

(7) The aggregate services contracted for do not exceed those which are reasonably necessary to accomplish the commercially reasonable business purpose of the services.

For purposes of paragraph (d) of this section, an agent of a principal is any person, other than a bona fide employee of the principal, who has an agreement to perform services for, or on behalf of, the principal.

Citation: 42 CFR 1001.952(d).

As described in Situation #3, a nurse practitioner arranging the annual state conference may arrange for pharmaceutical manufacturers to:

1) Purchase booth space in the exhibit hall at which they will distribute information and items of minimal value, such as pens or note pads.
2) Provide unrestricted grants for general conference overhead, in return for a listing as sponsor on the program.
3) Fund specific speakers, including speaking fee, travel, slides and handouts, as long as the information the speakers provide is educational and consistent with patient safety.

However, the manufacturer should not purchase expensive books as gifts for attendees. A book is likely to be more than trivial in value, and acceptance of the book could diminish, or appear to diminish the objectivity of professional judgment of the recipient nurse practitioner. Nor should the pharmaceutical company fund the travel expenses of high volume prescribers.

Situation 4

It may be ethical to try to save the patient money, but it is illegal—fraud—to diagnose depression in a patient whose mood is normal, so that the clinician can prescribe Wellbutrin for smoking cessation so that the prescription will be covered by insurance.

Fraud is defined as: "an intentional deception or misrepresentation which the individual knows to be false or does not believe to be true, and the individual is aware that the deception could result in some unauthorized benefit to him/herself or some other person."

Citation: 18 USC §§ 1341, 1343 and 1347.

Is it fraud if you diagnose "smoking," and prescribe Wellbutrin? Probably not, because you are not deceiving anyone. However, the insurer is likely to deny payment for the Wellbutrin.

Is it fraud if you diagnose "depression" and omit any reference to smoking? Yes. Is it fraud if you diagnose "depression" and "smoking" and prescribe Wellbutrin? Probably not. Ask yourself: Can you make the argument, with a straight face, that he is both depressed and a smoker, or that he is using nicotine to self-medicate for depression, or that he may be depressed about his smoking? Before taking that route, consider these factors: Unless a patient is truly depressed, you may not want to enter that diagnosis unless the patient agrees that he is depressed. In the future, the patient may want to authorize release of his medical record to a prospective employer. If that happens, you don't want the patient to be surprised and upset to find that he has a history of depression. Furthermore, are you ready to follow-up your diagnosis of depression by addressing that problem in subsequent visits by performing and documenting one of the depression scales? Are you prepared to follow the standard of care for treatment of depression; i.e., treat for 12 months?

A health plan in Wisconsin recently performed a medical chart audit to see how closely clinicians were following the health plan's Wellbutrin prescription guidelines. The plan's newsletter warned: "It is considered fraud to not disclose required information or to make entries into the record to enhance a patients condition."*

A clinician may have the best intentions—to relieve the patient's problem and save the patient money—but there is a risk to you that probably outweighs the benefits in these situations.

ETHICAL ANALYSES

In general, nurse practitioners might approach a situation with ethical considerations in the following manner:

- Gather information
    - Is this a legal, rather than ethical question?
    - Is there a law governing this situation?
        - Consider laws governing:
            - Scope of practice
            - Kickbacks
            - Patient privacy and confidentiality
            - Billing Medicare, Medicaid, and commercial insurers
            - Good Samaritan laws
            - End of life issues such as decision not to resuscitate

---

**Source:* Provider connection.Valley Health Plan Newsletter. 2002; 2: issue 4. Available at http://www.valleyhealth.biz/pconnect1202.pdf. Accessed July 2003.

Who is benefitting from this situation? How?
Who is being hurt or could be hurt by this situation? How?
Do I have a gut feeling about what is the right or wrong course of action in this situation?
Am I being swayed by what is beneficial to me or my group?
What would other, ethical practitioners do?
Does my state Board of Nursing have any guidance regarding this situation on their Web site?
Does my malpractice insurance cover me in this situation?

- Structure a plan.
  Identify the course of action you would like to take.
  Identify alternate approaches.
  Identify the pros and cons of the preferred course of action, and the alternative approaches.
- If it is a patient care matter, present the issue to the patient, if appropriate.
- Tell the patient that you would like him or her to direct you in this situation.
- If it is a business matter, consult with your partners, committee members, employer, and/or employees.
- If there is a code of conduct from a governmental agency, a professional society or your own institution which applies, follow the dictates of that code.
- Make a decision
  Prepare, for yourself, an argument that supports your decision. Carry out your plan.
- If you decide later that you made the wrong decision, learn from your mistake.

Of course, every situation is different and is accompanied by nuances that are beyond the scope of this book. To explore medical ethics and problem solving, an excellent reference is a recent book by Dr. Bernard Lo.[3]

NOTES

1. Department of Health and Human Servies, Office of Inspector General. Compliance Program Guidance for Pharmaceutical Manufacturers, April 2003. Available at: http://oig.hhs.gov. Accessed August 2003.

2. Pharmaceutical Research and Manufacturers of America, PhRMA Code on Interactions with Health Care Professionals, April 2002. Available at: http://www.phrma.org. Accessed August 2003.

3. Lo B. *Resolving Ethical Dilemmas: A Guide for Clinicians.* Philadelphia, PA: Lippincott Williams & Wilkins; 2000.

CHAPTER 17

Strategies for NPs

The difference between making do and advancing is the difference between eating all of what is put on one's plate and deciding what to have for dinner.

NPs faced with restrictive or outdated law sometimes report at professional meetings that they are proud of how they are able to function despite the law. For example, NPs who want to have their own businesses can construct a private practice that conforms to the law as long as they hire a physician consultant. NPs who want to prescribe but whose state laws require physician oversight can prescribe as long as a physician cosigns or does whatever else is necessary to conform to the state's requirements. NPs who cannot be designated as primary care providers (PCPs) and handle panels of managed-care patients actually perform the patient care, while a physician is designated as the PCP. The NPs say their reward is that the patients know that the NP is providing their care and appreciate the NP's efforts.

Although many NPs are making the best of existing law, in many states, the law is far from satisfactory. Only in Oregon, Alaska, Washington, Maine, Utah, New Mexico, Arizona, and New Hampshire are NPs free to practice their profession without mandated participation from physicians.

OPPORTUNITIES IN A CHANGING FIELD

In states where barriers to NP practice have been lifted and where reimbursement is attainable from third-party payers, there are opportunities for health care delivery systems that increase attention to preventive medicine, increase access to citizens, and provide alternatives to expensive physician-oriented systems.

Under a see-a-nurse-first system, patients initially would be seen by a registered nurse or NP. The nurses would take care of as many of a patient's health care problems as would be prudent, and would seek consultation and referral for those problems that exceeded the scope of their practice.

A see-a-nurse-first system is depicted in Figure 17-1.

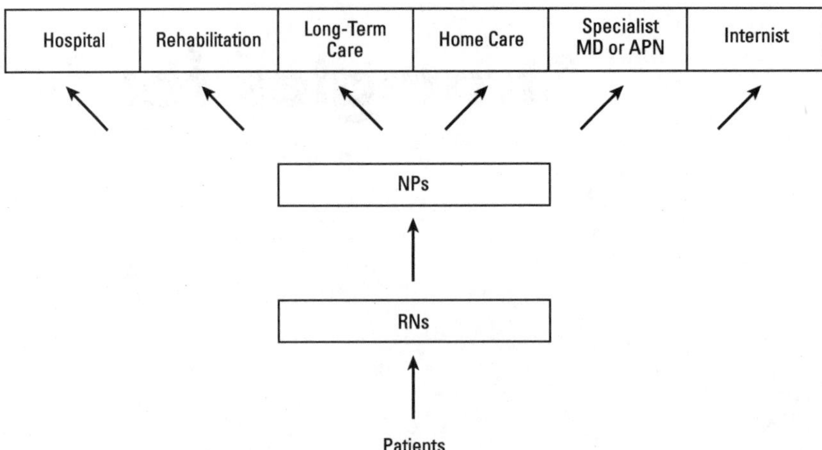

Figure 17-1. See-a-nurse-first primary care delivery system. *Source:* © Carolyn Buppert.

OPPONENTS OF A SEE-A-NURSE-FIRST SYSTEM

Physicians can be counted on to oppose a see-a-nurse-first system of health care delivery. The American Academy of Family Physicians (AAFP) has the following policy regarding NP practice: "The nurse practitioner should not function as an independent health practitioner. The AAFP position is that the nurse practitioner should only function in a collaborative practice arrangement under the direction and responsible supervision of a practicing, licensed physician.[1]

Some patients may be suspicious of a see-a-nurse-first system. For that reason, patients should be offered a choice of nurse and/or physician providers. Once the law offers a level playing field, both physicians and NPs will have incentives to improve their services to patients and will thereby advance their respective professions.

WHAT ARE THE CHALLENGES FOR NPs ATTEMPTING TO ADVANCE THE PROFESSION?

First, there is the matter of the energy required. NPs are accustomed to volunteer organizations. Now is the time to consider hiring professionals. Public relations experts, not volunteers, develop public relations campaigns for physician organizations. Physicians do not expect to see 30 patients at the office, stop by the hospital on the way home, and then get together at 8 PM to develop public relations campaigns. Physician organizations hire public relations firms or in-house staff whose sole job is to attend to the public image of physicians. NPs can hire professionals, too, and should. Much publicity can be gained with a small budget and creative public relations professionals.

Second, there is the challenge of publicizing the good in NPs and comparing NP services to physician services without denigrating physicians. The solution to that challenge is to continue to publicize the studies of the efficacy and quality of NPs that have shown that NPs are as competent providers of primary care as physicians.

Third, there is the phenomenon that every action generates a reaction. When physicians see NPs step up efforts to advance the profession, physicians may feel it necessary to react with more aggressive efforts. NPs who are intimidated by this thought should remember their goal and stay on course.

The major focus of physician arguments—that only physicians should have the authority to direct primary care—is the educational differential between NPs and physicians. The counterargument for NPs is: Physicians set their educational level. There has been no major study of physician education and training since 1910, when Abraham Flexner published a report commissioned by the Carnegie Foundation that called for medical training to be university-affiliated programs rather than eight-month programs where students came without a high school diploma.[2] There are no studies showing that the appropriate education for providing primary care is four years of medical school and three years of residency, which is the education for all physicians, whether they are brain surgeons, researchers into neurotransmitters, or providers of primary care. On the contrary, there are many studies showing that NPs are quite appropriate providers of primary care (see Chapter 13).

STRATEGIES TO IMPLEMENT COLLECTIVELY

NPs are familiar with the advantages of working collectively toward change. First, individuals can pool money to have more purchasing power than one individual NP. Second, groups are taken seriously by lawmakers and political parties.

Marshalling support of even homogeneous groups is no small accomplishment. In the case of NPs, a stumbling block to collective action is the heterogeneity of NPs, as not every NP has the same professional interests, the same viewpoint, or the same goals. For example, NPs who are professors have professional goals that include getting government funding for educational programs for NPs. NPs who are clinicians do not have educational funding as a top-priority goal. Instead, they have the goal of being able to practice with few barriers.

Nevertheless, organizations are necessary for the advancement of the NP profession. NPs inspire, encourage, and rejuvenate other NPs, all of which is necessary when the goals are long term.

TEN ORGANIZATIONAL STRATEGIES

The following ten strategies are suggested for NPs who want to advance the profession and/or their own opportunities:

Set a Goal

For example, one NP set herself a goal of being a "primary care provider," credentialled with health plans. She built up a base of loyal patients, became an excellent clinician, and worked with the state's organization of NPs to change the law so that an NP could be designated by a health maintenance organization as a PCP. She succeeded.

Of course, NPs work not only in primary care, but in specialty practices and tertiary care. In every setting, NPs need to choose an achievable and reasonable goal, one that would affect not only themselves, but other NPs.

Analyze the Law for Barriers

There is much ignorance and confusion about the law as it affects NPs. Some NPs say, "The law says we need to be supervised, but we really practice independently." By participating in a practice situation where the law is stretched, NPs are taking a risk. In some states, the law puts responsibility squarely on the NP for ensuring that supervisory requirements are met. Clinics, hospitals, and medical groups have had little to lose by providing little or no supervision and letting the NP go as far as the NP's willingness for intellectual adventure and professional judgment allows. NPs are bringing in at least $120 per hour and getting paid about $30 per hour. If an NP makes few mistakes and no one enforces the law, everything runs smoothly. However, the better an NP does with independent decision making, the more momentum builds for more independence, and pretty soon the NP is out on a limb, with no physician available to answer telephone calls to help, much less supervise. As soon as an NP makes a mistake, the burden is back on the NP for not seeking supervision. If the NP is a practice owner making $120 per hour and willing to take the risk, that is one thing, but if the NP is an employee earning $30 per hour, the risks outweigh the benefits.

Some NPs have argued that current law and custom permit NPs to practice in a satisfying manner, so "why open a can of worms" by attempting to change the law? This argument not only offends a sense of legal "neatness," where law and current practice jibe, but condones a timidity that is incongruent with the level of assertion needed to perform as an NP. Why would NPs participate in life-and-death decisions for patients and yet retreat from challenging statutory omissions that relegate NPs to the invisible category of "others" or "nonphysicians"?

Every NP needs a copy of every law that affects the NP's practice. That includes law that does not mention NPs but that affects NPs because of the omissions. For example, every NP needs a copy of the scope of practice for an NP in the state where the NP is licensed and practicing.

National NP organizations need fact sheets that include federal law regarding:

- Delegation of duties in nursing home care.
- Direction of the care of hospitalized patients.
- Anti-kickback laws.
- Definition of medical care and medical care provider.
- Application for Drug Enforcement Administration (DEA) numbers.
- Reimbursement by Medicare and Medicaid.

- Coding and billing of Medicare and Medicaid visits.
- Documentation guidelines.
- Definition of collaboration.

Because the officers and board members of NP organizations change from year to year, NP organizations should maintain a current file of the relevant law for each new officer to review at the start of the term. Much anxiety will be avoided if NPs have copies of the exact language of the law.

Lobby for Eradication of the Barriers

Once the barriers are known, organizations can enlist lobbyists to help eradicate the barriers. NPs may make progress in one area, such as convincing managed-care organizations to admit NPs to panels, only to find that there is some phrase in state law that a state administrator interprets as barring NPs from becoming PCPs.

NPs should not expect to win passage of new legislation the first time it is introduced. Each time an issue is lobbied, more information comes out about NPs, and the idea of NPs becomes more comfortable to lawmakers.

NPs may argue that if certain issues are brought up, NPs may lose ground in the law rather than gain ground. NPs ask: What if we introduce a law, but it is amended and passed at the last minute, and our authority to prescribe is lost? The counterargument is: that is a possibility, but not a probability. Compare the situation an NP faces every day in clinical practice: a patient arrives complaining of low back pain. In 99 percent of cases, the back pain will be due to musculoskeletal strain and will respond to rest and nonsteroidal anti-inflammatory drugs. In one case out of 100, the back pain will be something else, and in a very minuscule percentage of cases, the low back pain will be cancer. Does the NP rush all patients who complain of low back pain to magnetic resonance imaging at the first visit? No. Likewise, the chances that NPs, by introducing legislation to advance the profession, will actually fall backward is minuscule, for the following reasons. First, NPs are valuable to medical groups, hospitals, HMOs, and health departments. Second, a good lobbyist, as well as the sponsor of a bill, is going to follow a bill very closely. It is unlikely that a bill that was introduced on behalf of NPs will be amended without the knowledge of the NPs' lobbyist. Because the lobbyist is hired by an NP organization, it is unlikely that a lobbyist will be caught unaware or will fail to rally the NP organization client when necessary. Third, there is virtually no opposition to NPs as health care providers other than from organized physician groups, and then only when NPs are striving to release the legal apron strings that tie NPs to physicians.

NPs should hire lobbyists to advise the NPs on strategies for getting a particular bill passed (see Chapter 12 for more about specific legislative strategies).

NPs should not be deterred by the prospect of introducing a bill five times before it is passed. If it takes five years to get a bill passed, so be it. It will take five years to get the bill passed if NPs wait five years to introduce it, and then ten years will have passed.

Sell MCOs and Purchasers of Health Services on NPs as PCPs

NPs can offer MCOs and the employers who purchase health care services for their employees quality services at a reasonable cost. However, NPs cannot depend on health plan purchasers to know what NPs can do unless NPs educate the purchasers.

MCOs and business executives are used to listening to business presentations from those who want to sell services. NPs are not used to giving business presentations, but they can learn. Alternatively, NP organizations can hire the services of professionals who make business presentations to do the work for the NPs.

The basic message of a business presentation on why MCOs and businesses should contract with NPs as PCPs is that NPs give high-quality care for a reasonable price. The message should be supported by data demonstrating the quality of NPs and numbers demonstrating the rationale of the pricing schedule. Finally, MCOs and businesses need to know how they can contract with NPs, that is, where the NPs are located and whom to contact.

Promote NPs to the Public

Individuals who have experienced the care of an NP have been satisfied with NPs. However, there are still a great many people who have never experienced the care of NPs. Promotional efforts need to be aimed at the unconvinced segment of the population.

Further, some individuals who have experienced the care of NPs and been satisfied may not know that NPs are responsible for the care NPs provide. People may believe that NPs simply relay what a physician has decided and that NPs are simply physician helpers. NPs will need to establish themselves as experts. That can be done through newspaper articles where NPs give advice on health care topics, through talk radio, through television public service announcements, through paid advertising, through presentations at community events, and through one-to-one interactions between NP and patient.

Work the Data

All studies done of the care given by NPs are supportive of NPs. This includes many studies done by physicians and operations researchers, as well as studies done by nurses. NPs need to cite and recite the data in language that a layperson can understand. NPs need to compile their own data on the effectiveness of their own care. For example, electronic medical record systems now allow clinicians who treat diabetes to produce data that compare the effectiveness of individual clinicians at controlling patients' HgAlc. While physicians are hashing and rehashing the educational differences between NPs and physicians, NPs need to be repeating the data that say: NPs give good care. Therefore, the educational differential, while significant, must not be relevant. To date, physicians have no data to prove that their additional years of education make them better PCPs than NPs.

Hire Professionals To Do the Association's Work

It is time to hire professionals and time for NP associations to act like businesses. It is time for board members to be relieved of the hands-on "doing" of association business so they can do what board members are supposed to do: decide how the association money is spent and evaluate the performance of the hired help.

Why? Because NPs are operating in an industry where changes are coming fast. NPs stand to gain ground, but progress will not come easily. Other professional groups are spending large sums to have experts monitor changes and ensure that their members' interests are represented when policy is made, law is enacted, and contracts are signed.

NPs have great potential because they combine nursing and medical knowledge. In volatile times, there are great opportunities. However, no laws are going to be enacted to designate NPs as PCPs unless bills are drafted expertly, hard lobbying is done successfully, and public relations efforts are increased and well targeted. No state regulations are going to be changed in NPs' favor without carefully drafted, persistent requests to state agencies. No health plans are going to open themselves to additional providers unless they can be shown how it will benefit the company.

How are NP organizations going to fund all this expert help? By developing revenue streams other than membership dues. Each NP organization that does not have an annual continuing-education conference for which the registration fee is at least $150 per day should have one. Putting on a conference may require hiring a part-time conference coordinator. The budget for a conference should support a conference coordinator, the speakers' time, and the expenses of room rental and coffee, and should make a profit. Each organization should charge for the use of its name and the use of its directory. When files of laws are sent out on request, the organization should charge for that service.

NP organizations need public relations specialists, lobbyists, and attorneys, either on retainer or on a per-project basis. Each organization needs a paid executive director who answers to the board of directors.

Volunteer officers, board members, and committee chairs of NP organizations are running themselves ragged and burning out. These volunteers are making the day-to-day decisions about their organizations; often they also are talking with newspaper reporters, trying to recruit new members, trying to make sense of laws, folding flyers, licking stamps, and answering nonstop questions from individual NPs.

At a time when NPs are defending themselves, in the press and in the legislatures, and fighting for their spot in the managed-care landscape, NPs need to be hiring expert assistance, not relying on do-it-yourself operations. It's time to hire professionals and to get appropriate service.

Don't Be Timid

Nurses have been timid in the past. NPs are trying to overcome barriers that were erected long before NPs were in existence, barriers that resulted from a history of timidity in nursing. For example, in 1955, the American Nurses Association's model definition of nursing stated that nursing "shall not be deemed to include any acts of diagnosis or prescription of therapeutic or corrective measures."[3] In 1955, nurses were performing acts that clearly were within the definition of diagnosis and prescription of corrective measures. Nevertheless, by 1967, 22 states had incorporated the ANA model language into state law.[4] To cover hospitals and agencies where nurses were doing "acts of diagnosis or prescription of therapeutic measures," joint statements of hospital, medical, and nursing associations were written that allowed nurses to perform certain acts, such as venipuncture or initiating IV fluids.[5] The joint statements were contrary to the law, yet no one challenged the law or the policy statements.

Today, NPs find that they can practice independently, meaning that they make decisions about patient care without consulting physicians. However, if state and federal regulations call for collaboration and define collaboration as supervision, NPs who push the envelope without also pushing for changes in legal language that supports their independent practice will be going nowhere.

It is time for NPs to be affirming, "NPs are experts in primary care," or "I am an expert in managing diabetes," rather than "NPs do primary care in collaboration with physicians."

Erase *Collaboration* from the Legal Vocabulary

NPs, like any other health care providers, cannot function without collaboration with other experts. Nevertheless, nurses are virtually the only profession that has "collaboration" as a legal mandate.

NPs have considered the word *collaboration* as an improvement on the word *supervision*. However, a close reading of federal law reveals that the law defines *collaboration* to mean supervision.

When arguing for erasure of barriers to NP practice, NPs have had difficulty convincing legislators of the difference between collaboration and supervision, and with good reason. Although there is a difference in the definitions of the two words—the dictionary defines collaborate as "work jointly with others" (and alternatively as "cooperate with an enemy force occupying one's country")[7p95] and supervision as "oversee, superintend"[6p493]—a legal mandate to collaborate suggests that the group given the mandate is not the final authority on a matter. Although NPs are not so arrogant as to consider themselves final authorities on all matters of health care, certainly NPs can and should consider themselves final authorities on primary care and other areas of medicine where an NP has specialized and extensive education and experience.

Consultation, yes. A legal requirement of collaboration, no.

Insist upon Legal Clarity of NP Authority To Practice

Compare laws A and B on NP scope of practice:

Law A:

> The board recognizes advanced and specialized acts of nursing practice as those described in the scope of practice statements for nurse practitioners certified by national certifying bodies recognized by the board.
>
> *Citation:* ALASKA ADMIN. CODE tit. 12, § 44.430.

Law B:

> The nurse practitioner provides holistic health care to individuals, families, and groups across the life span in a variety of settings, including hospitals, long term care facilities, and community-based settings. Within his or her specialty, the nurse practitioner is responsible for managing health problems encountered by the client and is accountable for health outcomes. This process includes:
>
> a. Assessment;
> b. Diagnosis;
> c. Development of a plan;
> d. Intervention;
> e. Evaluation.
>
> The nurse practitioner is independently responsible and accountable for the continuous and comprehensive management of a broad range of health care, which may include:
>
> a. Promotion and maintenance of health;
> b. Prevention of illness and disability;
> c. Assessment of clients, synthesis and analysis of data, and application of nursing principles and therapeutic modalities;
> d. Management of health care during acute and chronic phases of illness;
> e. Admission of his/her clients to hospitals and long-term care facilities and management of client care in these facilities;
> f. Counseling;
> g. Consultation and/or collaboration with other care providers and community resources;
> h. Referral to other health care providers and community resources;
> i. Management and coordination of care;

j. Use of research skills;
k. Diagnosis of health/illness status;
l. Prescription and/or administration of therapeutic devices and measures including legend drugs and controlled substances as provided in OAR 851-050-0131 and dispensing drugs as provided in OAR 851-050-0133, 0134, and 0145, consistent with the definition of the practitioner's specialty category and scope of practice.

The nurse practitioner is responsible for recognizing limits of knowledge and experience, and for resolving situations beyond his/her nurse practitioner expertise by consulting with or referring clients to other health care providers. The nurse practitioner will only provide health care services within the nurse practitioner's scope of practice for which he/she is educationally prepared and for which competency has been established and maintained. Educational preparation includes academic course work, workshops or seminars, provided both theory and clinical experience are included.

Citation: OR. ADMIN. R. 851-050-0005.

There is no question what an NP in law B can do. Many questions are left unanswered by law A. For example: What is "advanced and specialized acts of nursing practice?" Do such acts include medical services, or is an advanced practice nurse the same as a registered nurse? While law B is specific and permissive of NP practice, law A is unclear.

NPs need to insist upon clarity. Without clarity, other groups may decide what the law addressing NPs means.

NOTES

1. American Academy of Family Physicians. Policy Statement 2002. Available at (http://www.aafp.org) Accessed July 2003.
2. Starr P. *The Social Transformation of American Medicine.* New York, NY: Basic Books; 1992: chapt 3.
3. ANA Board approves a definition of nursing practice. *Am J Nurs* 1955; 55:1474.
4. Phillips RS. Nurse practitioners: their scope of practice and theories of liability. *J Leg Med* 1985; 6:391–414.
5. Bullough B. The first two phases in nursing licensure. In *The Law and the Expanding Nursing Role,* vol 7. New York, NY: Appleton-Century-Crofts; 1975.
6. *New Merriam-Webster Pocket Dictionary.* New York, NY: Pocket Books; 1972.

Index

A

AANA (American Association of Nurse Anesthetists), 16t
AANP (American Academy of Nurse Practitioners). *see* American Academy of Nurse Practitioners
Abandonment, patient, and good Samaritan acts, 461–462
Abbottsford Community Health Center, 424
Abuse, reporting, 144
Accreditation, 443
ACNM (American College of Nurse Midwives), 16t
Adams v. Kreuger, 238–239
Admitting privileges, hospital, 227–234, 431
Advance for Nurse Practitioners, 301
Advanced pratice nurses (APNs), 3, 16t
Advanced registered nurse practitioner (ARNP), 6
Age Discrimination Act of 1967, 145
Agency for Healthcare Research and Quality (AHRQ), 243, 445–446, 452
Alabama
- definition of nurse practitioner, 18
- educational and licensing requirements, for NPs, 117
- physician collaboration requirements, 75–77
- physician involvement requirements, 44
- prescriptive authority in, 184, 185, 188–189
- regulatory agency for NPs, 114
- scope of NP practice, 41, 47–48
- titles for nurse practitioners, 33

Alaska
- definition of nurse practitioner, 18
- educational and licensing requirements, for NPs, 117
- physician collaboration requirements, 44, 77, 469
- prescriptive authority in, 184, 185, 189–190
- regulatory agency for NPs, 114
- scope of NP practice, 48, 477
- titles for nurse practitioners, 33

American Academy of Family Physicians, 8–9, 13t, 283, 405, 470
American Academy of Nurse Practitioners (AANP), 5
- standards of care, 438–441
- statement on scope of practice, 37–38

American Academy of Physician Assistants, 11, 12, 13t
American Association of Colleges of Nursing, 425
American Association of Nurse Anesthetists (AANA), 16t
American College of Nurse Midwives (ACNM), 16t
American College of Nurse Practitioners, 7
American Medical Association (AMA), 430
- Council on Medical Service Report, 431
- Current Procedural Terminology *(CPT)*, 263, 270–271, 279, 281

"Documentation Guidelines for Evaluation and Management Services", 138, 146–181, 264, 282t
Guidelines for Physician/Physician Assistant Practice, 11
public relations, 405, 417
American Nurses Association (ANA), 476
American Nurses Credentialing Center (ANCC), 5, 13t, 16t
Americans With Disabilities Act (ADA), 145
APRN (advanced practice registered nurse), 6
Arizona
definition of nurse practitioner, 19
educational and licensing requirements, for NPs, 117–118
physician collaboration requirements, 77, 469
physician involvement requirements, 44
prescriptive authority in, 184, 185, 190–192
regulatory agency for NPs, 114
scope of NP practice, 41, 48
titles for nurse practitioners, 33
Arkansas
definition of nurse practitioner, 19
educational and licensing requirements, for NPs, 118
physician collaboration requirements, 44, 77
prescriptive authority in, 184, 185, 192
regulatory agency for NPs, 114
scope of NP practice, 48
titles for nurse practitioners, 33
ARNP (advanced registered nurse practitioner), 6
Attorney, retaining, 263
to fight barriers to practice, 407, 410–412, 475–476
Audits, by CMS, 283
Avorn, J., 421–422, 423
Azzolino v. Dingfelder, 240–241

B

Battery, 255–256, 259
Benefits, employment, negotiating, 302
Billing
Medicare and Medicaid, 263–264, 270–271. *see also* Coding, for Medicare billing
rejected, 284
self-paying patients, 284
Boards of nursing, state
appearing before, 261–263, 442
Colorado, 461
Bono, Sonny, 403
Bonus formulas, employment, 293–295
Budget Reconciliation Bill of 1997, 137, 138
Burton v. Brooklyn Doctor's Hospital, 257
Business plan
sample agreement, 377–392
table of contents, 379
writing, 338–343
resources for help with, 342–343
sections of, 341–342
top 20 questions, 341
Business risk management, 264–265
Business structures, for practice, 331, 335–337

C

Califano, Joseph, Jr., 403
California
barriers to practice in, 401
definition of nurse practitioner, 2, 19
educational and licensing requirements, for NPs, 118
informed consent laws, 260–261
malpractice case in, 238
physician collaboration requirements, 77–80
physician involvement requirements, 44
prescriptive authority in, 183, 184, 185, 192–194
regulatory agency for NPs, 114
scope of NP practice, 48
titles for nurse practitioners, 33
Call, coverage for, 359, 366
CANP (certified advanced nurse practitioner), 6
Canterbury v. Spence, 258–259, 260
Capitated practices, 325
and NP salary, 300

Cardiovascular exam, documentation of, 159–161
Carnegie Foundation report, 471
Center for Medicare and Medicaid Services (CMS, formerly Health Care Financing Administration), 135–136, 138, 264, 269
auditing procedures, 283
"Documentation Guidelines for Evaluation and Management Services", 146–181
"Physicians' Referrals to Health Care Entities With Which They Have Financial Relationships", 140–141
resource-based relative value scale (RBRVS), 270–271
Web site, 138, 281, 283
Certification requirements
for nurse practitioners, 13t
for physician assistants, 12, 13t
Certified advanced nurse practitioner (CANP), 6
Certified geriatric nurse practitioner (CGNP), 6
Certified nurse midwife, 3
Certified pediatric nurse practitioner (CPNP), 6
Certified registered nurse anesthetist (CRNA), 16t
lawsuit against, 245
Certified registered nurse practitioner (CRNP), 6
CGNP (certified geriatric nurse practitioner), 6
Chaperones, for patient visits, 359–360
Chiropractors, and hospital privileges, 232
Civil Rights Act of 1964, 145
CLIA (Clinical Laboratories Improvement Act), 365, 369
Clinical errors, 235
risk of, 249–250
Clinical Laboratories Improvement Act (CLIA), 135, 140, 365, 369
and patient confidentiality, 144
Clinical nurse specialist (CNS), 3, 15, 414
Clinton, Bill, 401
CMS 1500 form, 279, 424
CMS (Center for Medicare and Medicaid Services, formerly Health Care Financing Administration). *see* Center for Medicare and Medicaid Services (CMS)
CNS (clinical nurse specialist), 15, 414
Code of Federal Regulation, 2
"Code on Interactions with Health Care Professionals" (pharmaceutical industry), 463–464
Coding, for Medicare billing, 263–264, 270–271, 279–285
comparison of five levels of visit, 282t
general guidelines, 280–281
Collaboration, with physician, 434. *see also* Supervision, by physician
federal definition, 138
and hospital privileges, 228–229, 232
laws affecting, 401, 469
working to remove, 476–477
Medicare requirements, 136–137, 137–138
in NP-owned practice, 329, 362–363, 371, 393–398
and NP salary, 299–300
and patient satisfaction, 423
practice agreements for, 304–305
sample agreement, 306–309
and prescriptive authority, 184
state laws, 44–45, 75–110, 469
Collaborative agreement, sample, 306–309
Colorado
definition of nurse practitioner, 19–20
educational and licensing requirements, for NPs, 118
physician collaboration requirements, 44, 80–81
prescriptive authority in, 184, 185, 194–195
regulatory agency for NPs, 114
scope of NP practice, 41, 49
state board of nursing, 461
titles for nurse practitioners, 33
Communication, with patients, 244, 252–253
Competition
among providers, 8–9
from other nurses, 414
with physician assistants (PAs), 414

with physicians, 413–414
and hospital privileges, 227–228, 229, 406–407
and legal system, 8–9, 38, 39, 404–405
and PCP designation, 349–350, 404–405, 430
Computer system, for practice, 360
Confidentiality, patient, 142–145, 359, 360
access to records for litigation, 144
breaching, risk of, 253–255
disclosure of information, 144
federal regulations, 142–145
in hospital setting, 232
maintaining, 360
Connecticut
definition of nurse practitioner, 20
educational and licensing requirements, for NPs, 118–119
physician collaboration requirements, 44, 81–82
prescriptive authority in, 184, 185, 195
regulatory agency for NPs, 114
scope of NP practice, 41, 49–50
Consent, right to informed, 255–259
exceptions, 259
and low intelligence patient, 266
patients with guardianship, 364
Controlled substances
definition, 183
prescribing, 142, 186–187
Controlled Substances Act, 183
Cooper v. Roberts, 257
Cornfeldt v. Tongen, 260–261
Corporate practice of medicine doctrine, 337
Corporation, 336–337, 359
"Council on Medical Service Report" (AMA), 431
CPNP (certified pediatric nurse practitioner), 6
Credentialing
of MCO providers, 275–276
standards for, 446–447
Credentialing information, 431–432
for employees, 361
for prescriptive authority, 361
typical application, 286–288
CRNA (certified registered nurse anesthetist), 16t
lawsuit against, 245
CRNP (certified registered nurse practitioner), 6
Current Procedural Terminology (CPT) (American Medical Association), 263, 270–271, 281

D

DEA (Drug Enforcement Administration), 135, 142, 361
definition of mid-level practitioner, 2
registration, 186
Decision making, documentation of complexity of
and amount/complexity of data reviewed, 177
and number of diagnoses or management options, 177
and risk of complications, 177–180
Delaware
definition of nurse practitioner, 20
educational and licensing requirements, for NPs, 119
physician collaboration requirements, 44, 83
prescriptive authority in, 184, 185, 196
regulatory agency for NPs, 114
scope of NP practice, 41, 50–51
titles for nurse practitioners, 33
Demographics
of nurse practitioners, 7
of physician assistants, 11
Dentists, and hospital privileges, 232, 406–407
Denton Reg. Med. Center v. LaCroix, 245
Department of Health and Human Services, 143
Department of Social Services (DSS), 362
Diagnoses, missed, 238–240, 252
Disabilities, patients with, 361–362
Disabled, antidiscrimination laws, 145
Disciplinary action, risk of, 261–263
Disclosure, and informed consent, 258–259
Discrimination, Federal laws prohibiting, 145, 361
District of Columbia, 10
definition of nurse practitioner, 20–21

educational and licensing requirements, for NPs, 119
informed consent laws, 258–259
physician collaboration requirements, 44, 83–84
prescriptive authority in, 184, 185, 196
prescriptive rights in, 183
regulatory agency for NPs, 114
scope of NP practice, 41, 51
titles for nurse practitioners, 33
Documentation
for compliance, 454–455
definition, 148
of evaluation and management services (E&M), 149–150
general principles, 149
importance of, 148
"Documentation Guidelines for Evaluation and Management Services", 138, 146–181, 264
complexity of medical decision making, 176–180, 283
for encounter dominated by counseling or coordination, 180, 284
examination, 154–176, 283
cardiovascular, 159–161
ear, nose, mouth, and throat, 161–163
eye, 163–164
general multi-system, 155–156, 156–159
genitourinary, 164–166
hematologic/lymphatic/immunologic, 166–168
musculoskeletal, 168–170
neurological, 170–171
psychiatric, 171–173
respiratory, 173–174
single organ system, 156
skin, 174–175
five levels of visit, 282t
history, 150–154, 281
chief complaint, 151
past, family, social, 153–154
present illness, 151–152
review of systems, 152–153
time, 284
Drug Enforcement Administration (DEA). *see* DEA (Drug Enforcement Administration)
Drugs. *see* Pharmaceuticals; Prescriptive authority
Duke University Medical Center, 12
Duty of care, 237
and good Samaritan acts, 461

E

E&M services (evaluation and management)
codes, 279–285. *see also* Coding, for Medicare billing
documentation guidelines, 146–181
online, 283
key components of, 149
levels of, 149–150, 282
Ear, nose, mouth, and throat exam, documentation of, 161–163
Educational requirements
for advanced practice nurses (APNs), 16t
for nurse practitioners, 5, 13t, 16t, 424–425, 433
by state, 117–133
for physician assistants, 11–12, 13t
for physicians, 13t, 14
for registered nurses, 15
Emergency plan, for practice, 363
Employee management, in NP-owned practice, 344–348
credentialing information, 361
Employee rights, 344
Employee, vs. independent contractor, 345–347
Employees, in NP-owned practice
injured at work, 362
NPs as, 366
Employer responsibilities, 344, 363
Employer rights, 345
Employment
agreement, sample, 310–319
by contract, 289–305
benefits of, 290–291
bonus formulas, 293–295
negotiating, 296–303
in NP-owned practice, 344, 347
and restrictive covenants, 291–293
termination from, 295, 296
interviewing for, 303
responsibilities of, for NP, 303

at will, 289, 291
in NP-owned practice, 344
Equal Pay Act of 1963, 145
Ethical dilemmas, 459–468
analyses, 467–468
good Samaritan, 459–460
and insurance fraud, 460, 466–467
and pharmaceutical companies, 460
Ethics in Patient Referral Act of 1989, 140
Evaluation of NPs performance, by employer, 304
Eye exam, documentation of, 163–164

F

Fact sheet on NPs, sample, 433–436
Family Practice Management, 283
Federal laws, 399
antidiscrimination, 145
ensuring compliance with, 454–455
on hospital privileges, 232
on medical laboratories. *see* CLIA (Clinical Laboratories Improvement Act)
on patient confidentiality, 142–145
precedence over state laws, 135
on preparation and licensing, 5
on prescriptive authority, 142
on reimbursement, 10
on reporting abuse, 144
Fee-for-service practices, 325
and NP salary, 300
Fein v. Permanente Med. Group, 238, 251–252
Final Rule, 143
Flexner, Abraham, 471
Florida
definition of nurse practitioner, 21
educational and licensing requirements, for NPs, 119
physician collaboration requirements, 44, 84
prescriptive authority in, 184, 197
regulatory agency for NPs, 114
scope of NP practice, 41, 51–52
titles for nurse practitioners, 33
Flow charts, 454–455
sample, 457–458
Ford, Loretta C., 7
Foundation for Accountability (FAcct), 431, 452
Fraud, 136, 138–139, 263, 280–281
definition, 466
prescription, 466–467

G

Gagino v. Harvard Community Health Plan, 241–242
Gates v. Jensen, 260
General multi-system exam, documentation of, 156–159
Genitourinary exam, documentation of, 164–166
Geographic Practice Cost Indexes (GPCIs), 270–271
Georgia
definition of nurse practitioner, 21
educational and licensing requirements, for NPs, 119
physician collaboration requirements, 44, 84
prescriptive authority in, 184, 185, 197
regulatory agency for NPs, 114
scope of NP practice, 41, 52
titles for nurse practitioners, 33
Good Samaritan acts, ethical dilemma, 460–462
Good Samaritan, ethical dilemma, 459–460
Guam, 10
Guidelines for Evaluation Management Coding (Center for Medicare and Medicaid Services), 279
Guidelines for Physician/Physician Assistant Practice, 11
Guidelines, for prescribing, 186–187
Guillaume, Carole, 283

H

Hall, J., 421, 423
Harrocks, S., 422, 423
Hawaii
definition of nurse practitioner, 21–22
educational and licensing requirements,

for NPs, 120
physician collaboration requirements, 44, 84–86
prescriptive authority in, 184, 197–200
regulatory agency for NPs, 114
scope of NP practice, 52–53
titles for nurse practitioners, 33
Hazardous waste removal, for practice, 364, 370–371
Health Care Financing Administration (HFCA, now the Center for Medicare and Medicaid Services), 136
"Documentation Guidelines for Evaluation and Management Services," 146–181
Health care reform, 401
Health care system, 403–405
Health Insurance Portability and Accountability Act (HIPAA), 143
Health Plan Employer Data and Information Set (HEDIS). *see* HEDIS (Health Plan Employer Data and Information Set)
Health policy, 400–401
Health Resources Services Administration, 7
HEDIS (Health Plan Employer Data and Information Set), 261, 330, 431, 444–445, 451–452, 454–455
Hematologic/lymphatic/immunologic exam, documentation of, 166–168
History, legal, of nurse practitioners, 6–7
HIV testing, and informed consent, 257
HMOs (health maintenance organizations), 274. *see also* MCOs (managed care organizations)
Hospital privileges, 227–234
application for, 233
definition, 232
denial of, 233
economics of, 230
expense of, 233
granting of, 230–321
levels of, 232–233
necessity of, for practice, 229–230
New York, 406–407
for nurse midwives, 231
Hospitalists, 227, 228
Hospitals, as locations of NP practice, 135–137
and lawsuits, 245
Housekeeping, for practice, 364

I

Idaho
definition of nurse practitioner, 22
educational and licensing requirements, for NPs, 120
malpractice case in, 238–239
physician collaboration requirements, 44, 86
prescriptive authority in, 184, 185, 200–201
regulatory agency for NPs, 114
scope of NP practice, 41, 53
titles for nurse practitioners, 33
Illinois
definition of nurse practitioner, 22
educational and licensing requirements, for NPs, 120
malpractice case in, 239
physician collaboration requirements, 44, 86–87
prescriptive authority in, 184, 185, 201–202
regulatory agency for NPs, 114
scope of NP practice, 41, 54
titles for nurse practitioners, 33
Indemnity insurers, reimbursement from, 273–274
Independent contractors
vs. employees, 345–347
sample agreement, 372–376
termination of, 347
Indiana
definition of nurse practitioner, 22
educational and licensing requirements, for NPs, 121
physician collaboration requirements, 44, 87–88
prescriptive authority in, 184, 185, 202–203
regulatory agency for NPs, 114
scope of NP practice, 41, 54–55
standards of care, 441–442
titles for nurse practitioners, 34

Information, release of, 144
  sample authorization form, 254–255
Information sheets, for patients, 364
Informed consent, 255–259
  and HIV testing, 257
  and low intelligence patient, 266
  negligent nondisclosure, 258–259, 260–261
  origins in law, 255–256
  state laws, 256–259
Initials, as NP designations, 6
Injury to patient, causation, 237–238
Institute of Medicine, 9, 10
Insurance
  fraud, 460, 466–467
  malpractice, 246–247
  for NP-owned practice, 365
    malpractice, 366
Internal Revenue Service (IRS), 345, 346, 347
International Classification of Diseases, 9th revision (ICD-9), 270
Interviewing, for employment, 303
Iowa
  definition of nurse practitioner, 23
  educational and licensing requirements, for NPs, 121
  physician collaboration requirements, 44, 88
  prescriptive authority in, 184, 185, 203
  regulatory agency for NPs, 115
  scope of NP practice, 55–56
  titles for nurse practitioners, 34

J

Jenkins v. Payne, 239–240
Johnson & Johnson, 143
Joint Commission on Accreditation of Healthcare Organizations (JCAHO), 431, 452
  standards of care, 443
Judicial system, the, 400, 443

K

Kansas
  definition of nurse practitioner, 23
  educational and licensing requirements, for NPs, 121
  physician collaboration requirements, 44, 88–89
  prescriptive authority in, 185, 204–205
  regulatory agency for NPs, 115
  scope of NP practice, 41, 56–57
  titles for nurse practitioners, 34
Karlsons v. Guerinot, 257
Kentucky
  definition of nurse practitioner, 23
  educational and licensing requirements, for NPs, 121
  physician collaboration requirements, 44, 89
  prescriptive authority in, 184, 205
  regulatory agency for NPs, 115
  scope of NP practice, 41, 57
  titles for nurse practitioners, 34
Kickbacks. *see* Stark Acts

L

Laboratories, 135, 140. *see also* Stark Acts for NP-owned practice, 365
Lauderdale v. United States, 260
Laundry, for practice, 365
Law Office of Carolyn Buppert, Web site, 145
Lawmaking, and health policy, 399–415
Laws. *see also* Federal laws; State laws
Laws, and health policy, 399–415
  changing, 401, 408–415
    analyzing barriers, 408, 472–473
    communication, with legislators, 410–412, 473–474
    goals and strategies, 408, 471–472
    legislative testimony, 411
    monitoring, 409
    role, of professional organizations, 475–476
    testimony, legislative, 409–410
  the judicial system, 400
  regulations, 399–400
  statutes, 399
Lawsuits, against nurse practitioners, 235–246, 436
  for battery, 256
  and disciplinary action, 261–263, 442
  examples of, 238–242
    failure to refer, 240–241, 241–242

hospital practice, 245
missed diagnosis, 238–240
importance of legal representation, 263
liability of collaborating physicians, 244–246
for negligence, 256
preventing, 244, 252–253
procedures for defendant in, 244
Legal challenges to NPs scope of practice, 39
Legal representation
for contract negotiations, 298
for lawsuits, 263
Library, for NP-owned practice, 365–366
Licensing boards, state, standards of care, 442
Licensing requirements
laws affecting, 401
for NPs, 5, 117–133
for physician assistants, 12
Limited liability company (LLC), 336, 359
Litigation, and patient confidentiality, 144
Litigious patient, and risk management, 266
Lobbying, for legislative change, 410–413, 475–476
do-it-yourself, 409–410, 412
Locations of practice, for nurse practitioners, 17
Louisiana
definition of nurse practitioner, 23–24
educational and licensing requirements, for NPs, 122
informed consent laws, 257
physician collaboration requirements, 44, 89–91
prescriptive authority in, 184, 185, 205–206
regulatory agency for NPs, 115
scope of NP practice, 41, 57–59
titles for nurse practitioners, 34

M

Madsen v. Park Nicollet Medical Center, 257
Maine
clinical nurse specialist, definition, 15
definition of nurse practitioner, 24
educational and licensing requirements, for NPs, 122–123
physician collaboration requirements, 44, 91, 469
prescriptive authority in, 184, 185, 206
regulatory agency for NPs, 115
scope of NP practice, 41, 59–60
titles for nurse practitioners, 34
Malpractice, 135, 235–248, 446
definition, 250
drug-related, 186
elements of, 236–238, 250
and good Samaritan acts, 461
insurance, 246–247, 366, 432
lawsuits. *see* Lawsuits, against nurse practitioners
records of, 361. *see also* National Practitioner Data Bank (NPDB)
risk management. *see* Risk management
Managed care organizations (MCOs), 271, 273, 274–279, 401–404
applying for membership, 275, 364
applying for provider status, 348–354
carrying out contract, 278–279
contract negotiation, 276–277
denial of provider status, 277–278
group vs. practice models, 274–275
negotiating contract with, 354–357
performance reports, 423–424
rejection of request for, 354
Managed care, stages of, 402–403
Marketing. *see also* Public relations
of NP-owned practice, 326, 327, 366, 367, 371
of nurse practitioners, as PCPs, 405
and patient confidentiality, 143, 144
of physicians, 417
Maryland
definition of nurse practitioner, 24
educational and licensing requirements, for NPs, 123, 434
informed consent laws, 257
NPs as primary care providers, 9–10
physician collaboration requirements, 44, 91
prescriptive authority in, 184, 185, 206
regulatory agency for NPs, 115
reimbursement in, 436
scope of NP practice, 41, 60, 434
titles for nurse practitioners, 34

Massachusetts
definition of nurse practitioner, 24
educational and licensing requirements, for NPs, 123
physician collaboration requirements, 44, 91–92
prescriptive authority in, 184, 185, 206–207
regulatory agency for NPs, 115
scope of NP practice, 41, 60
titles for nurse practitioners, 34
MCOs (managed care organizations). *see* Managed care organizations (MCOs)
Medicaid, 138, 405
fraud, 263–264
and NP-owned practice, 321
and nursing homes, 138–139
reimbursement, 273, 436
screening for eligibility, 362
Medical Economics magazine, 325, 422
Medical errors, 235
risk of, 249–250
Medical Group Management Association (MGMA), 301
Medicare, 135–139
Center for Medicare and Medicaid Services. *see* Center for Medicare and Medicaid Services (CMS)
fraud, 136, 138–139, 263–264, 280–281
"incident to" relationship, 137
and nursing homes, 138–139
provider status, applying for, 272
reimbursement, 137–139
capitated, 271, 273
coding for, 279–285
fee-for-service, 270–271
"incident to" services, 271
indemnity insurers, 273–274
screening for eligibility, 362
Medicare Carriers Manual, 138
Michigan
definition of nurse practitioner, 24–25
definition of registered nurse, 14
educational and licensing requirements, for NPs, 123
and patient privacy, 143
physician collaboration requirements, 92
prescriptive authority in, 183, 185, 207
regulatory agency for NPs, 115
scope of NP practice, 41, 61
titles for nurse practitioners, 34
Mid-level practitioners, definition, 2–3
Minnesota
definition of mid-level practitioner, 2
definition of nurse practitioner, 25
educational and licensing requirements, for NPs, 123–124
informed consent laws, 257, 257–258, 260
physician collaboration requirements, 44, 92
prescriptive authority in, 185, 207–208
regulatory agency for NPs, 115
scope of NP practice, 61
Missed diagnoses, 238–240, 252
Mission statement, for NP-owned practice, 368
Mississippi
definition of nurse practitioner, 25
educational and licensing requirements, for NPs, 124
physician collaboration requirements, 44, 92–93
prescriptive authority in, 184, 208
regulatory agency for NPs, 115
scope of NP practice, 61
scope of physician practice, 43
titles for nurse practitioners, 34
Missouri
definition of nurse practitioner, 25
educational and licensing requirements, for NPs, 124
physician collaboration requirements, 44, 93–96
prescriptive authority in, 184, 208–210
regulatory agency for NPs, 115
scope of NP practice, 61
supreme court, 39
Montana
definition of nurse practitioner, 25–26
educational and licensing requirements, for NPs, 124
physician collaboration requirements, 44, 96–97
prescriptive authority in, 183, 184, 185, 210–211
regulatory agency for NPs, 115
scope of NP practice, 41, 61–62

standards of care, 441
titles for nurse practitioners, 34
Multisystem failure, patient, 265
Mundinger, M., 422–423, 423
Musculoskeletal examination, documentation of, 168–170

N

National Academy of Sciences' Institute of Medicine, 7
National Certification Board of Pediatric Nurse Practitioners and Nurses (NCBPNPN), 5, 16t
National Certification Corporation (NCC), 5, 16t
National Committee on Quality Assurance (NCQA), 402, 444–445, 450, 453–455
HEDIS (Health Plan Employer Data and Information Set). *see* HEDIS (Health Plan Employer Data and Information Set)
National Practitioner Data Bank (NPDB), 135, 142, 235, 242–243, 361
NCC (National Certification Corporation), 16t
Nebraska
definition of nurse practitioner, 26
educational and licensing requirements, for NPs, 124–125
physician collaboration requirements, 44
prescriptive authority in, 184, 185, 211–212
regulatory agency for NPs, 115
scope of NP practice, 41, 62
titles for nurse practitioners, 34
Negligence, 235–248
Negligent nondisclosure, 257–258, 260–261
Negotiating employment contracts
benefits, 302
preparation for, 296–297
salary, 298–301
methods of payment, 299
work environment, 302–303
Negotiating managed care contracts, 354–357
preparation for, 354–355
Nelson v. Patrick, 257
Neurological examination, documentation of, 170–171
Nevada
definition of nurse practitioner, 26
educational and licensing requirements, for NPs, 125
physician collaboration requirements, 44, 97–98
prescriptive authority in, 184, 185
state law, 212
regulatory agency for NPs, 115
scope of NP practice, 41, 62–63
titles for nurse practitioners, 34
New Hampshire
definition of nurse practitioner, 26
educational and licensing requirements, for NPs, 125
physician collaboration requirements, 44, 98, 469
prescriptive authority in, 184
state law, 213
regulatory agency for NPs, 115
scope of NP practice, 41, 63–64
titles for nurse practitioners, 34
New Jersey
definition of medical practice, 12
definition of nurse practitioner, 26
educational and licensing requirements, for NPs, 125–126
physician collaboration requirements, 44, 98–99
prescriptive authority in, 184, 185
state law, 213–214
regulatory agency for NPs, 115
scope of NP practice, 41, 64
titles for nurse practitioners, 34
New Mexico
definition of nurse practitioner, 26–27
physician collaboration requirements, 44, 99, 469
prescriptive authority in, 184, 185
state law, 214
regulatory agency for NPs, 115
scope of NP practice, 41, 64
titles for nurse practitioners, 34
New York
definition of nurse practitioner, 27
educational and licensing requirements, for NPs, 126
hospital privileges in, 230–231, 406–407

informed consent laws, 256
physician collaboration requirements, 44, 99–100
prescriptive authority in, 184, 185, 215
scope of NP practice, 41, 65, 406–407
scope of practice, 430
titles for nurse practitioners, 34
New York Times, 241
Noncompliant patient, and risk management, 266
North Carolina
definition of nurse practitioner, 27
educational and licensing requirements, for NPs, 126
physician collaboration requirements, 44, 100
prescriptive authority in, 184, 185, 215
regulatory agency for NPs, 115
scope of NP practice, 41, 65
titles for nurse practitioners, 34
North Dakota
definition of nurse practitioner, 27
educational and licensing requirements, for NPs, 127
physician collaboration requirements, 100–101
prescriptive authority in, 184, 185, 215
regulatory agency for NPs, 115
scope of NP practice, 41, 42, 43, 65–66
scope of RN practice, 14, 42–43
titles for nurse practitioners, 34
Novak v. Texada, Miller, Masterson, and Davis Medical Clinic, 257
NPDB (National Practitioner Data Bank), 135, 142, 235, 242–243
Nurse anesthetist, 3, 16t
Nurse midwives, 16t, 231
Nurse practitioner, definition, 1–2, 3
Nurse practitioners
collaboration with physicians. *see* Collaboration, with physician
compared to physician assistants, 10
compared to physicians, 12, 13t, 421–425, 452–453
compared to registered nurses, 14–15
demographics, 7
educational requirements, 16t, 117–133
licensing requirements, 117–133
locations of practice
hospitals, 135–137. *see also* Hospital privileges
nursing homes, 138–139
new graduates, 300–301
as primary care providers (PCPs), 227–228, 229–230
protocols for, 44, 45
scope of practice. *see* Practice, scope of
services provided by, 3–5
Nurse psychotherapist, educational requirements, 16t
Nursing homes, 138–139

O

OBRA (Omnibus Budget Reconciliation Act of 1993), 140
Office of Inspector General (OIG), "Federal Register Notice on the Compliance Program Guidance for Pharmaceutical Manufacturers," 464, 465–466
Ohio
definition of nurse practitioner, 27–28
educational and licensing requirements, for NPs, 127
physician collaboration requirements, 101
prescriptive authority in, 184, 185, 215–216
regulatory agency for NPs, 115
titles for nurse practitioners, 34
Oklahoma
definition of nurse practitioner, 28
educational and licensing requirements, for NPs, 127
physician collaboration requirements, 44, 101
prescriptive authority in, 184, 185, 216
regulatory agency for NPs, 115
scope of NP practice, 39, 41, 66–67
titles for nurse practitioners, 35
Omnibus Budget Reconciliation Act of 1993 (OBRA), 140
On-call, coverage for, 359, 366
Optometrists, and hospital privileges, 232, 406–407

Oregon
definition of nurse practitioner, 28
educational and licensing requirements, for NPs, 128
hospital privileges in, 231
physician collaboration requirements, 101, 469
prescriptive authority in, 184, 185, 216–217
regulatory agency for NPs, 115
scope of NP practice, 10, 41, 41–42, 67–68, 406, 477–478
scope of physician practice, 43
titles for nurse practitioners, 35
OSHA (Occupational Safety and Health Act), 344
compliance, in practice, 367
Osteopaths, and hospital privileges, 232
Ownership, of practice. *see* Practice, NP-owned

P

Partnership, in practice, 335–336, 359
risks of, 264–265
Patient satisfaction
with NPs, 422, 423, 430, 431, 435
standards for, 447
Patients
with disabilities, 361–362
high-risk, 265–266
litigious, 266
screening for Medicaid, 362
Patients rights
confidentiality. *see* Confidentiality, patient
informed consent, 255–261
refusal of treatment, 261
Pennsylvania
definition of nurse practitioner, 28–29
educational and licensing requirements, for NPs, 128
informed consent laws, 257
physician collaboration requirements, 44, 101–102
prescriptive authority in, 184, 185, 217
regulatory agency for NPs, 115
scope of NP practice, 39–40, 41, 68
titles for nurse practitioners, 35
Performance
research on, 452–453
steps for good evaluation, 454–455
Performance evaluation
of employees, 347
of NP, by employer, 304
Performance, measures of, 449–455
housekeeping, 451
National Committee on Quality Assurance (NCQA), 451–452
patient ratings, 453
peer review, 453
productivity, 450–451
quality, 449
utilization, 453–454
Perry, K., 423
Pharmaceutical companies, and ethics, 460, 462–466
Pharmaceutical industry, "Code on Interactions with Health Care Professionals," 463–464, 464–465
Pharmaceuticals. *see also* Drug Enforcement Administration (DEA); Prescriptive authority
in NP-owned practice, 367–368
PHOs (physician-sponsored organizations), 274. *see also* MCOs (managed care organizations)
Physician assistants (PAs), 10–12
competition with nurse practitioners, 414
educational requirements, 13t
as physician extenders, 10
Physician extenders, 2, 10
Physician Insurers Association of America, 186
Physicians
collaboration with NPs. *see* Collaboration, with physician
compared to NPs, 12, 13t, 421–424, 452–453
compared to physician assistants, 13t
competition with nurse practitioners. *see* Competition, with physicians
education, 13t, 424–425
involvement with physician assistant practice, 11
portrayal on TV, 417

scope of practice, 43
shortages, 7, 12
Physician's Desk Reference, 186
"Physicians' Referrals to Health Care Entities With Which They Have Financial Relationships" (CMS), 140
Planned Parenthood v. Vines, 241
Podiatrists, and hospital privileges, 232, 406–407
Policies, legal, 400
Policy, definition, 400
Polypharmacy of patient, and risk management, 266
Positive review of systems, and risk management, 266
Practice, NP
areas of, 6
primary care, 7–8, 9
secondary and tertiary care, 10
barriers to, 401, 404–407, 469, 470–471
fighting, 407–415, 471–478
Practice, NP-owned, 321–371
advantages, 321–322, 404
barriers to, 322
business plan
sample agreement, 377–392
writing, 338–343
business structure, 331, 335–337, 359
checklist for setting up, 358–371
administration, 358
billing, 358–359
business structure, choosing, 359
chaperones, 359–360
confidentiality, maintaining, 360
coverage for on-call, 359
credentialing information for employees, 361
office equipment, 360, 361
choosing location, 328–329
and collaboration requirements, 371
collaboration, with physicians. *see* Collaboration, with physician
compared to physician-owned, 325–326, 327, 328
considerations in, 322–325, 343
coverage for on-call, 366
employee management, 338, 344–348
equipment for, 365–366
expenses, 324–327, 345–347
funding, 370
guidelines, writing, 243
hours of operation, 364
management, 330–331
marketing, 326, 327, 348, 366, 367, 371. *see also* Public relations
OSHA compliance, 367
performance evaluation, 455
pharmaceuticals in, 368, 369
physical plant, 368
purchasing, 368
quality assurance, 329–330, 368
record-keeping forms, 363–364
referrals, 368–369
reimbursement, 347–357
responsibilities of, for NP, 343–344
security, 369
standard of care, 369
supplies, 370
support staff, 370
systems for running, 337
types of, 366
Practice, scope of
importance of defining, 37, 38, 39–40, 477–478
legal challenges to, 39
New York, 430
nurse practitioner, 10, 433
compared to registered nurse, 40, 42, 43
laws affecting, 401
state laws, 47–74
registered nurse, 14, 40
state laws, 37–38, 39–40, 405–406
Pratt v. University of Minnesota, 257, 257–258
Prescribing, guidelines for, 186–187
Prescriptive authority, 183–187, 368
credentialing information, 361
federal regulations, 142
forms of, 184
and insurance fraud, 460, 466–467
origination of, 7
physician involvement requirements, 184, 185
state-by-state, 188–226
and substance abusing patient, 266
Primary care, definition, 7–9
Primary care providers

NPs as, 9–10, 404–406, 435, 469–471
and hospital privileges, 227–228, 229–230
in managed care organizations, 274, 349
removing barriers, 405–415, 474
physicians as, 8–9
Privacy, patient, 142–145, 359
Professional relationship, existence of, 250–251
Protocols, for NPs, 44, 45
writing, 243
Provider status
applying for, 348–353, 353–354, 358–359
arguments to MCOs for, 350–352
arguments to other NPs for, 352–353
arguments to physicians for, 349–350
arguments to practice managers for, 350–352
Medicare, 272
rejection of request for, 354, 359
denial of, 277–278
PSOs (provider-sponsored organizations), 274. *see also* MCOs (managed care organizations)
Psychiatric examination, documentation of, 171–173
Psychologists, and hospital privileges, 232
Psychotherapy, and confidentiality, 144
Public perceptions
of healthcare providers, 405
of NPs, 417
Public relations, 417–426, 474–476. *see also* Marketing; Public perceptions
data collection for, 421–424
barriers to, 424
dealing with unfavorable facts, 424–426
importance of, 426
message, 420–421
talking points, 430–432
plan, 418–420
sample, 428–429
specialists, 475–476
Purchasing, for NP-owned practice, 368

Q

Quality of care, laws affecting, 401

R

RBRVS (resource-based relative value scale), 270–271
Record-keeping, 457–458
for compliance, 454–455
Referrals, directory for, 368–369
Registered nurse
definition, 14
educational requirements, 15
scope of practice, 40, 42–43
Registered nurse, certified specialist (RN, CS), 6
Regulations, definition, 399–400
Regulatory agencies for NPs, state-by-state, 114–116
Reimbursement, 269–288
fee-for-service, 270–271
and good Samaritan acts, 461–462
laws affecting, 401
Medicaid, 436
Medicare, 137–139. *see also* Coding, for Medicare billing; E&M services (evaluation and management)
for NP-owned practice, 323–325, 347–357, 369
contracts, 348
indemnity insurers, 348
Managed care organization (MCO), 348
self-paying patients, 347–348
rejection of request for, 284
resources, 285
systems, 300
Respiratory system, documentation of exam, 173–174
Rhode Island
definition of nurse practitioner, 29
educational and licensing requirements, for NPs, 129
physician collaboration requirements, 44, 102
prescriptive authority in, 184, 185, 217–218
regulatory agency for NPs, 116
scope of NP practice, 41, 68
titles for nurse practitioners, 35
Rights
employee, 344

employer, 345
patient. *see* Patients rights
Risk, diagnostic, table of, 177–180
Risk management, 249–267
of disciplinary action, 261–263
failure to refer, 265
and high-risk patients, 265–266
by limiting patient relationships, 251
Medicare fraud, 263–264
negligent nondisclosure, 260–261
and patient communication, 252–253
and patient confidentiality, 253–255
and perception as poor-quality provider, 253
right to informed consent, 255–259, 266
standard of care, 265, 266
RN, CS (registered nurse, certified specialist), 6

S

Salary
median, for NP, 301–302
negotiating, 298–301
Salkever, D. S., 421, 423
Secondary and tertiary care, role of NPs, 10
See-a-nurse-first system, 469–470
Self-evaluation, 456
Self-referral. *see* Stark Acts
Serementis, Stephanie, 403
Sermchief v. Gonzales, 39
Silver, Henry K. 7
Single organ system exam, documentation of, 156
Skin, documentation of examination, 174–175
Snow v. A. H. Robins Co, Inc., 241–242
Social Security Act, 136, 138, 140, 141, 232
Sole proprietorship, 335, 359
South Carolina
definition of nurse practitioner, 29
educational and licensing requirements, for NPs, 129
and patient privacy, 143
physician collaboration requirements, 44, 103
prescriptive authority in, 184, 185, 218–219
regulatory agency for NPs, 116
scope of NP practice, 41, 68–69
titles for nurse practitioners, 35
South Dakota
definition of nurse practitioner, 29–30
educational and licensing requirements, for NPs, 129
physician collaboration requirements, 44, 103–105
prescriptive authority in, 184, 185, 219
regulatory agency for NPs, 116
scope of NP practice, 41, 69–70
titles for nurse practitioners, 35
Standard of care, 237, 251–252, 369
definition, 437
and JCAHO, 443
keeping current with, 446
measures of, 446–447
monitoring, 437–446
by professional societies, 438–441
by the state, 441–443
state laws, 441–443
Stark Acts, 135, 140–142
State Laboratory Administration, 365
State laws
conflict with federal laws, 135
ensuring compliance with, 454–455
on informed consent, 256–258
on prescriptive authority, 188–226
scope of NP practice, 37–38, 404
standards of care, 441–442
Statute, definition, 399
Stead, Eugene, 12
Substance abusing patient, and risk management, 266
Supervision, by physician. *see also* Collaboration, with physician
Medicare requirements, 137–138
state-by-state requirements, 44–45
Surgery, informed consent for, 255, 256

T

Tennessee
definition of nurse practitioner, 30
educational and licensing requirements, for NPs, 129–130

physician collaboration requirements, 105
physician involvement requirements, 44
prescriptive authority in, 184, 185, 219–220
regulatory agency for NPs, 116
scope of NP practice, 70
titles for nurse practitioners, 35
Termination, from employment, 295, 296
in NP-owned practice, 347
Texas
definition of nurse practitioner, 30
educational and licensing requirements, for NPs, 130
lawsuit in, 245
physician collaboration requirements, 44, 105–106
prescriptive authority in, 184, 185, 220–221
regulatory agency for NPs, 116
scope of NP practice, 41, 70–71
titles for nurse practitioners, 35
Third-party payers, 269–282
billing, 279–282
Title VII, Civil Rights Act of 1964, 145
Titles, for nurse practitioners, by state, 33–35
Tommasino, Joseph, 403–404
Topp v. Logan, 239
Torresi, D., 424
Truman v. Thomas, 260–261

U

United States Department of Health and Human Services, 242
United States Justice Department, 138, 263
United States Office of Civil Rights, 253
University of Colorado, 7
Upcoding, 263, 280–281
Utah
definition of nurse practitioner, 30
educational and licensing requirements, for NPs, 130
physician collaboration requirements, 44, 106–107, 469
prescriptive authority in, 184, 185, 221
regulatory agency for NPs, 116
scope of NP practice, 41, 71
titles for nurse practitioners, 35

V

Vermont
definition of nurse practitioner, 31
educational and licensing requirements, for NPs, 130
physician collaboration requirements, 44, 107
prescriptive authority in, 184, 185, 221
regulatory agency for NPs, 116
scope of NP practice, 41, 71–72, 405–406
titles for nurse practitioners, 35
Virginia
definition of nurse practitioner, 31
educational and licensing requirements, for NPs, 131
physician collaboration requirements, 44, 107–108
prescriptive authority in, 184, 185, 221–223
regulatory agency for NPs, 116
scope of NP practice, 72
titles for nurse practitioners, 35

W

Washington State
definition of nurse practitioner, 31
educational and licensing requirements, for NPs, 131–132
informed consent laws, 256–257, 260
physician collaboration requirements, 44, 108, 469
prescriptive authority in, 184, 185, 224
regulatory agency for NPs, 116
scope of NP practice, 41, 72–73
titles for nurse practitioners, 35
Web sites
Agency for Healthcare Research and Quality (AHRQ), 243
Center for Medicare and Medicaid Services, 281
Health Plan Employer Data and Information Set (HEDIS), 261, 445, 452
West Virginia
definition of nurse practitioner, 31–32
physician collaboration requirements, 44, 108–109

prescriptive authority in, 184, 185, 224–225
regulatory agency for NPs, 116
scope of NP practice, 73
titles for nurse practitioners, 35
Wisconsin
definition of nurse practitioner, 32
educational and licensing requirements, for NPs, 132
fraud in, 467
prescriptive authority in, 184, 185, 225–226
regulatory agency for NPs, 116
scope of NP practice, 41, 73–74
titles for nurse practitioners, 35
Women's Health Program, Mount Sinai Medical Center, 403
Work environment, negotiating, 302–303
Workers' compensation, 362
Workers' Compensation Commission, 347
Wyoming
definition of nurse practitioner, 32
educational and licensing requirements, for NPs, 132–133
physician collaboration requirements, 44, 109–110
prescriptive authority in, 184, 185, 226
regulatory agency for NPs, 116
scope of NP practice, 41, 74
titles for nurse practitioners, 35